PHYSICAL ENHANCEMENT

with an Edge

S. HOMINUK

(1ST EDITION: JAN. 1997)

ISBN# 0-9681647-0-6

NOTICE

No liability is assumed by Q.F.A.C. Publishing, or the author for any information contained within this book. This book has not been intended to be a guideline, catalogue, or an exact pricelist regarding the administration of anabolic/androgenic steroids, diuretics or related pharmaceuticals and veterinarian products. The intention of this book has not been to encourage or endorse the use of steroidal substances in athletic sports, but instead, to provide general information only. Medical advice regarding adventitious dosage and administration has not been provided; as these recommendations have been based upon speculative values. Proper clinical usage of these substances have been obtained from medical journals, including the "PDR", "CPS", and other related books, and also from the Veterinarian Compendiums, and have been stated within each individual compound description. However, specific clinical advice should only be obtained from a licensed physician. The information contained within this book has not been intended to promote anabolic/androgenic steroids which have been available in the country of Mexico in regards to potential illegal possession, trafficking, importing, or exporting. The author also strongly disapproves of inappropriate administration and illegal purchase of these substances, and warn that attempting to remove anabolic/androgenic steroidal compounds from the country of Mexico is illegal, and may result in severe penalties. This book also does not contain legal advice, but general legality information relevant to the steroid issue. Specific legal advice should be obtained by proper legal counsel.

This book has been intended for a mature reading audience. Readers younger than the age of 18 must seek parental consent.

SPECIAL ACKNOWLEDGEMENT:

Stephen C. Reeves -
Executive Contributing Advisor/Anabolic, Training and Health Consultant/Executive photographer.

Dr. Esteban Ortis Pavon -
Head of Surgeons, Acapulco, Mexico/Medical Anabolic Consultant.

Michael Dawson - Co-author of World Anabolic Review 1996/Anabolic Consultant.

Dean Clifford, Rachelle Artibise, Kelly Michulak
Barb & Craig Fisher - Photography, scans and layouts.

Bill & Joyce Hominuk - Financial and moral support.

Special thanks to all the "athletes" who had in one way or another contributed to the completion of the first edition of "Physical Enhancement with an Edge".

TABLE OF CONTENTS

MEXICAN HUMAN ANABOLIC STERIOD DESCRIPTIONS:

MEXICAN VETERINARIAN STERIOD DESCRIPTIONS:

MACRONUTRIENTS:

INTRODUCTION

Many bodybuilders, powerlifters, wrestlers, athletes of all sports, ranging from the professional ranks to that of an amateur status, may have at one time or another, either anticipated, or participated in the enhancement of anabolic/androgenic steroids. However, even though an estimated 4 million of these individuals may have had actually had entertained these pharmaceutical and veterinarian items, it had been done so, at their own discretion. Unfortunately, the medical profession had often not been supportive or even knowledgeable in the administration of these compounds, which had frequently left many individuals at the mercy of perhaps a coach, peer, but usually, their own self-estimation.

This book has been compiled to have offered some information about these pharmaceutical and veterinarian products, which many individuals have been dangerously self-administering, and possibly, may have been endangering their health. Foul language and cartons will not be found within the following text, as self-prescribing and self-administering prescription and veterinarian pharmaceutical drugs without the supervision of a qualified physician, has been a very serious matter, and if not appropriately considered, may be very dangerous.

Instead, "a-matter-of-fact" approach has finally been taken to try and offer information to many oblivious athletic individuals, who individually have chosen to have entertained the self-administration of steroidal compounds. "Athletes" has often been referred to solely within this book for mere simplicity, as this term has been intended to have included all "steroidal substance using individuals". The adventitious dosages has varied, as a common, average measure amongst steroid users has been attempted to have been documented. Therefore, this text has been gathered from several medical documentations, journals, "med-lines", encyclopedias, physician, veterinarian and pharmaceutical desk references, manufacturing companies, physicians, veterinarians, law books, lawyers, Custom agents, peace officers, and several athletes themselves in efforts to have provided the most accurate information possible.

As anabolic/androgenic steroidal substances have become a controlled substance in many countries, many individuals have felt that perhaps traveling abroad to a country where they are still "legal", may have been their only alternative in attempts to obtain such compounds. Mexico, of course, has currently been one of the countries where a written prescription from a physician, has allowed an individual to acquire steroidal compounds for personal utilization. However, again, many Mexican physicians also have not been knowledgeable with respect to these substances, and most of the time, have not been able to provide medical assistance (even if English had been spoken). On the other hand, veterinarian suppliers have often readily sold these items without the requirement of a prescription, which had been easier and cheaper for several athletes to acquire.

Obviously, pretending the issue of practicing self medicine does not exist would have still left many individuals available to possibly unknowingly, endanger their health, and possibly violate the law; due to ignorance. Therefore, avoiding the steroid issue will not retard the utilization of these products, nor will the sensationalism or exaggerating of possible damaging or fatal side effects.

Despite the controversy regarding the issue of steroids for athletic enhancement, and instead of ignoring this problem, the possibility of educating potential, and present steroidal users, in attempts to; if not dissuade the use of anabolic/androgenic steroids, then to possibly provide a better knowledge and understanding of these pharmaceuticals, and the possible consequences resulting from their application both "clinically", and "legally" has been highly desired.

In the United States and Canada, steroidal compounds have been illegal to possess, however, they are, and will continue to be, used without medical supervision regardless of legal application.

HOW SYNTHETIC STEROIDAL COMPOUNDS WORK IN THE BODY:

Exogenous synthetic steroidal compounds are introduced into the system in several various techniques. Administration can accomplished by intramuscular injection, which requires a needle and syringe to transport the compound directly into the muscle; orally, which is taken by the mouth and swallowed, or sometimes if applicable, transdermally, which is administered through the skin's surface. Different techniques permit the compounds to be absorbed by the body differently; injectables and transdermal patch compounds are dispersed directly into the bloodstream, and oral compounds initially pass through the gastrointestinal tract, through the liver, then into the bloodstream.

Once a steroidal compound enters the bloodstream, it develops into a molecule which has a specific message to deliver to destined cells throughout the entire body. Each individual message is delivered to particular areas containing receptor sites, which only recognize distinct signals transmitted by steroids. Therefore, some receptor sites ignore these steroidal molecules, while others acknowledge them, such as the optimal muscle cell. Unfortunately, several of the receptor sites which also accept steroid messages are hair follicles, (premature balding) oil and skin sebaceous glands, (acne) certain endocrine glands, and the brain. However, the type and concentration of a particular cell receptor, will determine the degree which an organ may be affected by a certain steroid. Also, if an individual has a genetic predisposition for some of these adverse effects, then these effects become usually more pronounced. Therefore, preventable measures such as dosage moderation and duration requires valid consideration, in order to avoid potential ill effects.

A steroid molecule combined with a receptor site connect, forming cellular cytosol, which is the liquid area encompassing a cell. This combination progresses to the nucleus of the cell, which interprets the message, and then performs the specific designated request. If by coincidence this was a muscle cell, the transmitted steroid message would order an increase in the production of RNA, that generates an increase of protein synthesis, which results in increased muscle mass and strength.

Administering steroidal compounds can increase muscle mass, as muscles are created primarily from protein. Also, the production of Creatine Phosphate which is a nitrogenous compound, also increases, which promotes the storage of particular muscle cells enzymes, namely ATP (adenosine Triphosphate). ATP is the actual fuel which allows the movement of muscles. Glycogen is the usable fuel which results from the metabolism of carbohydrates, which is also increased and withheld within a cell. An increase in muscle mass and endurance is additionally experienced with increased glycogen storage.

As commonly experienced with some types of steroids, a strength increase may result, unaccompanied by usual associated weight or muscle gains. Consequently, steroidal compound administration often is associated with fluid retention; which, ultimately enables an extra supply of nutrients to be provided to the cell. Nitrogen (a component of protein), retention is also increased by a muscle cell, and if this amount exceeds the amount released, a positive nitrogen balance state occurs. This state is synonymous with muscle growth.

Evidence of steroidal effectiveness can be measured when the muscle tissues consumes less cortisol. This creates an anti-catabolic state, as cortisol decreases muscle mass due to catabolic characteristics. It is automatically produced by the body, therefore, the anabolic effects of steroidal administration is amplified when the system tries to prevent cortisol from entering the muscle tissue.

Steroid Effectiveness

All steroidal compounds usually perform similarly in the system, however, may produce different results in different individuals, due to the concentration of receptors. Genetics are responsible for certain individuals to possess a high quantity of muscle cells, which permit a greater amount of steroid molecules to become attached. This allows steroid signals to be transmitted more intensely, which of course can result in increased muscle mass when enhancing compounds such as exogenous anabolic steroids are administered. Unfortunately, an individual's receptor site quantity cannot be altered to allow for potential higher gains, however, certain precautions can aid steroid receptor states to remain active for longer durations. This can be accomplished by the limitation of steroidal cycles, which allow the receptor sites to become rejuvenated and once again, susceptible to steroid signals. Increasing the dosage amounts of steroidal compounds will only produce a decrease of receptor's acceptability to the desired signals. Therefore, moderate dosages administered for limited intervals, (average 2 to 12 weeks), with abstinence breaks between cycles, will accomplish the most optimal, desired results.

Steroidal compounds also produce a greater effect on younger individuals, benefiting those primarily between the ages of 18 to 22. As the age increases, the effects of steroidal compounds slightly decreases. Consequently, younger individuals who administer steroids can accomplish greater results at lower dosage amounts, than older individuals who use greater dosages to acquire the same outcome. Consequently, for the initial two weeks of administration in all individuals, the steroidal compound will be producing purely anabolic effects, as it will be attaching itself chiefly to the same areas on the muscle cells, the receptors; which natural Testosterone attaches to. This period produces the greatest muscle increases. After these two weeks, the body's cortisol effect will become blocked by a limited amount of the steroid, which will slow down the anabolic effects, and ultimately results in slower development.

TESTOSTERONE

Biochemists have been artificially synthesizing many hormones in the laboratory, since the early 1940's. One of these alterable hormones was Testosterone, as it was discovered that it had the capability to provide a much more powerful action. Henceforth, the discovery and birth of anabolic and androgenic steroids, which would later lead to much controversy in both athletic and political fields.

Testosterone is primarily the sex hormone which is produced by the testes and is responsible for controlling a great number of metabolic functions in men. It has both anabolic and androgenic effects. Anabolic effects refer to those effects which enable muscle tissue to grow, and is considered by most athletes, as the most desirable reason for engaging in a steroid regime. Androgenic effects refer to the secondary sexual characteristics which are primarily related to men such as maturing of the voice (deepening), facial hair, sexual organ development, as well as aggression. These androgenic effects are primarily sought after for clinical purposes, but to some extent, are also welcomed by some athletes. Strong athletes are fond of androgens due to the excitability of the nervous system, as it has receptors for androgens, which consequently, enables the possibility of using high loads of this compound. Unfortunately, the possibility of producing an anabolic steroid without the unwanted effects of androgens, has, and continues to be undiscovered. Previously, and currently, anabolic steroids still produce a certain androgenic effect; similarly as androgenic steroids are able to produce anabolic characteristics. However, there has been the invention of Testosterone derivatives which have a lessened androgenic effect when administered. Consequently, the separating characteristics of anabolic and androgenic steroids, involves the amount of Testosterone each possess. Steroidal compounds which are less "androgenic", are referred to as "Anabolic steroids", and the steroids which are more "androgenic", are referred to as "Androgenic steroids". However, most synthetic steroidal compounds have both characteristics.

Females also possess a certain amount of Testosterone naturally in their bodies, just as males naturally produce a certain amount of Estrogen, which is the female's primary sex hormone. Testosterone and Estrogen are essentially what separates women from men. When females start taking Testosterone or Testosterone derivatives, they begin acquiring male characteristics. Consequently, when males administer Estrogen, they start developing female characteristics. Oddly enough however, if a male induces too much Testosterone into his system, the effect can rebound, and instead of producing desired male characteristics, the system produces more Estrogen to compensate for too much of a sudden influx of Testosterone. This of course, leads to feminizational traits, such as further development of breast tissue, which inevitably develops into a condition known as gynecomastia.

Testosterone in plasma is approximately 98% bound to a specific Testosterone-Estradiol binding globulin. The percentage of free and bound Testosterone is determined generally by the amount of binding globulin concentration; and determination of of half-life is determined by free

Testosterone. There are may considerable variations in the half-lives of Testosterone, which range from 10 to 100 minutes. For example, MethylTestosterone, which is a Testosterone derivative, has a half-live of 2.5 to 3 hours, while oral Fluoxymesterone's half-life is approximately 8 days. The inactivation of Testosterone primarily occurs in the liver where approximately 90% of the administrated dose is excreted in the urine (as conjugates of Testosterone and its metabolites), and approximately 6% in the feces.

Different Testosteronal Applications:

Oral Testosterones:

These forms of Testosterone are available in a tablet form, and are taken via the mouth, to be swallowed. Oral Testosterone is metabolized by the gastrointestinal system, and the liver abruptly and almost entirely eliminates pure Testosterone through a process called first-pass elimination, where 44% is cleared. To prevent this from happening, other pharmacologic conversions are required to keep the compounds in circulation longer, without the potential of being eliminated. This of course, led to the 17-a Alkylated steroids such as Stenox (Fluoxymesterone), Android (MethylTestosterone), (currently, not available in Mexico), and Anapolon (Oxymetholone). These synthetic androgens are more suitable than Testosterone for oral administration as they are less extensively metabolized by the liver and have longer half-lives. Peak serum concentrations are acquired approximately two hours after oral administration. These compounds are very androgenic, and therefore are considered to be the most toxic compounds that are available in the steroid market. Oral administration of Testosterone may also cause gastro- intestinal upset. These oral compounds have also been associated with liver toxicity, cholestatic jaundice, and a typical pattern of virilization in female users. Therefore, their consumption should be very limited and not abused, while special attention should be focused on potential harmful side effects.

Buccal Testosterones:

These forms are placed under the tongue or between the gum and cheek area. They are not to be chewed or swallowed, but allowed to be absorbed by salvia; and no solids, liquids or smoking should take place while buccal tablets are being dissolved. The buccal administration permits MethylTestosterone to be absorbed directly into the tissues, and has approximately twice the potency of oral MethylTestosterone. Peak serum concentrations are attained approximately one hour after buccal administration.

Injectable Testosterones:

There are several injectable (intramuscular) Testosterone preparations. These synthetic versions include both water (aqueous) and oil-based diluents. Testosterone esters are less polar than free Testosterone, and are slowly absorbed from the lipid phase.

Testosterone Cypionate:

This has both high androgenic and anabolic effects. Testosterone Cypionate, which is an oil-based compound, aromatizes very easily, which makes water retention a potential problem for many individuals. It is only moderately toxic to the liver, however, it is able to disturb the body's own endogenous production of male hormones. Testosterone Cypionate has about a 5 to 7 day life in the system therefore, requires to be re-injected intramuscularly, at least once every seven days to maintain optimal effects. Also, when used in physiologic replacement dosages, Testosterone Cypionate does not raise dihydroTestosterone (DHT) levels.

Testosterone Enanthate:

The primary difference between Testosterone Enanthate and Cypionate, is that Enanthate has a longer life, and a lessened amount of impact upon the system. Testosterone Enanthate, which is also an oil-based compound, usually only requires to be administered intramuscularly once every 10 to 14 days, which of course, provides for a much greater convenience, and is usually more cost efficient. An average life of Testosterone Enanthate is anywhere from 10 to 20 days in the system.

Several compounds include either Testosterone Cypionate or Testosterone Enanthate versions as both are considered to be the most efficacious, due to their capabilities of existing in the system, for longer durations. Possessing a longer half-life also enables for a much lessened injection requirement. This of course, is very desirable as this option decreases both the pain, and scar tissue possibilities which are often associated with frequent, multiple injections.

Testosterone Decanoate, Isocaproate, Phenylpropionate, and Propionate:

These Testosterone preparations, also all procure an oil as the diluent to extend their half-lives. It has been discovered that the slow absorption from the oil depot rather than slow de-esterification of these compounds are what establishes the half-life characteristics once administered into the system. The short term of existence however, markedly reduces the potential liver toxicity, and the production of normal patterns of virilization. Testosterone Decanoate, Isocaproate, Phenylpropionate, and Propionate, have a very short life in the system, existing anywhere from 1 to 3 days. This also of course, requires more frequent intramuscular injections which are uncomfortable and inconvenient.

Testosterone Suspension (Aqueous):

Testosterone Suspension is another injectable Testosterone however, it is "suspended" in a water solvent. This product is one of the oldest androgens still available, and remains very popular amongst athletes due to fast acting characteristics. As Testosterone Suspension is a water-based compound, it is able to enter the bloodstream very quickly, usually within a matter of hours. It also has a life of approximately a day or two, which permits it to be only effective for about 24 hours, therefore, allowing it to be impractical in long-term clinical hypogonadal treatment. Due to Testosterone Suspension's characteristic of possessing a short-life in the system, this compound has to be administered frequently, therefore, more intramuscular injections have to be endured. Another negative characteristic of Testosterone Suspension, is due to the increased frequency of injections, can also often lead to not only a very uncomfortable cycle, but to potential scar tissue buildup in the injection site. Still, many athletes sacrifice comfort to profit from the dramatic gains in size and strength, which are often affiliated with Testosterone Suspension administration.

Testosterone Undecanoate:

Testosterone Undecanoate is an oral administration compound, which is available in capsule form. These capsules are to be swallowed by the mouth combined with a liquid, and do not require to be crushed or chewed. Testosterone Undecanoate absorption varies greatly, and is largely dependent upon the percentage of the fat content in the diet. The intestinal mucosa is known to sometimes de-esterify this compound, preventing it from entering the lymphatics. This characteristic makes it difficult to occasionally achieve therapeutic levels, even with extremely high dose administration. Currently, another somewhat unique oral compound of Testosterone, which is formulated with oleic acid, has been able to aid in Testosterone Undecaonate absorption into the lymphatics, as opposed to being processed by the liver, by normally entering the hepatoportal circulation. Unlike most other oral compounds, this is not 17-a-alkylated, which is advantageous in the prevention of inducing liver toxicity. Unfortunately, this is still being extensively studied, due to extreme discrepancies in results experienced within the same tested dependent.

However, when Testosterone Undecanoate is properly absorbed, it can increase DHT levels significantly, without exacerbating benign prostatic hyperplasia. Another common disadvantage of Testosterone Undecanoate is frequent gastric irritation. It also has an extremely short half-life, therefore, as it produces inadequate levels at night, it requires to be administered several times a day. This steroidal compound can prove to be expensive, due to the quantity required for effectiveness, and the cost associated with each capsule. Clinically, Testosterone Undecanoate has not produced impressive results in the application of hypogonadism treatment.

Scrotal Transdermal Patch:

Testoderm, is a product which administers Testosterone through absorption of the scrotal skin, due to this area's characteristic of being 5 times more permeable than regular non-scrotal skin. The stratum corneum of scrotal skin is thinner, with an increased superficial vasculature than non-scrotal skin, which leads to more effective absorption of large molecules such as Testosterone. However, a previous inhibiting factor was the relatively small quantities of substance which could be maximally delivered by a transdermal patch over time, as the clinical required amount of Testosterone is between 50 and 100 times that of the Estrogens in the comparable patch for menopausal women. This problem has been recently solved, enabling the Testosterone transdermal application to be very efficacious. Consequently the Testosterone transdermal system will not produce an adequate serum Testosterone concentration if it is applied to nongenital skin.

Ensuing placement of a Testosterone scrotal transdermal patch, the serum Testosterone concentration rises to a maximum at 2 to 4 hours; which returns towards initial values within approximately 2 hours after the patch is removed. Serum levels reach a plateau at 3 to 4 weeks, and Testosterone levels which can be achieved are generally within the range for normal men.

Clinically, patients initiate therapy with a 6 mg/day system which is placed on scrotal skin daily. If the scrotal area is inadequate, a 4 mg/day system is used instead. The patch is placed on dry, clean, dry-shaved, scrotal skin for optimal skin contact, (The use of chemical depilatories should be avoided), and applied under warm conditions, with warm hands, to warm scrotal skin. This provides a more even expansion of scrotal skin, which allows for greater adherence of the patch, which is pressed onto the scrotal skin and held in place for 10 seconds, (fastening to the skin usually can occur without the necessity of using tape). Assurance of immobilization of the patch can be additionally acquired by tight-fitting underwear .

The Testosterone transdermal system requires to be worn 22 to 24 hours on the scrotal surface. Peak absorption is arrived at in a few hours after application, which approximates the circadian peak of Testosterone in young, healthy male individuals. Abstinence from wearing the patch for two hours enables the blood levels to decrease to slightly below normal levels, which mimics the natural, endogenous rhythm. After approximately 3 to 4 weeks of continued daily compliance, plateau levels are achieved which indicate clinical effective Testosterone levels, which can be maintained for an optimal six years. Blood screenings should be obtained to determine levels of serum total Testosterone, approximately 3 to 4 weeks of continued daily use. Consequently, due to possible variances in analytical values amongst different diagnostic laboratories, these blood screening tests should be performed at the same laboratory.

The scrotal transdermal application of the Testosterone patch, has several advantages over other administration techniques. Primarily, the Testosterone which is absorbed into the system, is pure and identical to the hormone Testosterone, which is naturally produced by the body. This allows successful mimication of the natural circadian rhythms; and avoids supraphysiologic peaks and subnormal depression of injectable preparations. Determination of the reduction of psychic changes may possibly be achieved by proper timing of a particular dose. Several other studies have indicated that the pulsatile delivery of other hormones may indeed enhance target organ responsiveness and efficacy. This would ensue the restoration of the normal circadian rhythms, which may help maintain normal sleep quality and quantity.

Unfortunately, there are also several disadvantages associated with the scrotal transdermal patch. Temporary incidences of irritation (approximately 7 %) sometime occur in compliant administration, which diminish over time. The possibility of cellulitis may result from dry-shaving, or possible associated laceration, and constant contact of the patch to the scrotal skin surface. Sufficient scrotal size must also be present to allow for adequate application of the transdermal patch, however, this can sometimes be applied to the penile shaft in order to achieve results. Utilization of this scrotal patch has also resulted in abnormal DHT levels, which often were greater than ten times higher than normal values. However, this may be attributed to the characteristic of scrotal skin, which possesses a markedly increased amount of cells with a 5-a reductase activity, which converts Testosterone to DHT locally, while it is being absorbed through the skin. Regular prostate screenings may rule out potential prostatic adverse effects, due to DHT increases.

Non-Scrotal Transdermal Patch:

Androderm is a recent available product, which works similarly to the scrotal patch, but has an exclusive characteristic which can enhance non-scrotal skin absorption of Testosterone. Each patch contains 12.8 mgs of pure Testosterone and over a 24 hour period, can deliver approximately

4 to 7 mgs. Two patches are placed on any shaved area of the arms, legs or trunk of the body, and is worn by an individual on a daily basis, for a 24 hour duration. Consequently, the absorption of this patch is slightly slower than the scrotal application, which therefore, requires individuals to administer these patches at approximately 10:00 p.m., in order to achieve reproduced peak levels in approximately six hours, which occur naturally by the system, in the morning. Plateau levels are usually achieved in approximately four weeks of daily compliance. The transdermal Androderm patch has clinically demonstrated excellent responses in hypogonadal individuals in regards to sexual function, as well as increased libido, energy and in the maintenance of pyschic regularity.

The primary advantage of the Androderm patch is that it does not elevate DHT (DihydroTestosterone), Estrogen, or SHBG (sex hormone binding globulin) levels, which can lessen the probability of premature balding, and prostatic changes. It can also be used by individuals who have inadequate scrotal size, as this does not require this area for strict application to be efficacious. The only disadvantage, which is only slightly temporarily bothersome, is the possibility of local skin irritation or cellulitis.

Conclusively, in comparison to all possible Testosterone administration applications, the Androderm transdermal patch appears to be the foremost supplemental system currently available, with the most effective delivery of Testosterone, in relation to side effects, and in mimicking the natural circadian rhythms.

THE FOLLOWING TRADE NAMES CAN BE FOUND UNDER THE FOLLOWING CHEMICAL NAMES:

Trade Name Found	*Common Trade Name*	*Chemical Name*
Human:		
Aldactone	Aldactone	Spironolactone.
Anapolon	Anadrol	Oxymetholone.
Novegam Spiropent	Clenbuterol	Clenbuterol Hydrocloride.
Omifin Serofene	Clomid	Clomiphene Citrate.
Maxibol	Co-Enzyme B12	Co-Enzyme B12.
Fertodur	Cyclofenil	Cyclofenil.
Cynomel	Cytomel	Liothyronine Sodium.
Deca-Durabolin	Deca-Durabolin	Nandrolone Decanoate.
Dyazide	Dyazide	Triamterene HCI.
Stenox	Halotestin	Fluoxymesterone.
Gonadotropyl Gonakor Profasi	HCG	Chorionic Gonadotropin.
Glucophage	Glucophage	Metformin.
Biotropin	Human Growth	Somatropin.

Genotropin Humatrope Norditropin Saizen	Hormone	
Protropin	Human Growth Hormone	Somatrem.
Beriglobina*P Humulin Seroglubin	Insulin	Human Biosynthetic Insulin.
Lasix	Lasix	Furosemide.
Eutirox Tiroidine	L-Thyroxine	Levothyroxine Sodium.
Madecassol	Madecassol	Centella Asiatica Extract.
Naxen	Naprosyn	Naproxen.
Nolvadex	Nolvadex	Tamoxifen Citrate.
Nubain	Nubain	Nalbuphine HCI.
Debeone	Phenformin	Phenformin HCI.
Primobolan Depot	Primobolan Depot	Methenolone Enanthate.
Primobolan Tablets	Primobolan Tablets	Methenolone Acetate.
Proviron	Proviron	Mesterolone.
Sten	Sten	Testosterone Pro- pionate, Testosterone Cypionate, Dihydro- testerone.

Sostenon 250	Sustanon	Testosterone Propionate, Testosterone Phenylpropionate, Testosterone Isocaproate, Testosterone Decanoate.
Primoteston Depot	Testosterone Enanthate	Testosterone Enanthate.
Neurofor	Vitamin B12	Cyanocobalamin.

Veterinary:

Norandren 50	Deca-Durabolin	Nandrolone Decanoate.
Metandiabol Reforvit-B	Dianabol	Methandrostenolone/ Methandienone.
Equi-Gan* Crecibol Maxi-Gan	Equipoise	Boldenone Undecylenate.
Laurabolin 20 & 50 Fortabol	Laurabolin	Nandrolone Laurate.
Ralgrow	Ralgrow	Zeranol.
Synovex*-H	Synovex*-H	Testosterone Propionate, Estradiol Benzoate.
Deposterona*	Sustanon	Testosterone Acetate, Testosterone Valerate, Testosterone Undecanoate.

Testosterona 200	Testosterone Enanthate	Testosterone Enanthate.
Testosterona 25 & 50	Testosterone Propionate	Testosterone Propionate.
Super Vitamina B12 5500 Hdroxo & Cyano	Vitamin B12	Cyanocobalamin.

MEXICAN HUMAN PHARMACEUTICALS

ALDACTONE

Chemical Name: Spironolactone.

Common Generic Name: Aldactone.

Other Trade Names Found in Mexico: Currently, just Aldactone.

Manufacturers: Aldactone - Searle.

Dosage Form: Aldactone "100" - 30 tablets.
Aldactone "A" - 30 x 25 mg tablets.

Storage: Aldactone should be stored at room temperature in a tightly closed, light-resistant container, below 30 degrees C or (86 degrees F).

Price Range: Aldactone "100" - approx. $107.20 pesos for 30 tablets.
Aldactone "A" - approx. $37.00 pesos for 30 x 25 mg tablets.

Type of Drug: Mild Diuretic and Antihypertensive.
Aldosterone Antagonist.

Ingredient: Spironolactone.

Drug Identification:

Aldactone **"100"** - for oral administration, is available in a white to off-white, round, standard, tablet, with SEARLE impressed on one side, and the other side has been scored. There are two silver packages with the 10 x 100 mg tablets, for a total of 20 tablets, available on each sheet contained within individual push-see-through blisters. The back of Aldactone*100, is silver with the product's entities written in navy blue ink. The Registration # 87911 and Lot # 4960585, and expiration date can also be found on the back. The accompanying package is bluish in color, with the products entities written in black and white. There is also a UPC code on the front of the package itself.

"Aldactone*-A" - is similarly available in a white to off-white, round, standard, oral administration tablet, with SEARLE impressed on one side, and the other side has been scored. There are also three silver packages with 10 x 25 mg tablets, for a total of 30 tablets, available on each sheet contained within individual push-see-through blisters. The back of Aldactone*-A, is also silver, with the product's entities written in navy blue ink. The Registration # 58500 and Lot # 4940252, along with the expiration date can be also found on the back. The packaging accompanying these tablets is bluish in color, with the product's entities written in black and white.

*****Please refer to the photographs of Aldactone "100" and Aldactone "A" for full color references.***

Drug Description:

Aldactone is a diuretic; which belongs to a subgroup of potassium-sparing diuretics, that had been often used clinically for the treatment of high blood pressure. Aldactone is an anti-androgen since it also had been able to have reduced the androgen levels. It additionally had been able to have influenced Aldosterone (the body's own hormone released from the adrenal gland), which had accelerated the excretion of potassium, and in turn, had reduced the excretion of sodium and water. The utilization of Aldactone significantly had also reduced the Aldosterone level, so that an increased excretion of sodium and water had occurred, while potassium had been reabsorbed at the same duration.

Potassium-sparing diuretics had generally been the most mildest of class of diuretics, and had often been used in combination with thiazides, such as Dyazide, or loop-agent diuretics such as Lasix, in efforts to offset the increased electrolytes which had been sometimes lost by the body.

As Aldactone had been a milder diuretic compound, many athletes had engaged in it's administration approximately 5 to 6 days prior to competition, in attempts to have eliminated remaining subcutaneous water. However, dehydration or "flattening" of the muscles had always been a great possibility, although it had not been as extreme as with the use of a loop-agent diuretic, such as Lasix.

Many female athletes had also utilized the compound of Aldactone for it's anti-androgen entities, in attempts to have reduced the androgen levels; in efforts to have minimized virilization symptoms that had sometimes been experienced both during and after steroid treatments. Even several natural bodybuilders had frequently used potassium-sparing agents such as Aldactone, which had often indicated this compound's subtlety as a prescription diuretic. Consequently, over-the-counter substances such as herbal preparations had been a possibility for athletes who had not wished to have taken last minute risks with prescription diuretics, and had the required time allotment for such mild agents to have been effective.

Usual Clinical Recommendation:

The usual recommendations for clinical administration had usually been approximately 400 mg/day for 3 to 4 days. This of course, had been under the care and supervision of a qualified physician.

Adventitious Dosage and Administration:

Aldactone tablets have been intended for oral administration, which had implied that they should have been swallowed by mouth. Many athletes had claimed that these tablets had produced the best results, when they had been consumed with water. They did not require to have been crushed or chewed. Aldactone tablets had allegedly produced more effective results if they had been taken all at once, first thing in the morning. The effects of Aldactone had been extremely mild, and sometimes had not been physically apparent upon initial administration. A common dosage regime of some athletes, has been discussed in the following:

Pre-contest bodybuilders had discovered the compound of Aldactone to have been useful in reducing excess water from abnormally high Estrogen levels in their systems. It had generally been utilized almost exclusively during the last week prior to competition. Before and during consumption of diuretics, most athletes had also often ingested higher than recommended amounts of calcium, magnesium, and potassium. This of course, had been easily accomplished by proper combinations of whole foods only, not by supplementation.

Females:

Female athletes had frequently administered Aldactone for it's anti-androgenic characteristics, as it had the ability to have reversed the effects of androgens. This had proven to have been rather useful for females who had used steroidal compounds, and had began to have suffered from virilization effects. If this had occurred, female athletes frequently had terminated the administration of the problematic compounds, and had administered Aldactone until such time the androgens had returned to within an acceptable range.

This had been usually anywhere from 1 to 3 tablet (25 to 75 mgs) range, which had been taken daily, totaling a dosage which had not exceeded more than 2 to 4 tablets, (50 to 100 mgs). This dosage had frequently been administered for a time period which had not extended past 3 to 5 consecutive days. If Aldactone "100" had been administered, then only 1 tablet per day, had been sufficient, as this had been the equivalent to 100 mgs.

Males:

Male athletes generally had administered Aldactone only for a few days at a time, as this substance had been able to have lowered the androgens so significantly, that painful nipples and potential gynecomastia had often become very problematic.

Aldactone had usually been frequently administered over 3 to 5 consecutive days, in a dosage of 4 tablets (100 mgs) daily. Five tablets, or 125 mgs of Aldactone, in any one given day had never been exceeded, nor had it been administered longer than 5 days. If Aldactone "100" had been administered, 1 tablet (equivalent to 100 mgs) per day had been sufficient for all male administering athletes.

If athletes had experienced these dosages of Aldactone to have been ineffective, instead of having increased the dosage amount, often a second diuretic such as Hydro-Diuril (of the thiazide family, which is currently not available in Mexico), had been additionally utilized. This practice had often had proved to have been tremendously advantageous, as a potassium-sparing diuretic and a thiazide together in lower dosages, generally had lowered the overall excretion of calcium. This had allegedly appeared to have been more effective than a single dose of a single compound item, such as using Aldactone as a sole entity.

Cautious athletes had been also extremely careful in not additionally having had administered any type of prescription potassium supplements in conjunction with potassium-sparing diuretics such as Spironolactone or Triamterene (currently, not available in Mexico).

Side Effects:

Several athletes had generally claimed that the side effects of potassium-saving diuretics such as Aldactone, had been relatively low compared to thiazides and furosemides. However, some of the side effects which had been experienced both clinically and in athletic application with this compound's utilization had included those of cramping, diarrhea, drowsiness, dizziness, dry mouth, headache, increased urination, rash, nausea, restlessness, vomiting or weakness, anxiety, clumsiness, confusion, fever, increased hair growth, muscle cramps, numbness or tingling in the hands, feet, or lips, palpitations, rapid weight gain, stomach cramps, unco-ordinated movements or unusual tiredness or weakness.

Side effects which had sometimes been especially troublesome to females athletes had included possible deepening or hoarseness of the voice, enlarged or swelling of the breasts, menstrual disturbances, and postmenopausal bleeding.

Some male athletes had occasionally encountered additional problems such as potential problematic side effects such as gynecomastia and impotence.

However, other adverse effects may have had been experienced by athletes who had self-administered Aldactone, but unfortunately, may not have been recognized, and therefore, had not been documented.

WARNING:

Most athletes had been very cautious in making certain that no additional potassium had been taken while they had administered Aldactone; as an increase in the serum potassium level could have proven to have been life-threatening. Also, the administration of Spironolactone had caused hyperkalemia (high levels of potassium in the blood).

Clinically, it had been advised that diuretics should not have been used for more than two or three days in a row, unless it had been administered and monitored under competent physician supervision, and/or for treatment of a medical condition.

If cardiac irregularities or possible other medical conditions had existed, the use of diuretics had never been self-administered by athletes, but instead, had been supervised by a physician. Possible fatal results had sometimes resulted when self-administration of diuretic compounds had been practiced by an athlete.

Rating:

Based on a 1 to 5 star scale, with 1 considered low, and 5 considered high, this compound of Spironolactone, had rated as the following:

	MALES	FEMALES
Contest Preparation	**	**
Anti-Estrogen/Androgen	--	***
Side Effects	***	***
Cost Efficiency	*	*

ANAPOLON

Chemical Name:	Oxymetholone.
Common Generic Name:	Anadrol.
Other Trade Names Found in Mexico:	Anapolon (presently manufactured only for institutional use). Genabol (N.L.M.).
Manufacturers:	Anapolon - Syntex.
Dosage Form:	Anapolon - 50 mgs tablets.
Storage:	Anapolon tablets should be protected from light and moisture, (keep in the blisters until contents are used), and stored at controlled room temperature 15 to 30 degrees C (59 to 86 degrees F).
Price Range:	Anapolon - Currently, since this steroidal compound is only available for institutional use, there is no market price available.
Type of Drug:	Potent Anabolic and Androgenic steroid.
Ingredient:	50 mgs of Oxymetholone.

Drug Identification:

Anapolon - Is available in tablet form for oral administration; each tablet contains 50 mgs of the steroid Oxymetholone. It is available presently only for hospital use, and can be found in 5 packages of 20 pink tablets, which are packaged in an individual plastic push-see-through blisters, with a silver foil punch through backing, and most often grouped together with an elastic band. The pink tablet is scored, allowing it to be further broken down if required. The other side is plain. On the back, Oximetolona, Anapolon 50, Syntex, Lot # 065142, Registration # 75521, and the clave 1709 is printed in black. There is no packaging accompanying these tablets, as they are often purchased by the institutions on a "bulk" basis.

****Please refer to the photographs of Anapolon for full color references.***

Drug Description:

Anapolon has been the strongest, oral steroidal compound, which is a derivative of dihydrotestosterone, that has been currently only available for institutional use in Mexico. Clinically, Anapolon had been often prescribed in efforts to have treated anemias which had been caused by deficient red cell production. The androgenic and high anabolic properties of Anapolon have been substandard of Testosterone, which had permitted this compound to have also been a dramatic muscle building product. Many athletes had claimed that strength and weight increases had been very substantial within a relatively short period of time. This characteristic had allowed the compound of Anapolon to have been a very popular choice of oral steroidal compounds amongst many athletes, primarily those of the male gender.

Most athletes had frequently experienced a general weight increase of approximately 10 to 15 lbs or more, within two weeks with the administration of this compound. This of course, had been largely attributed to the tremendous amount of water retention which had immediately increased the muscle diameters, which in turn, had permitted a rapid increased size appearance. Consequently, this retained amount of water in the muscle cells and joints, had also additionally provided a smooth appearance, as the size increase had been quantitative, not qualitative. An advantageous effect of the water retention however, had been the ability to have eliminated, or having soothed associated joint problems, which had been due to this side effect's subsequent lubricating quality. This had often been appreciated by most athletes, as this characteristic had frequently allowed for intense workouts, which had often been previously somewhat restricted, due to associated aggravated pain in the joints.

The Anapolon oral steroidal compound, had further increased the number of red blood cells, which in turn, had enabled the muscles to have absorbed more oxygen. This had generally resulted in the muscle being able to have endured more physical stress, which had been due to the significant increase in blood volume. A "pump" effect had often been experienced when training particular muscles, and had even become somewhat painful to the extent, that the performed exercise had frequently been required to have been abandoned, in order to have alleviated this sensation.

However, this perception of increased strength and power had commonly been desired by all athletes who had practiced the self-administration of this compound, as this sensation had usually been indicative that the compound of Anapolon had indeed, been performing to it's full capacity. Several athletes had also claimed that another distinguishing trait of Anapolon, had been the increased training durations, as this compound had been able to have stimulated the regeneration of the body, which often had enabled further muscle-building progress, and had stalled the possibility of over-training.

However, although the substance of Anapolon had been powerful, it unfortunately, also had *imposed the highest threat for serious adverse reactions out of any oral or injectable steroidal compounds.* A few athletes had experienced excessive water retention which had sometimes resulted in high blood pressure. Anapolon has very high DHT levels, and had been very toxic to the liver, due to the characteristics of being a C-17 alpha-alkylated steroid.

Although the Anapolon steroidal compound had been known for quick strength and mass gains, it's utilization had not been suitable for novices, and had only been used by some athletes after a certain development had been achieved; or consequently, the prior use of weaker steroidal compounds had been experienced.

Anapolon had the most side effects reported out of all of the anabolic or androgenic steroids available.

Usual Clinical Recommendation:

The recommended daily dose in both children and adults had been 1 to 5 mgs/kg of body weight per day. The usual effective dose had been 1 to 2 mg/kg/day, but higher doses have been required, therefore, the dosage had been usually individualized.

Adventitious Dosage and Administration:

Anapolon tablets had been intended for oral administration, which had implied that they should have been swallowed by mouth. Several athletes had claimed that these tablets had produced the best results, when they had also been consumed with water, and had always been taken with meals. They did not require to have been crushed or chewed. A common dosage regime of some athletes, has been discussed in the following:

Females:

Primarily, female athletes generally had not engaged in the administration of Anapolon, due to the fact that it had usually been poorly tolerated, and simply "too powerful" for most women. The usage of Anapolon had frequently resulted in virilization effects, even on what had been considered to have been a low tolerable dose.

However, some adventurous female athletes still had chosen to have risked utilizing this compound in efforts to have achieved great gains in mass. An usual regime mostly had often consisted of a half of a 50 mg tablet (25 mgs), every two days, combined with a milder injectable anabolic such as Primobolan Depot, at approximately 2 to 2 1/2 x 50 mg ampules (100 to 150 mgs) on a weekly basis.

If virilization side effects had become a problem, then the options of either having discontinued Anapolon, or possibly having added a half of a Proscar tablet (currently, not available in Mexico), a day to the regime, had been sometimes utilized by these female athletes, in efforts to have calmed the adverse effects.

Consequently, most female athletes had usually chosen to have avoided the Anapolon steroidal compound, as there had been other more tolerable anabolics that had been able to have rendered similar results, without the encounterment of harmful adverse effects.

Males:

Many male athletes had claimed that the administration of Anapolon had been excellent for dramatic gains in strength and muscle mass, as well as a weight increase. The usual effective dosage had generally consisted of 0.5 to 8 mg/kg/day. However, higher doses had sometimes been required, and perused; but had usually always been individualized accordingly.

The usual range in dosages had been anywhere from 1 to 4 tablets (50 to 200 mgs) per day. Most male athletes had been cautious not to have exceeded more than four tablets (or 200 mgs) in any one given day; as up to three tablets (or 150 mgs) usually had sufficed for desired gains in both weight and strength increases.

When male athletes had initiated a cycle, they most often had begun with one 50 mg tablet once a day for one week. On the second week, this had been increased to two 50 mgs tablets taken once in the morning, and once in the evening. Then, this had once again been increased to three tablets a day for the third week. After the third week, the cycle had been reversed by having repeated three tablets a day for one week, two tablets a day for the next week, and then finally, one tablet a day for the last week. This had totaled a cycle of 6 weeks. These athletes had been careful to have always administered the compound of Anapolon with their meals.

Several athletes had reported that after discontinuing Anapolon, a drastic reduction in weight and strength had usually been experienced. In efforts to have prevented this from occurring, many athletes had continued a steroid treatment with another compound such as Sostenon 250, or Primoteston Depot 250, for several weeks. Another feasible common stack had consisted of Anapolon x 100 mg +/day, Parabolan (currently, not available in Mexico), and Sostenon 250 at 500+ mgs (or 2 cc's) per week.

Anapolon had generally been used in precontest preparation, even though it had maintained muscle mass and enabled intense training regimes. However, in many untested competitions, it had been used up to a week previously, with the aid of anti-Estrogens such as Nolvadex and Proviron, to counteract the problematic water retention. These compounds along with diuretics, had often allowed the muscles to have maintained a full and hard appearance, which of course, had been ultimately desired by athletes, especially competing bodybuilders.

Side Effects:

There had been several side effects that had been experienced both clinically and in athletic application, that had been associated with the administration of Anapolon. A few of which that had occasionally been experienced by some athletes had included; nausea, vomiting, changes in skin color, ankle swelling, muscle cramps, edema, decreased glucose tolerance, insomnia, increased or decreased libido, water retention, high blood pressure, hairloss, jaundice, discoloration of fingernails, or eyes, and a general feeling of ill-feeling.

Anapolon also had a notorious reputation as a cause of hair loss in chronic abusers. Most importantly, since Anapolon had been considered to have been ***the*** most harmful steroid, there had also been general pathological changes in liver values; which had generally often had become evident even after only a week's administration. Also, if liver enzymes of GOT and GPT had become elevated, which usually had indicated hepatitis, liver infection had also been a possibility. If high dosages of Anapolon had been taken over a prolonged period of time, liver damage had become inevitable. Athletes often had their liver values checked periodically by a competent physician, to have ensured that their levels had been within an acceptable range.

Potential side effects which female athletes had especially experienced, had been those of virilization, such as hoarseness or deepening of the voice, increased facial and body hair, male pattern baldness, acne, clitoral enlargement, menstrual irregularity, even censation of periods. Most of these side effects once obtained, had not been reversible. The compound of Anapolon had very androgenic to females, and the possibility of these potential side effects had been very high and probable.

Several male athletes had additionally experienced gynecomastia, inhibition of testicular function, testicular atrophy, deficient amount of spermatozoa in seminal fluid, impotence, chronic priapism (abnormal, painful and continued erection of the penis due to disease, not sexual desire), epididymitis, bladder irritation, and a decreased seminal fluid.

Of course, other side effects may have had been experienced, which had not been recognized by the athlete, therefore, had not been documented.

WARNING:

Anapolon had been the only anabolic/androgenic steroid which had been linked to liver cancer. Cautious athletes usually had not administered Anapolon for prolonged periods of time, and always routinely had liver values such as GOT, GPT, bilirubin, gamma-GT, and alkaline phosphatase (AP), and LDH/HBDH checked.

Rating:

Based on a 1 to 5 star scale, with 1 considered low, and 5 considered high; a -- symbol is indicative of no value. This compound of Oxymetholone had rated as the following:

	MALES	FEMALES
Strength Increase	*****	**
Mass & Weight Increase	*****	**
Contest Preparation	***	*
Side Effects	*****	*****
Cost Efficiency	??	??

(CLENBUTEROL)

Chemical Name:	Clenbuterol Hydrocloride.
Common Generic Name:	Clenbuterol.
Other Trade Names Found in Mexico:	Novegam (N.L.M.) Spiropent.
Manufacturers:	Novegam - Chinoin (N.L.M.) Spiropent - Promeco.
Dosage Form:	Novegam - 120 ml solution (N.L.M.) 20 tablets (N.L.M.) Spiropent - 120 ml solution. 20 tablets.
Storage:	Novegam and Spiropent tablets should be protected from light and moisture, (keep in the blisters until contents are used), and stored at controlled room temperature 15 to 30 degrees C (59 to 86 degrees F). The liquid should also be stored in this manner.
Price Range:	Novegam - approx. $23.20 pesos for 120 ml solution. - approx. $29.20 pesos for a box of 20 tablets. Spiropent - approx. $60.20 pesos for 120 ml solution. - approx. $67.90 pesos for a box of 20 tablets.
Type of Drug:	Nonsteroidal. Beta-2-symphatomimetic. Anti-Catabolic.

Ingredient: 0.02 mg Clenbuterol.

Drug Identification:

Spiropent - as an oral administration tablet, is a white tablet with the Promeco company logo impressed on one side, and scored on the other side, allowing the dosage to be broken down into half strengths. It is packaged in a clear individual plastic blister, with a silver foil punch through backing. It is available in 2 sheets of 10 tablets, totaling 20 per box. On the back, Spiropent, Tableta 0.02 mg, with Promeco's company logo is printed repeatedly in black throughout the backing. The Lot # is 143601.

Spiropent - as an oral solution administration, is somewhat of a clear syrup, with a pleasant "minty" taste. It is available in 120 ml bottle solution, in 0.2 mg strength. The bottle is dark brown with a screw on/off white lid. The white label has the product's entities written in navy blue ink, accompanied by a yellow, and navy blue stripe. Instructions for usage as a bronchodilator is indicated on the back of the label in Spanish. A measuring cap is also found on the top of the bottle, and is marked for easy measuring identification. It is suggested to gently shake the bottle before usage. The accompanying package is identical to the bottle itself.

Novegam - as an oral administration tablet, and ***Novegam*** as an oral solution administration, could not be obtained for illustration and identification purposes; as most Farmacias had heavily stocked their shelves with the ever popular "Spiropent" versions.

The manufacturers of the compound "Novegam", had recently stopped producing both the oral and solution products. However, some farmacias may still have a few of these products still located upon their shelves. Novegam may be difficult to find, and will be obsolete in the near future.

*****Please refer to the photographs of Spiropent for full color references.***

Drug Description: *** Spiropent and Novegam have been commonly referred to as Clenbuterol for simplicity measures in the following text.*

Clenbuterol had first surfaced in the athletic fields early in 1988. Clinically, it is a beta-two symphatomimetic, which had been utilized in the treatment of asthma. Clenbuterol has very little beta-3 stimulation, and until there is a new synthetic beta-3 agonist commercially available, it will continue to be the preferred beta agonist. Consequently, there has been a stronger research chemical that has been currently available in the United States, referred to as Cimaterol. The administration of Clenbuterol had been becoming very popular over the last few years, therefore, this substance had also been added to the banned substance list of the U.S. Olympic Committee, and other sporting federations, even though it has not been a steroidal item per se. Clenbuterol has been available in other countries in such forms as syrups, drops, liquids, and dosing Clenbuterol Hydrocloride, and also in veterinarian forms such as Ventipulmin.

Clenbuterol's effects on fat tissue had been wondrous, as a well known effect of beta agonist therapy, it had appeared to have worked by directly having had aroused lipolysis in the fat tissue (although this had not been proven in all laboratory testing done in animals). Therefore, decreased bodyfat had been probably due to an increase of fatty acid mobilization, and also a decrease in fat production. The administration of Clenbuterol had also been known to have increased the body's ability to have burned calories in heat production, and this may have been the reason why there had often been an increase in perspirational entities. Furthermore, there had been different receptor sites in skeletal muscle and adipose tissue, and muscle receptors had downgraded much quicker than those of fat tissue receptors. The compound of Clenbuterol appeared to have had caused hypertrophy, but not the muscle growth in animal studies.

Consequently, the utilization of Clenbuterol had decreased the rate at which protein had been reduced in muscle cells, which in turn, had caused them to have enlarged; which had additionally resulted in a strong anticatabolic effect. Clenbuterol had also caused significant qualitative muscle hypertrophy and strength gains. Several athletes had utilized the compound of Clenbuterol after the termination of a steroid regime, in efforts to have stabilized the resulting catabolic phase, and to also have obtained maximum strength and muscle mass. The compound of Clenbuterol had been very popular amongst female athletes, as it had been able to have provided a hard, qualitative muscle gain and strength, with the addition of having had accelerated the burning of bodyfat. These characteristics had frequently been ultimately desired by the female athlete gender, as these gains had not generally been associated with negative adverse effects, such as those that had primarily been obtained by other enhancement products. However, it had also been apparent that unless Clenbuterol had been administered continuously, and diet regimes had been somewhat adjusted, any lean body mass had often quickly reverted back to previous states. Clenbuterol had frequently been able to have burned bodyfat without the necessity of extreme dieting, as it had been slightly able to have increased the body temperature, which in turn, had forced the body to have burned fat for energy. Currently, in research, this effect had been repeatedly proven in numerous studies of all species, except in human beings.

To date, there have been no clinical human studies available on the administration of Clenbuterol's anabolic and fat burning entities. Also, no clinical investigations into long-term cardiovascular side effects have been undertaken. The only available data on Clenbuterol had been conducted on animals in laboratories, and slaughter stocks. However, the rate of extrapolation obtained from animal studies to unsupervised human usage has been steadily increasing, but physicians still require accurate information regarding Clenbuterol in human studies for purposes such as mentioned in this text; other than solely as a broncholilator.

Many athletes have abandoned the administration of other compounds such as Ephedrine, (currently, not available in Mexico), Cynomel, Eutirox, and Tiroidine, as they had generally claimed that the utilization of Clenbuterol had been much more effective in lipolysis, strength and highly qualitative muscle increases. However, these effects of Clenbuterol had appeared to have been only temporary, as they had only been able to have been experienced for a short duration, due to the down regulating of the receptor sites. Therefore, these effects had been most apparent upon the initial two week administration of the Clenbuterol substance.

Usual Clinical Recommendation:

The only recommendations for Clenbuterol administration had been documented as instructions pertaining to utilization as a bronchodilator.

As previously stated, there had been no studies performed pertaining to the clinical human administration for fat burning or muscle increase entities. Therefore, as a broncodilator, the recommended dosage had been usually 1 to 2 tablets, or 1 to 2 doses of syrup, four times a day, with the warning of not having exceeded this recommended dosage.

Adventitious Dosage and Administration:

Spiropent and Novegam tablets had been intended for oral administration, which have implied that they had been designed to have been swallowed by mouth. Both female and male athletes had claimed that these tablets had produced the best results, if they had also been consumed with water, prior to meals. They did not require to have been crushed or chewed. The solutions had been administered in much the similar manner, without the requirement of having to have swallowed water. A common dosage regime of some athletes, has been discussed in the following:

Pre-contest bodybuilders had discovered that the compound of Clenbuterol had been useful in burning bodyfat. Therefore, this had been utilized primarily a month prior to competition for acquiring a desired "ripped" appearance. Also, Clenbuterol had also been often administered after a steroid cycle in efforts to have balanced the resulting catabolic phase; while having obtained maximum strength and muscle mass. The administrated dosage had been dependent upon the bodyweight, and by additionally having had measured personal body temperature, many athletes had been able to have accelerated these results.

It had appeared to have been important that the athlete had started the initiation of the Clenbuterol compound by having taken only one tablet on the first day, then having increased this dosage by one tablet each of the following days, until the desired maximum dosage had been reached for two weeks. Then usually, Clenbuterol had then been administered on a two day on, two day off cycle.

Ideally, many athletes had administered this compound for a period of approximately three weeks, and then had abstained for a duration of six weeks, in efforts to have prevented abatement of the receptor sites. However, many athlete's cycles had ranged anywhere from a 3 to 6 week interval, which had mostly been dependent upon if the emphasis had been placed on fat burning, or on strength, muscle growth and fat burning entities.

Several athletes had engaged in the regime of having stacked Clenbuterol with Cynomel 25 mcg (1 tablet), and Zaditen 10 mg (currently not available in Mexico), each day after the cycle of Clenbuterol had been discontinued, for three weeks, in efforts to have possible further enhanced the thermogenic effect.

Anabolic effects of Clenbuterol had generally diminished after as little as 18 days if it had been administered continuously, due to rapid receptor downgrading. This had been shown to have had an equal effect on both female and male athletes, as well as have had an equal effect on both a high or low calorie diet regiment.

Females:

Female athletes generally had administered approximately 80 to 100 mcgs (2 to 4 tablets) daily, in divided equal dosages. Again, this had been largely dependent upon bodyweight and desired goals.

Males:

Male athletes had primarily administered approximately 100 to 140 mcgs (5 to 7 tablets) daily, in divided dosages, again which had been dependent upon bodyweight, and also desired goals.

Side Effects:

Side effects which had frequently been associated with the administration of Clenbuterol, had not been considered to have been serious, when it had been used within conservative amounts. However, some adverse effects had been significant enough to have prohibited some athletes from administering it; as many could not have tolerated the associated headaches or tremors which this compound had appeared to have induced.

The compound of Clenbuterol did not have typical anabolic steroid side effects, as it had not been a hormone compound. Some of the known side effects which had been occasionally experienced by some athletes had included restlessness, palpitations, involuntary trembling of the fingers (tremors), headaches, increased perspiration, insomnia, possible muscle spasms, increased blood pressure and nausea. However, approximately 48 hours after the practice of having discontinued the administration of Clenbuterol, had often resulted in the cessation of these side effects.

Other possible adverse effects may have been experienced by athletes who had self-administered Clenbuterol, which may not have been recognized, or documented.

WARNING:

Athletes who had suffered from hypertension (high blood pressure), asthma, diabetes, heart irregularities, or any other health disorder, had not engaged in the self-administration of Clenbuterol.

Also, athletes who had been sensitive to moderate central nervous system stimulants such as Ephedrine or caffeine, had frequently experienced an increased sensitivity to this compound.

As previously mentioned, there have been no human studies available, therefore, there may have been many more side effects which may have been encountered, but not yet diagnosed. There have also been no long term studies available on Clenbuterol's administration for prolonged periods of time.

Rating:

Based on a 1 to 5 star scale, with 1 considered low, and 5 considered high, a -- symbol is indicative of no value. This compound of Clenbuterol Hydrocloride had rated as the following:

	MALES	FEMALES
Strength Increase	***	***
Mass & Weight Increase	***	***
Fat Burner	*****	*****
Contest Preparation	****	****
Appetite Depressant	***	***
Side Effects	**	**
Cost Efficiency	***	***

(CLOMID)

Chemical Name: Clomiphene Citrate.

Common Generic Name: Clomid.

Other Trade Names Found in Mexico: Omifin
Serofene.

Manufacturers: Omifin - Hoechs.
Serofene - Serono.

Dosage Form: Omifin - 30 x 50 mgs tablets.
Serofene - 10 x 50 mgs tablets.
- 30 x 50 mgs tablets.

Storage: Clomid tablets should be protected from light and moisture, (keep in the blisters until contents are used), and stored at controlled room temperature 15 to 30 degrees C (59 to 86 degrees F).

Price Range: Omifin - approx. $104.60 pesos for 30 x 50 mgs tablets.
Serofene - approx. $ 30.00 pesos for 10 x 50 mgs tablets.
- approx. $ 80.95 pesos for 30 x 50 mgs tablets.

Type of Drug: Synthetic Estrogen. Non-steroidal.

Ingredient: 50 mgs of Clomiphene Citrate.

Drug Identification:

Omifin - Is available in tablet form for oral administration; each tablet is round, white, one side has a "M" within a "double circle", while the other side has been scored, allowing the tablet to be broken into a half strength, if required. These tablets are packaged in an individual plastic see-through blister, with a silver foil punch-through backing, available in 3 sheets of 10 tablets, for a total of 30 tablets within a package. On the back of the silver backing, Omifin, Registration # 65748 and Lot # can be found written down the center in navy blue ink. The package itself is quite basic, a medium bluish color with a white border, tops and sides. The product's entities are written in both white and navy blue ink.

Serofene - for oral administration, unfortunately could not be obtained for illustration and identification purposes. This product however, is still manufactured by Serono, but may be somewhat difficult to find, as most farmacias may have to specially order it in.

*****Please refer to the photographs of Omifin for full color references.***

Drug Description: ***Omifin and Serofene have been commonly referred to as Clomid for simplicity measures in the following text.*

Clomid is not only a synthetic Estrogen, but also functions as an anti-Estrogen as well. Clomiphene Citrate had been clinically utilized as a fertility enhancer in the female gender, as it had been able to have increased the rate of ovulation by having initiated the process of releasing hormones. This in turn, had been able to have stimulated the release of gonadotropins in females who had anovulatory cycles (cycles without the production of an ovum), and had been sterile as a result. The administration of Clomid had been able to have had improved the activity between the mid-brain, pituitary gland, and the ovaries, which in turn, had stimulated the hypophysis to have released more gonadotropin; which had resulted in a faster and higher release of follicle stimulating hormone (FSH), and Luteinizing hormone (LH).

Clomid however, had been ultimately unable to act as an anti-Estrogen in males, as clinically, it was not to have been administered for a prolonged period of time; which would have been required in efforts for Clomid to have an anti-Estrogenic property in male athletes. Consequently, males also had often experienced a stimulation of the hypophysis, which had generally been similar to that experienced by women, however, instead, this stimulation had increased the male body's own Testosterone levels. The compound of Clomid had been usually able to have normalized the Testosterone level and the sperm development within a time period of one to two weeks. One of the main reasons that it had a very low Estrogenic effect and strong Estrogen factor, had been generally due to the aromatization of steroids, which had often become blocked at the receptors. Therefore, as it had become unable to have attached to receptors, the increased Estrogen had not prevented the administered steroids from aromatizing.

Clomid had been principally utilized by male athletes after having had discontinued a steroid cycle, in efforts to have prevented a loss of strength and muscle, while at the same time, having elevated the Testosterone production back to normal levels.

Usual Clinical Recommendation:

Clinically, many female patients had frequently responded to 50 mgs of Clomid taken daily, for five days. The dosage and duration of therapy beyond 100 mgs a day for 5 days, had never have been further increased.

Adventitious Dosage and Administration:

Omifin and Serofene tablets had been intended for oral administration, which had implied that they had been designed to have been swallowed by mouth. Many male athletes had reported that these tablets had produced the best results if they had also been consumed with water and meals. They did not require to have been crushed or chewed. A common dosage regime of some athletes has been discussed in the following:

Females:

Female athletes usually had not employed the administration of Clomid in efforts to have enhanced athletic or bodybuilding properties. If females had utilized the compound of Clomid, it had usually been for clinical reasons to have treated infertility.

Males:

Several male athletes had occasionally administered the compound of Clomid for it's properties as a Testosterone stimulant, while having had terminated a steroid cycle. A common dosage of 50 to 100 mgs (1 to 2 tablets) a day had been often taken for two weeks, then the dosage had been gradually decreased after the fifth day, down to 50 mgs (1 tablet). However, if several tablets had been taken, they had been evenly administered throughout the day, and always had been consumed with meals. The compound of Clomid had never been administered for a time period more than two weeks, as it had allegedly usually been able to have increased the endogenous production of Testosterone well within this period.

Several male athletes had claimed that having had combined Clomid with Gonadotrophyl-C, Gonakor, or Profasi (HCG), or having administered Clomid after a cycle of (HCG), generally had enhanced the stimulation of Testosterone. The main differences between Clomid and (HCG) had been that the compound of Clomid had regenerated the entire regulating cycle, as it had a direct effect on the hypothalamus and the hypophysis, whereas, (HCG) could only have imitated the effect of the Luteinizing hormone (LH) to have stimulated the Leydig's cells in order to have produced more Testosterone. Therefore, many male athletes had often chosen to have administered (HCG) prior to the utilization of Clomid, as it had been able to have reached distinct elevated plasmatestosterone levels; usually within a few hours after it had been administered.

Side Effects:

If Clomid had been utilized by male athletes in conservative dosages, side effects had usually been very rare. However, some of the side effects known to have been associated with the administration of this compound had included those of bloating, stomach or pelvic pain, jaundice, blurred vision, headaches, nausea and vomiting, dizziness, and lightheadedness. Although the possibility of liver functions becoming inadequate had been slight, it had still been somewhat of a possibility.

Some side effects which particularly had been especially bothersome to females, had included those of ovarian enlargement and breast discomfort. The administration of Clomid may had also have aggravated the potential of multiple fetuses in one particular birthing incident.

Of course, there may have been other adverse effects which had been experienced by athletes who had self-administered Clomid, which may not have been recognized, therefore, had not been documented.

WARNING:

If athletes had experienced visual disturbances, they had discontinued the use of Clomid, and had intelligently sought the advice of a competent physician.

Rating:

Based on a 1 to 5 star scale, with 1 considered low, and 5 considered high, a -- symbol is indicative of no value. These compounds of Clomiphene Citrate had rated as the following:

	MALES	FEMALES
Testosterone Stimulant	***	--
Anti-Estrogen	****	--
Side Effects	***	**
Cost Efficiency	**	**

(CYCLOFENIL)

Chemical Name: Cyclofenil.

Common Generic Name: Cyclofenil.

Other Trade Names Found in Mexico: Fertodur.

Manufacturer: Fertodur - Schering.

Dosage Form: Fertodur - 200 mgs x 16 tablets.

Storage: Fertodur tablets should be protected from light and moisture, (keep in the individualized foil wrap until contents are used), and stored at controlled room temperature 15 to 30 degrees C (59 to 86 degrees F).

Price Range: Fertodur - approx. $100.00 pesos for 16 x 200 mg tablets.

Type of Drug: Mild Anti-Estrogen.

Ingredient: 200 mgs Cyclofenil.

Drug Identification:

Fertodur - tablets are welded in an individualized silver aluminum foil wrap, with 8 tablets per sheet. There are two sheets in each box, for a total of 16 tablets. The foil wrap has Fertodur Tabletas, the Reg. #, 62945 the Lot #, Schering Mexico, S.A. DE CV written across in black. The accompanying package is white, with an orangy-beige color vertical stripe near the right corner of the box, displaying the Schering company logo. The product's entities are displayed in black ink. This product may be difficult to find in most farmacias, however, it is available.

*****Please refer to the photograph of Fertodur for full color references.***

Drug Description:

Fertodur, much like Clomid, also belongs to the group of sex hormones, and is not an anabolic or androgenic steroid. Fertodur not only has acted as an anti-Estrogen property, but also has been able to have increased the body's own Testosterone levels at the same duration.

The compound of Fertodur has been similar to Omifin and Serofene (Clomid) and Gonadotrophyl "C", Gonakor, and Profasi (HCG), as it also had been able to have increased the endogenous Testosterone production, by having stimulated the testes. Most male athletes who had completed a steroid cycle, generally had wished to have elevated their own body's Testosterone levels; therefore, had often administered Fertodur in efforts to have increase these levels back up to a previous normal level. Frequently after a steroid cycle, many male athletes generally still had maintained a high level of Estradiols, while their own levels of Testosterone had been suppressed. Since the administration of anabolic/androgenic steroidal compounds had been terminated, the percentage of Estradiol to Testosterone had often remained elevated. Male athletes had been most sensitive to Estradiol conversion when the required accompanied administration of an anti-Estrogen had been concluded. However, the administration of the Fertodur compound, had occupied the Estrogen receptors, which had prevented the stronger Estrogens from having bonded and becoming active, which had permitted for a low Estrogen maintenance during a steroid cycle.

The main difference between Fertodur and Gonadotrophyl "C", Gonakor, and Profasi (HCG), had been that although Fertodur had been considered to have been not as effective; the chances of having developed gynecomastia had also not been as likely to have occurred. Fertodur had been primarily utilized in preparations for drug tested competitions, drug-free training, and both during and after steroid cycles.

Fertodur had been often recognized by male athletes primarily for it's advantageous characteristics of having had increased strength, moderate weight gains, faster recuperation time, increased energy levels, and for the reduction of gynecomastia and water retention. These results had been imperious especially in athletes and bodybuilders, who had only a slight experience with some steroidal substances, or sometimes, none at all.

Usual Clinical Recommendation:

The usual clinical dose at 100 mgs once a day, had often increased Testosterone levels up to 110 mgs to 120 mgs, which would have normally been at 50 mgs to 60 mgs. This had represented an average increase of 115%.

Adventitious Dosage and Administration:

Fertodur tablets had been intended for oral administration, which had implied that they had been designed to have been swallowed by mouth. Several athletes had claimed that these tablets had produced the best results, if they had been also consumed with water, usually prior to meals. They did not require to have been crushed or chewed. A common dosage regime of some athletes, has been discussed in the following:

The additional administration of the compound of Fertodur, generally had permitted the male athlete to have achieved a harder appearance to the muscles. However, the compounds of Nolvadex or Proviron had been frequently utilized instead of Fertodur, due to the fact that it had allegedly sometimes had been "too mild", and it's effects had not been apparent enough for some male athletes. Consequently, when Fertodur had been administered, it had been done so either during a steroid cycle, or after the termination.

Females:

Most female athletes had generally not utilized the compound of Fertodur, as it had appeared to have been ineffective when it had been administered within the female hormonal system, for athletic enhancement endeavors.

Males:

Many male athletes had usually perused high dosages of approximately 400 to 600 mgs, (2 to 3 tablets) a day, as lower dosages generally had not provided appeasing results. Cycles had frequently been entertained for a six week period, followed by anywhere from a six week, up to three month abstinence interval. The administration of Fertodur usually had taken approximately a week before it had become effectual. Slight acne and an increased sex drive had been general indicative signs that this compound had been effective.

Side Effects:

Although the side effects of this compound had been considered to have been very minimal, there had been a few associated with the administration of the Cyclofenil compound, primarily amongst male athletes. These adverse effects had included those of a slight acne, increased libido, and hot flashes. Sometimes, when Fertodur had been discontinued, the side effects of a depressed mood, and possible decreases in strength had been also experienced.

Again, there may have been other adverse side effects that had been experienced by the self-administration of Fertodur, which may have not been acknowledged, or documented.

WARNING:

Male athletes who have had self-administered Fertodur for anti-Estrogen purposes during a steroid cycle, may have actually had caused a backfire effect once it had been discontinued. High dosages of Fertodur had been able to have increased both Testosterone and Estrogen production, which had often been able to have converted into Estradiols in the peripheral body tissues. This of course, had frequently resulted in feminization effects, such as gynecomastia.

Rating:

Based on a 1 to 5 star scale, with 1 considered low, and 5 considered high, a -- symbol is indicative of no value. This compound of Clomiphene Citrate had rated as the following:

	MALES	FEMALES
Strength Increase	**	--
Mass & Weight Increase	**	--
Testosterone Stimulant	***	--
Anti-Estrogen	***	--
Side Effects	**	--
Cost Efficiency	***	***

CYNOMEL

Chemical Name: Liothyronine Sodium.

Common Generic Name: Cytomel.

Other Trade Names Found in Mexico: Currently, just Cynomel.

Manufacturer: SmithKline Beecham.

Dosage Form: Cynomel - 100 x 25 mcg tablets.

Storage: Cynomel tablets should be protected from light and moisture, (keep in the blisters until contents are used), and stored at controlled room temperature 15 to 30 degrees C (59 to 86 degrees F).

Price Range: Cynomel - approx. $10.40 pesos for 100 x 25 mcg tablets.

Type of Drug: Thyroid Hormone.

Ingredient: 25.9 ug of Liothyronine Sodium.

Drug Identification:

Cynomel - as an oral administration tablet, is distributed in a dark brown glass bottle. It has a white screw on and off lid, with a safety plastic seal with black writing around it. The bottle has a white sticker, with the product's entities written in a reddish-brown ink. There are 100 x 25 mcg tablets in each bottle. The tablets and accompanying package had not been obtained for illustrational and identifying purposes.

*****Please refer to the photograph of Cynomel for full color references.***

Drug Description:

Cynomel is a synthetically form of the natural thyroid hormone 3, 5, 3' -triiodothyronine, which has all the pharmacologic activities of the natural substance. Clinically, Cynomel had been often utilized in efforts to have treated Hypothyroidism, which is a thyroid insufficiency, as well as other secondary symptoms such as obesity, metabolic disorders, and fatigue. Thyroid hormones had been characteristically believed to have been able to have exerted most of their actions through the control of protein synthesis. When moderate amounts of Thyroid hormones had been administered, they had been able to have increased the synthesis of RNA and protein, which had often been followed by an increased basal metabolic rate; as well as having stimulated the oxidative enzyme systems. This, in turn, had enhanced the release of free fatty acids from adipose tissue, and had increased the intestinal absorption and peripheral utilization of glucose. When higher concentrations had been apparent, this had generally resulted in the decrease of protein synthesis, and in the increase of the breakdown of glycogen, lipids and protein.

The Cynomel compound closely had resembled the natural thyroid hormone, Tricodide-thyronine (L-T3), and under normal circumstances, the thyroid usually had produced two hormones, L-thyroxine (L-T4) and L-triiodine -thyronine (L-T3). However, the latter hormone, had been much stronger and more effective of the two, and had been approximately 4 times as potent as L-T4 on a weight basis.

When Cynomel had been administered orally, it had been readily available to the body tissue with approximately 95% of the dose being absorbed within 4 hours from the gastrointestinal tract. The biological half-life of Cynomel had been approximately two and a half days, with the maximal pharmacologic response having occurred within 2 or 3 days. This characteristic had also provided for an early clinical response, as the onset of activity had usually occurred within a few hours.

Several self-administering athletes had generally claimed that the synthetic compound of Cynomel had been ablc to have produced the same processes in the body, as if the thyroid had been able to have to produced more of the hormone. Consequently, this entity had allowed Cynomel to have been more effective than the compound of Eutirox or Tiroidine, which had been other commercially available L-T4 compounds that had been currently available in Mexico.

Many athletes had taken advantage of these characteristics which had been able to have stimulated the metabolism, which in turn, had resulted in a faster conversion of the macronutrients of carbohydrates, proteins, and fats. Bodybuilders, had been especially interested in increased fatburning (lipolysis) entities of the compound of Cynomel. Cynomel had been often utilized by competing bodybuilders several weeks prior to competition, as it had aided in having maintained an extremely low fat content, without the extremes of a starvation diet. This distinctive feature also had made it very popular amongst female athletes, due to the fact that women generally had slower metabolisms than men. Administration of Cynomel had allegedly allowed for the ridding of bodyfat, without a drastic caloric restriction. This also had permitted many athletes to have been able to have remained on high calorie diets with the added advantage of having maintained a "ripped" appearance. Athletes who had utilized Cytomel over several weeks, often had experienced a decrease in muscle mass, which had been discovered to have been avoidable or at least delayed, by the simultaneous intake of steroidal compounds, and by the consumption of a protein rich diet.

Another advantage which several athletes who had administered low dosages of Cynomel had claimed to have experienced, had been that the simultaneous intake of steroidal compounds had appeared to have become more effective. This possibly may have occurred as a result of the faster conversion of protein. Although some athletes still had utilized the administration of Cynomel, it had not been nearly as popular as it had once appeared to have been. Spiropent, and Ephedrine (the latter is currently not available in Mexico), had emerged to have had employed the same accelerating metabolism effects, with other added advantages such as possible strength and muscle increases. The combination however, of Cynomel and Spiropent, or Ephedrine (the latter is currently not available in Mexico), had allegedly appeared to have had enormously accelerated lipolysis.

Usual Clinical Recommendation:

Dosages had usually been determined by the clinical response of the patient, and by the findings of the laboratory results.

Small doses such as 5 ug taken on a daily basis, had been effective in some individuals. However, often a satisfactory clinical response had not been achieved until the recommended dosage levels had been exceeded. Therefore, sometimes dosages of up to 150 ug, had been occasionally well tolerated in a few resistant individuals.

In the treatment of mild hypothyroidism for example, the usual starting dosage had consisted of 25 ug daily, which if it had been required, had been increased by 125 or 25 ug every 1 to 2 weeks. The usual maintenance dosage then had consisted of 25 to 75 ug daily. Again, sometimes smaller dosages had been sufficient in some individuals, while others had sometimes required dosages of 100 ug or more.

Again, depending on the disorder that the individual had been treated for, had been a deciding factor in the application of Cynomel.

Adventitious Dosage and Administration:

Cynomel tablets had been intended for oral administration, which had implied that they should have been swallowed by the mouth. Many athletes had claimed that these tablets had produced the best results, when they had been also consumed with water and meals. They did not require to have been crushed or chewed. A common regime of some athletes, has been discussed in the following:

Prior to having attempted the utilization of this synthetic thyroid hormonal substance of Cynomel, most athletes had undergone laboratory evaluations to have ensured that they had not had a pre-existing thyroid problem. However, this had been sometimes clinically difficult to have detected, as substances such as androgens, corticosteroids, Estrogens, Estrogen-containing oral contraceptives, iodine-continuing preparations and salicylates, often had interfered with accurate thyroid function readings.

If no abnormalities had been clinically detected, the athletes who had proceeded to have self-administered the compound of Cynomel, had usually been very careful with this strong, highly effective thyroid hormone substance. Therefore, it had been extremely important that they had begun with a low dosage, and had increased the amount of Cynomel slowly, and evenly over the course of several days.

Most athletes had often accomplished this by first having consulted a physician to have ensured that no thyroid hyperfunction had pre-existed; then usually had initiated a Cynomel cycle by having administered one 25 mcg tablet per day, and then slowly had increased this dosage by one additional tablet, every 3 to 4 days. A dose higher than 100 mcg (or 4 tablets) a day, had often not been necessary and therefore, definitely had not been generally perused by most athletes.

Some athletes had claimed that having divided this amount into three smaller individual doses over the day, instead of taking these tablets all at once, had appeared to have been more effective. Athletes who had administered Cynomel usually had only administered this compound for 6 weeks, and then practiced an abstinence period of approximately two months in-between cycles. Many athletes also had stated that it had been just as important that the dosage had been slowly and evenly reduced, by having administered fewer tablets, when having completed a cycle. Many athletes had been very careful in not having terminated the consumption of Cynomel tablets abruptly, which would have ultimately had resulted in the disruption of the function of the thyroid. Also, if the initiation of Cynomel had increased too quickly, accompanied by a high dosage, this often had resulted in clinical hyperfunction of the thyroid.

Other athletes who had engaged in high dosages of Cynomel for prolonged periods of time, had been at a great risk of having developed a chronic thyroid insufficiency, which would have required the possible administration of thyroid medication for the duration of life.

Females:

Female athletes generally had administered 25 to 50 mcgs (1 to 2) tablets daily for a 6 week interval, with an abstinence of a two month duration which had followed. Allegedly, the best results had appeared to have resulted from the administration of this dosage, which had been divided into smaller, three dosages throughout the course of the day.

Males:

Male athletes usually had administered 50 to 100 mcgs (2 to 4) tablets daily for a 6 week interval, again with the abstinence of a two month duration which had followed. Again, the most effective results had been apparent when these dosages had been further divided into three smaller dosages spread evenly throughout the day.

Side Effects:

Athletes who had safely self-administered the thyroid hormone compound of Cynomel in short intervals as discussed previously, usually had not experienced any adverse affects. However, athletes who had administered large amounts of Cynomel too rapidly at the initiation of the cycle, accompanied by prolonged durations, frequently had experienced the clinical symptoms of thyroid hyperfunction. These side effects had included, heart palpitation, trembling, irregular heartbeat, heart oppression, agitation, shortness of breath, headaches, nausea, excessive perspiration, excretion of sugar through the urine, diarrhea, weight loss, psychic disorders, and symptoms of hypersensitivity. Of course, other side effects may have been experienced which may not have been recognized by the athlete, therefore, had not been documented.

Some athletes however, had claimed that these negative side effects could have generally been eliminated by temporarily having reduced the daily dosage, before they had progressed to further detrimental stages.

Female athletes however, had been more prone to have suffered from thyroid side effects, often even without the added administration of these compounds. However, cautious female athletes had been able to have kept these potential health risks at a minimum, by not having exceeded the above mentioned dosages, and by having had obtained proper thyroid function testing by a physician.

WARNING:

The misuse or abuse of this thyroid hormone synthetic substance, can and has resulted in an individual having had to administer thyroid hormone medication for the duration of life, in order to have maintained euthyroidism (normal thyroid activity).

Also, having combined the administration of this thyroid hormone in addition to the use of an insulin or another oral hypoglycemic, may clinically have required an increase in insulin or oral hypoglycemic requirements.

Rating:

Based on a 1 to 5 star scale, with 1 considered low, and 5 considered high; a -- symbol is indicative of no value. This compound of Liothyronine Sodium had rated as the following:

	MALES	FEMALES
Fat Burner	****	****
Contest Preparation	****	****
Side Effects	*****	*****
Cost Efficiency	*	*

DEBEONE

Chemical Name: Phenformin Hydrochloride.

Common Generic Name: Phenformin.

Other Trade Names Found in Mexico: Currently, just Debeone.

Manufacturer: Debeone - Armstrong.

Dosage Form:

Debeone	25 mg tablets.
Debeone "DT"	50 mg capsules.

Storage: Debeone tablets and capsules should be protected from light and moisture, (keep in the carton until contents are used), and stored at controlled room temperature 15 to 30 degrees C (59 to 86 degrees F).

Price Range:

Debeone - approx. $ 8.70 pesos for 25 x 25 mg tablets.

Debeone "DT" - approx. $17.40 pesos for 50 x 25 mg tablets.

- approx. $15.30 pesos for 20 x 50 mg capsules.

Type of Drug: Biguanide (synthetic chemicals).

Ingredient: 25 mg or 50 mgs of Phenformin Hydrochloride.

Drug Identification:

Debeone - The tablets are in a white box with the shades of light blue descending into darker blue shades at the bottom. The compound's entities are written in black, along with the manufacturer Armstrong, and Armstrong's symbol. The tablets themselves have been unobtainable for identification and illustration purposes. Debeone is not a popularly stocked item in most farmacias, therefore, it may be a difficult product to generally obtain.

****Please refer to the photo of Debeone for full color references.***

Drug Description:

Debeone previously had been the only Biguanide to have been marketed in the United States, as an oral hypoglycemic agent. However, the FDA had removed this compound from public access in 1977 for approval of utilization, due to it's association with the development of lactic acidosis. The condition of lactic acidosis refers to a metabolic irregularity which had resulted in a mortality rate of 50 to 75%, and is currently still under investigation for cause and effect. In fact, the compound of Phenformin had only been presently available in most countries, including the United States and Canada, under the Investigational New Drug Application (IDN) exemption, under conditions which had been predetermined by the FDA. The compound of Phenformin, with the trade name of Debeone, however, had still been available by prescription, in a few select countries including Mexico, however, this product may have been somewhat difficult to find in most farmacias.

Clinically, biguanides had been used orally in the management of mild to moderately severe, stable, non-insulin dependent (Type II) diabetes mellitus, in patients who had been over the age of 40 years, obese, and most likely had this illness onset in adulthood. The use of Phenformin (in the U.S., and Canada), had been so restricted, that even if it had been utilized for investigational purposes, heavy documentation, and certain patient criteria must have been acquired, along with a informed consent from the patient before it had been prescribed by a physician.

Most athletes had indicated that they generally had not engaged in the entertainment of the administration of the Debeone (Phenformin) product, as Glucophage (Metformin) had been often preferred as the choice oral insulin mimicker. The compound of Glucophage had been in the same family as Debeone, but had differed chemically, which in turn, had a lessened effect of potency. This characteristic also had allowed for lessened potential associated risks with the administration. When the compound of Debeone had been utilized as opposed to Glucophage, it had been approximately 5 to 10 times more potent, on a milligram per milligram comparison.

Usual Clinical Recommendation:

The usual clinical recommendation had been 1 x 25 mg tablet, taken once or twice a day for 3 days, and then this amount had possibly increased to 2 x 25 mg tablets, depending on the patient's individual circumstance. A dosage of 150 mg had been used in very extreme cases, however, had been very closely monitored by a physician.

Adventitious Dosage and Administration:

Debeone tablets had been intended for oral administration, which had implied that they had been intended to have been swallowed by mouth. Several athletes had claimed that these tablets had produced the best results, when they had also been consumed with water, and always had been taken prior to meals. They did not require to have been crushed or chewed. A common dosage regime of some athletes, has been discussed in the following:

Primarily, both genders of athletes had usually not engaged in the administration of Debeone, due to the fact that it had been a potentially very dangerous substance if misused, or abused.

Females:

A few female athletes had sometimes employed the administration of Debeone for a total of 75 mg (3 tablets) on a daily basis. This amount had been divided into 3 individual doses of 25 mgs taken three times a day.

Males:

Some male athletes also had chosen to have risked having utilized this compound in efforts to have achieved a pump, and vascularity due to the mimicked insulin effect. An usual regime mostly had often consisted of three 50 mg tablets, administered three times a day. This had been equivalent to 150 mg of Phenformin in total.

Side Effects:

There had been several side effects associated with the administration of the compound of Phenformin; Debeone. A few of which that had occasionally been experienced both clinically, and athletically had included epigastric discomfort, nausea and vomiting, a metallic taste in the mouth, diarrhea and anorexia. Most of these adverse effects had been transient, and several athletes had been able to have brought these under control by having reduced the dosage, or even had discontinued the administration of Debeone altogether.

Lactic acidosis had been a very serious and often fatal metabolic complication, which had been commonly observed when the compound of Debeone had been administered in voluminous and long term dosages. This condition had often been characterized by decreased blood pH (acidosis); an electrolyte disturbance with an increased anion gap, and lactate level with altered lactate-pyruvate ratio. Azotemia may have also been present. Cautious athletes had been especially observant to have watched for these signs of indication of possible onset, in which case, they had abandoned the utilization of this product.

WARNING:

Many athletes had paid particular attention to short and long range complications, as the administration of the compound of Debeone had not prevented the development of complications which had been peculiar to diabetes mellitus. Therefore, periodic cardiovascular, opthalmic, hematological, hepatic and renal assessments had often been undergone by athletes who had utilized this compound.

Cautious athletes had ensured that they had not self-administered Debeone if they had an existing contraindication. If acidosis of any kind had developed, the administration of Debeone had been discontinued immediately.

The risk of lactic acidosis had increased with the degree of renal dysfunction, impairment of creatinine clearance, and the age of the athlete. Also, athletes who had serum creatinine above the upper limit of the normal range, had not engaged in utilization of Debeone.

Rating:

Based on a 1 to 5 star scale, with 1 considered low, and 5 considered high, a -- symbol is indicative of no value. This compound of Phenformin Hydrochloride had rated as the following:

	MALES	FEMALES
Fat Burner	***	***
Contest Preparation	***	***
Side Effects	*****	*****
Cost Efficiency	**	**

DECA-DURABOLIN

Chemical Name: Nandrolone Decanoate.

Common Generic Name: Deca-Durabolin.

Other Trade Names Found in Mexico: Norandren 50 (veterinary).

Manufacturer: Deca-Durabolin - Organon.

Dosage Form: Deca-Durabolin - 2 x 50 mg x 1 ml redi-jects.

Storage: Store at controlled room temperature 15 to 30 degrees C (59 to 86 degrees F). Do not permit to freeze. Protect from light. It is advisable to keep in packaging until use.

Price Range: Deca-Durabolin is approx. $153.10 pesos for 2 x 50 mg x 1 ml redi-jects.

Type of Drug: Anabolic Steroid.

Ingredient: 50 mgs of Nandrolone Decanoate.

Drug Identification:

Deca-Durabolin - is available in 2 x 1 ml, 50 mg redi-ject syringes. There are also two 20 gauge, sterile, packaged needles included in each box. The redi-jects themselves are packaged in a plastic see-through blister, with a silver foil punch-through backing. The printing on the syringes is in green ink. The backing consists of Deca-Durabolin, Nandrolona, 50 mgs, Organon, Reg. #53979, and Solucion Injectable written throughout in navy blue. The package accompanying the 2 redi-jects is quite basic, it is white with the product's entities written in black ink. The top of the box does contain some color of orange and blue.

*****Please refer to the photographs of Deca-Durabolin for full color references.***

Drug Description:

Deca-Durabolin is a sterile solution of Nandrolone Decanoate, which is a derivative of 19-Nortestosterone; considered to be a long acting anabolic agent. It is an oil-based (dileunt is sesame oil), intramuscular injectable. Both the human and veterinary versions of Nandrolone Decanoate, Deca-Durabolin and Norandren 50 (veterinarian product), had been considered to have been the most widely used steroids of choice amongst all athletes.

The substance itself, is a moderate androgen, and a highly anabolic preparation. The use of Deca-Durabolin had proven to have been an excellent product for having had promoted size and strength gains, as it had allowed the muscle cells to store more nitrogen than what had been released; so that a positive nitrogen balance had primarily been generally achieved. It had been well known that a positive nitrogen balance had been synonymous with muscle growth, as when the muscle cell had been in this phase, it had been able to have accumulated a greater amount of protein than usual. However, a positive nitrogen balance and the protein building effect which had often accompanied it, had occurred only if enough calories and protein had been supplied. Therefore, athletes had to have ensured that proper protein and caloric intake had been obtained, in efforts to have received the full benefits of the Nandrolone Decanoate compound.

Consequently, at the same time, various athletes had also experienced considerable water retention if they had administered high dosages of this drug, which had usually resulted in a smooth and watery-type appearance. However, if Deca-Durabolin had been utilized in conservative dosages, it dramatically had improved the nitrogen cortisone to have reached the muscle cells and the connective tissue cells. As Deca-Durabolin also had stored more water in the connective tissues, it had also temporarily eased, or even had frequently eased existing pain in joints; which often had allowed sore elbows, shoulders, knees etc., to have been alleviated. The administration of Deca-Durabolin not only had improved the nitrogen retention, but also had improved the recuperation time between training periods.

The exogenous administration of Deca-Durabolin did have an effect on the body's natural hormone levels, however, these effects had not been as great as those which had been generally experienced from Testosterones. Unfortunately, Nandrolone Decanoate had possessed very stubborn metabolites, which had often appeared in steroid testing, even as long as 18 months after it had last been utilized. This, along with the Deca Durabolin's vast popularity, had contributed to it's presence on steroid tests to have been greater than any other compound. Obviously, athletes had not administered Deca-Durabolin in competitions where drug testing had been prevalent. Consequently, it still had remained to have been the number one choice for selection of a steroidal compound; for athletes who had not required to have undergone substance testing.

Usual Clinical Recommendation:

A single intramuscular injection every 3 to 4 weeks for a continuous period of up to 12 weeks, had been generally practiced. A repeat course of therapy, which had followed a rest interval of 4 weeks, had been also administered if it had been necessary. The usual adult dosage had been 50 to 100 mgs, administered once a day.

Adventitious Dosage and Administration:

The use of Deca-Durabolin had been intended for deep intramuscular injection. The best site for this type of injection had been in the gluteus medius muscle area, which had been the upper outer portion of the buttock, approximately 2 to 3 inches below the hip bone (iliac crest). Most athletes had generally alternated injections from one side to the other, (first injection on the left side, the second time injection administered on the right, or vice versa) in efforts to have alleviated pain somewhat, which also had occasionally allowed the area to have slightly "healed". This practice had also often had prevented a thick scar tissue from having had potentially formed. However, the more injections that had been administered, the greater possibility of scar tissue had also increased. A common dosage regime of some athletes, has been discussed in the following:

Deca-Durabolin had generally been utilized by some athletes for "cutting and bulking"; and it had also been beneficial in the preparation for untested competitions. Allegedly, results had been evident from administration of 2 mgs/pound of body weight. If water retention had become problematic, it had usually been counteracted with the additional stack of Nolvadex, combined with Proviron.

Females:

Some female athletes had occasionally entertained the dosages of approximately 50 to 100 mgs (1 to 2 redi-ject ampules, or 1 to 2 mls) per week, or the combination of Deca-Durabolin at approximately 50+ mgs (1 redi-ject ampule, or 1 ml) weekly, with Oxandrolone (currently, not available in Mexico), at approximately 10+ mgs daily.

If dosages had been kept at a relatively low range, then potential masculization ill-effects had also been kept at a low minimum. Other popular stacks female athletes had often also administered had included Deca-Durabolin stacked with Winstrol tablets (currently, not available in Mexico), or the application of Primobolan tablets. If female athletes had experienced ill-effects even at a low dosage of Deca-Durabolin, they had often discontinued this compound, and had switched to a milder compound such as Durabolin.

Males:

The average dosage that many male athletes had generally administered had been in the area of 2 to 400 mg (4 to 8 redi-ject ampules, or 4 to 8 mls) per week. Deca-Durabolin had been successfully stacked with practically every other steroidal drug compound for positive results, as it had appeared to have been an excellent base drug on any cycle.

Other common perused stacks amongst many male athletes had included: Deca-Durabolin 200 to 400 mgs (4 to 8 redi-ject ampules, or 4 to 8 mls) a week, stacked with Metandiabol or Reforvit B 15 to 40 mgs (approximately 1/2 ml to 1 1/2 mls) daily, or Deca Durabolin 400 mgs (8 redi-ject ampules, or 8 mls) weekly and Sostenon 250 at 500 mgs (2 cc's or 2 mls) weekly.

Another more potent stack had often consisted of Deca-Durabolin 400 mgs (8 redi-jects, or 8 mls) weekly, with Sostenon 250 at 500 mgs (2 cc's or 2 mls), with Metandiabol or Reforvit B 30 mgs (just a little more than half of a cc, or half of a ml) daily, which had often produced rapid and strong increases in muscle mass.

The anabolic and buildup effect of Deca-Durabolin to a certain degree, allegedly had depended on the dosage. If more than 600 mgs a week had been administered, the risk/benefit factor had greatly been increased, which primarily had resulted in greater ill effects, than positive results.

Side Effects:

Some of the known side effects which had been occasionally experienced by both female and male athletes had included those of nausea, leukopenia, symptoms resembling those of a peptic ulcer, acne, edema, excitation, sleeplessness, chills, vomiting, diarrhea, hypertension, prolonged blood clotting time, and an increase in libido.

Some of the side effects which had been peculiar to especially females who had administered Deca-Durabolin in high, excessive amounts included virilization such as menstrual irregularities, post-menopausal bleeding, swelling of the breasts, hoarseness or deepening of the voice, enlargement of the clitoris, and water retention.

Some of the side effects which had been sometimes experienced by a few male athletes had included those of impotence, chronic priapism, epididymitis, inhibition of testicular function, oligospermia, and bladder irritability.

Deca-Durabolin's conversion to the dihydro form called dihydro-nandrolone (not Dihydrotestosterone), through the action of 5-alpha reductase, had caused it to have been less androgenic after it had been converted. This, had allowed it to have much less likely to have caused any hair loss, as Nandrolone Decanoate only had converted to Estrogen at about 20% of the rate which Testosterone had. This also had greatly reduced the potential for feminization effects such as gynecomastia. This compound also had minimal liver toxicity, and only had aromatized in excessive dosages.

The exogenous administration of the compound of Deca-Durabolin had an effect on the body's natural hormone level, however, it had not been nearly as pronounced as it had been with compounds such as Testosterone.

WARNING:

Caution had been practiced by athletes who had suffered from cardiac, renal or hepatic disease. Therefore, intelligent athletes had often undergone proper health testing to have ruled out possible health concerns before they had considered the self-administration of Deca-Durabolin.

Rating:

Based on a 1 to 5 star scale, with 1 considered low, and 5 considered high, a -- symbol is indicative of no value. This compound of Nandrolone Decanoate had rated as the following:

	MALES	FEMALES
Strength Increase	***	***
Mass & Weight Increase	***	***
Side Effects	***	***
Cost Efficiency	**	**

DYAZIDE

Chemical Name: Triamterene Hydrochlorothiazide.

Common Generic Name: Dyazide.

Other Trade Names Found in Mexico: Currently, just Dyazide.

Manufacturer: Dyazide - Armstrong.
- SmithKline Beecham.

Dosage Form: Dyazide - 50 x 50/25 mgs.

Storage: Dyazide tablets should be protected from light and moisture, (keep in the blisters until contents are used), and stored at controlled room temperature 15 to 30 degrees C (59 to 86 degrees F).

Price Range: Dyazide - approx. $32.20 pesos for 50 x 50/25 mgs.

Type of Drug: Combination Diuretic. Antihypertensive.

Ingredient: 37.5 mgs of Triamterene, 25 mgs of Hydrochlorothiazide.

Drug Identification:

Dyazide - Are available in oral administration tablets, each containing 37.5 of Triamterene, and 25 mgs of Hydrochlorothiazide. It is available in 2 packages of 25 round, flat, bevel-edged, peach-colored, compressed tablets, scored, which allows them to be further broken down into half strengths, with a "SB" impressed on the other side. They are packaged in individualized plastic see-through blisters, with a silver foil punch-through backing. On the back, Dyazide Triamterene/Hydrochlorothiazide,

50/25 mg Tabletas, SmithKline Beecham, along with Registration # and Lot # 39507, are printed throughout in black. The accompanying package is red and white.

****Please refer to the photographs of Dyazide for full color references.***

Drug Description:

Dyazide is a combination of a diuretic/antihypertensive which combines natriuretic (a drug which increases the rate of excretion of sodium in the body), and antikaliuretic (a drug which prevents the excretion of potassium in the urine). The onset of Hydrochlorothiazide's diuretic effect usually had occurred within two hours, with the peak action taking place in four hours, and the entire diuretic activity having had persisted anywhere from 6 to 12 hours. The Triamterene aspect of Dyazide had created it's diuretic effect by having increased the sodium excretion, while having reduced the excessive loss of potassium and hydrogen associated with Hydrochlorothiazide.

These types of diuretics had often acted similarly to loop agents such as Lasix, however, they had not caused as much calcium excretion, and had not been considered to have been as effective. Dyazide (from the Thiazide family) had been generally considered as an "in-between", as it had not been as powerful as a loop-diuretic, but had been generally stronger than that of potassium-sparing diuretics.

Clinically, Dyazide had most often been prescribed in efforts to have controlled hypertension. Many athletes had utilized the compound of Dyazide in attempts to have dislodged excess water which had often been obtained from several steroidal compounds, or to have possibly eliminated subcutaneous water prior to a competition. Dyazide had potassium sparing characteristics, which had not depleted muscle tissues as severely as a loop agent, such as Lasix.

Usual Clinical Recommendation:

Starting clinical dosage had generally been 1 tablet daily after meals. When dry weight had been reached, a maintenance dosage of 1 tablet daily usually had sufficed. One tablet every other day had sometimes been indicated for some patients. The usual dosage had been 1 to 2 capsules given once daily, with the appropriate monitoring of the serum potassium levels, and of the clinical effect. Maximum dosage had not exceeded 4 tablets.

Adventitious Dosage and Administration:

Dyazide tablets had been intended for oral administration, which had implied that they had been designed to have been swallowed by mouth. Many athletes had claimed that these tablets had produced the best results, if they had been ingested with water. They did not require to have been crushed or chewed. Dyazide tablets had produced more effective results, when they had been administered all at once, first thing in the morning. The effects of Dyazide had been somewhat moderate, but had not always been physically apparent upon the initial administration. A common dosage regime of some athletes, is discussed in the following:

Female & Males:

As Dyazide had been primarily utilized prior to competition in efforts to have released the body of the last layer of water beneath the skin, most athletes had administered 25 to 100 mgs (1 to 4 tablets) daily for approximately 4 days previously, while having constantly monitored the results; then had adjusted this dosages accordingly.

Similar to clinical dosages, athletes had been careful not to have had exceeded four tablets in any one given day. Well prepared athletes always had tried to have avoided having to have administered a diuretic compound before competition, as it had not always consistently guaranteed positive results. If diuretics had been used exceedingly or extensively, severe side effects and even death had been known to have sometimes occurred.

Side Effects:

Some side effects which had been associated with the administration of Dyazide had included rash, photosensitivity, low blood pressure (hypotension), diabetes mellitus, hypokalemia, jaundice, nausea and vomiting, diarrhea, constipation, abdominal pain, acute renal failure, muscle cramps, weakness, fatigue, dizziness, headache, dry mouth, transient blurred vision, respiratory distress, and exacerbation of lupus. Male athletes had also additionally occasionally experienced impotency.

WARNING:

Hyperkalemia (abnormal elevation of serum potassium levels). Warning signs had included numbness, prickling or tingling, sensations, muscular weakness, fatigue, flaccid paralysis of the extremities, bradycardia and shock. If hyperkalemia had been left untreated, it often had proven to have been fatal.

Most athletes had also been very cautious not to have administered potassium supplements or potassium salts in conjunction with this diuretic compound.

Rating:

Based on a 1 to 5 star scale, with 1 considered low, and 5 considered high; a -- symbol is indicative of no value. This compound of Triamterene Hydrochlorothiazide, had rated as the following:

	MALES	FEMALES
Contest Preparation	***	***
Side Effects	****	****
Cost Efficiency	**	**

EUTIROX

Chemical Name: Levothyroxine Sodium.

Common Generic Name: L-Thyroxine.

Other Trade Names Found in Mexico: Eutirox
Tiroidine.

Manufacturer: Eutirox - Merck.
Tiroidine - Rudefsa.

Dosage Form:

Eutirox - 100 x 100 mcgs tablets.
- 50 x 100 mcgs tablets.

Tiroidine - 100 x 100 mcgs tablets.
- 60 x 0.025 mcgs tablets.
- 40 x 0.050 mcgs tablets.
- 30 x 0.100 mg tablets.

Storage: Eutirox and Tiroidine tablets should be protected from light and moisture, (keep in the blisters until contents are used), and stored at controlled room temperature 15 to 30 degrees C (59 to 86 degrees F).

Price Range: Eutirox - approx. $42.60 pesos for 100 x 100 mcgs tablets.
- approx. $26.50 pesos for 50 x 100 mcgs tablets.

Tiroidine - approx. $83.30 pesos for 100 x 100 mcgs tablets.
- approx. $12.50 pesos for 60 x 0.025 mcgs tablets.
- approx. $16.65 pesos for 40 x 0.050 mcgs tablets.
- approx. $ 29.90 pesos for 30 x 0.100 mgs tablets.

Type of Drug: Synthetic Thyroid Hormone.

Ingredient: Synthetic, crystalline Levothyroxine Sodium.

Drug Identification:

Eutirox - tablets are available for oral administration, in 100 mcgs, uncoated, white tablets, scored for breaking down into half strengths, and the other side has the number "100" on it. There are two packages with 25 tablets per sheet in box for 50 tablets, and four packages with 25 tablets per sheet for 100 tablets. The tablets are packaged in individual see-through blisters, with a silver aluminum foil punch-through backing. On the back, Eutirox, Levotiroxina Tabletas 100 mcgs, Reg. # 297M89, Lot # (actually there had not been one indicated on the package), Merck, are printed throughout in black ink. The accompanying package is white, with a light purple stripe, and the product's entities are written in black ink.

Tiroidine - oral administration tablets are available in *0.025 mgs*, which contain 3 packages of 20 tablets apiece, for a total of 60 tablets. Reg. # 268M89. These tablets are small, off-white, and scored. They are packaged in individual see-through blisters, on a copper color front, with a silver foil punch-through backing. The *0.050 mg* tablets Reg. # 268M89, are available in 2 packages of 20 tablets each, for a total of 40 tablets within a package. These tablets are somewhat larger than the 0.025 mg version, and have a slight light green color, and are plain in appearance.

They are also packaged in individualized see-through blisters, on a copper color front, with a silver foil punch-through backing. The *0.100 mg* tablets Reg. # 268M89, are available also in two packages, however, one package contains 20 tablets, and the other contains only 10, for a total of 30 tablets within a package. These tablets are the same size as the 0.050 mg tablets, and are an off-white color, and are plain in appearance. They are also packaged in individualized see-through blisters, on a copper front, with a silver foil punch-through backing. All three strength's of Tiroidine packing are identical, with the difference in the strength of the tablet, indicated by the color. The 0.025 mg strength is indicated by a yellow color outlined with black ink, the 0.050 mg strength is indicated by a light blue color, also outlined with black ink, and the 0.100 mg strength is white, outlined by blue ink.

*****Please refer to the photographs of Eutirox and Tiroidine for full color references.***

Drug Description:

The principle effect of thyroid hormones had been generally to have had increased the metabolic rate of the body tissues. The compound of Eutirox and Tiroidine had been synthetic, and had been similar to the natural L-thyroxine in the thyroid gland. Levothyroxine is the monosodium salt of the levo-isomer of thyroxine (T4), which is the principal hormone that had been secreted by the thyroid gland. L-thyroxine together with L-triiodthyronine (L-T4 and L-T3), are two hormones which had been constructed in the thyroid. As L-T4 had been insubstantial to L-T3, the latter compound had been approximately 4 times as potent as L-T4, on a weight basis. Levothyroxine had been nearly totally bound to serum proteins, and had an elimination half-life of 6 to 7 days in individuals who had normal thyroid function.

Clinically, the administration of Eutirox or Tiroidine, had been utilized for specific replacement therapy for diminished or absent thyroid function which had originated from any type of etiology. It had been also indicated that the administration of substances such as Eutirox or Tiroidine, (Levothyroxine) for the treatment of obesity in individuals who had not been hypothyroid, had been ineffective, and actually had proven to have been potentially harmful.

Consequently, different levothyroxine products had usually not been interchangeable, due to the potential difference in potency and bioavailability of each compound. In other words, clinically, if stabilization had been obtained on a particular brand of levothyroxine, such as Eutirox, this did not necessarily mean that this would have been achieved by another levothyroxine substance such as Tiroidine.

However, several athletes had often used this synthetic compound of Eutirox or Tiroidine in attempts to have accelerated the metabolism of carbohydrates, proteins and fat. The administration of Eutirox or Tiroidine had generally permitted the body to have burned more calories than usual, therefore, this had often resulted in the burning of more fat, when greater amounts of calories had been consumed. However, increased dosages of more than 400 to 600 mcgs (4 to 6 tablets) of Eutirox or Tiroidine in a day, (which often had resulted in more carbohydrates and protein having been burned), had also provoked muscle loss if steroids had not also been used in conjunction with this compound.

Therefore, athletes instead, had generally preferred the utilization of the compound Cynomel, which is a synthetic substance of L-T3, Ephedrine, Triacana (both are currently not available in Mexico), or Spiropent for fat burning entities. Therefore, the use of Eutirox had been often utilized, if these other substances had not been readily available.

Usual Clinical Recommendation:

The dosage and rate of administration of Eutirox or Tiroidine had primarily been determined by the indication, and had been individualized according to the patient's response and laboratory results. However, the patient's age, general physical condition, severity and duration of hypothyroid symptoms may have also had determined the initial dosage, and the rate at which the dosage may have been increased, to the eventual maintenance dosage.

For the management of mild hypothyroidism in adults, the usual initial dose had been 50 ug once daily, with an increase in dosage in increments of 25 to 50 ug/day, at intervals of 2 to 4 weeks, until the desired clinical response had been obtained.

If patients had severe hypothyroidism, the usual initial administration dose had usually been 12.5 to 25 ug once daily. This dosage had been increased by increments of 25 to 50 ug/day, at intervals of 2 to 4 weeks, again until the desired clinical response had been obtained.

The usual maintenance dosage for full replacement therapy had been 100 to 200 ug/day, although certain patients had occasionally required higher dosages. It had been very rare for a patient not to adequately have responded to dosages which had exceeded 300 to 400 ug/day.

It had been currently recommended that excessive dosages not have been administered, as minimal brain damage had been reported to have had occurred in children with thyrotoxicosis during infancy, and also may have accelerated the bone age, and have caused premature cranio-synostosis.

Adventitious Dosage and Administration:

Eutirox and Tiroidine tablets had been intended for oral administration, which had implied that the tablets had been intended to have been swallowed by the mouth. Many athletes had generally claimed that these tablets had provided the best results when they had been ingested with water. They did not required to have been crushed or chewed. Athletes had claimed that having divided the dosage into three equal portions throughout the day had appeared to have been more effective than having administered the entire dosage all at once. A common dosage regime of some athletes, has been discussed in the following:

***Females
& Males:***

Both female and male athletes had usually initiated the use of Eutirox or Tiroidine by a small dose of 25 to 100 mcgs, (1/4 to 1 tablet) which had been taken for the first couple of days, and then had slowly and evenly been increased over several days. Athletes had often increased the dosage of Eutirox or Tiroidine up to 200 to 400 mcgs (0.1 to 0.2 mgs) daily, or (2 to 4 tablets) for up to 2 to 3 weeks, with a rest interval of approximately 1 to 2 months to have followed this cycle.

Most athletes had also been adamant that the dosage had to have been slowly tapered back down and evenly at the end of a cycle, similar to the method it had slowly been increased at the beginning; in attempts to have avoided the discontinuance of Eutirox abruptly. These measures allegedly had provided the most effective benefits from the administration of these L-T4 synthetic compounds.

Side Effects:

Athletes had claimed that if the Levothyroxine Sodium compound had been utilized properly, it had been relatively safe and had few side effects. However, dosages that had been too highly administered, and particularly, had been increased too quickly, too early at the beginning of a cycle, had often warranted some side effects such as trembling of the fingers, excessive perspiration, diarrhea, insomnia, nausea, increased heartbeat, inner unrest, angina pectoris, tachycardia, intolerance to heat, fever and weight loss.

Severe overdosage had been equivalent to a "thyroid storm", which often had been manifested by coma, cardiac decompensation, and even death, which had been secondary to cardiac dysrhythmia or failure. The effects of an acute overdosage had sometimes taken several days to have become apparent. Of course, other side effects may have been experienced which possibly had not been recognized by the athlete, therefore, had not been documented.

Athletes had claimed that these adverse side effects could often had been eliminated by temporarily having had reduced the daily dosage.

Clinically, in efforts to have had achieved a declination of these effects, Eutirox or Tiroidine had often been discontinued for 2 to 7 days, and then had been resumed by a treatment which had consisted of lower dosages.

WARNING:

If synthetic thyroid hormones had been taken in excessive, high dosages, over prolonged periods of time, thyroid hyperfunction had generally developed. Signs of thyroid hyperfunction had included heart palpitations, irregular heartbeat, heart oppression, agitation, shortness of breath, excretion of sugar through the urine, trembling, excessive perspiration, diarrhea, weight loss, psychic disorder, and possible symptoms of hypersensitivity. As a consequence, the possibility of having had to administer thyroid medication for the duration of life, had often proposed to have been a great probability.

Rating:

Based on a 1 to 5 star scale, with 1 considered low, and 5 considered high, a -- symbol is indicative of no value. This compound of Levothyroxine Sodium had rated as the following:

	MALES	FEMALES
Fat Burner	****	****
Contest Preparation	****	****
Side Effects	****	****
Cost Efficiency	**	**

GLUCOPHAGE

Chemical Name: Metformin Hydrochloride.

Common Generic Name: Glucophage.

Other Trade Names Found in Mexico: Currently, just Glucophage.

Manuf acturer: Glucophage - Co. Lakeside Farm.

Dosage Form: Glucophage Forte 40 x 850 mgs tablets.

Storage: Glucophage tablets and capsules should be protected from light and moisture, (keep in the carton until contents are used), and stored at controlled room temperature 15 to 30 degrees C (59 to 86 degrees F).

Price Range: Glucophage - approx. $ 37.70 pesos for 40 x 850 mg tablets.

Type of Drug: Oral Antihyperglycemic Agent. Biguanide derivative.

Ingredient: 850 mgs of Metformin Hydrochloride.

Drug Identification:

Glucophage - is available for oral administration. There are five packages of 8 uncoated, oblong ivory-colored tablets, for a total of 40 tablets in each box, each individually contained in plastic, push-see-through blisters. The backing of the package is silver, with the product's entities displayed throughout in black ink. The accompanying package is white with a medium colored blue strip across the top of the box containing the product name Glucophage Forte within. The product's entities are also written in black ink.

****Please refer to the photo of Glucophage for full color references.***

Drug Description:

Glucophage is a trade name for Metformin, which belongs to a class of drugs referred to as biguanides. Metformin, Buformin, and Phenformin, are all oral hypoglycemic agents which have been able to have increased the transport of glucose (blood sugar), into the muscle cells by directly having increased the insulin sensitivity. The main difference between Debeone (Phenformin) and Glucophage (Metformin) had been that the latter substance had been considered to be somewhat milder of a compound, which had not been greatly associated with the onset of lactic acidosis; as the administration of the compound of Debeone had been. However, both of these compounds typically had not caused hypoglycemia (low blood sugar), but had been able to have had inhibited the formation of sugar by the liver.

Glucophage is also a biguanide derivative, which had been able to have produced an antihyperglycemic effect only when there had been an insulin secretion. Consequently, this effect could have only been observed in man or in the diabetic animal.

Metformin, at therapeutic doses, had not caused hypoglycemia when it had been utilized alone, except when a near lethal dose had been administered. Therefore, many athletes had decided that this compound of Glucophage had been a much more conservative method of treatment, which had not been as potent as Phenformin, (Debeone). The utilization of Metformin had no effects on the pancreatic beta cells. Clinically, it had been concluded that Metformin might potentiate the effect of insulin, or possibly might have enhanced the effect of insulin on peripheral receptor sites; as this increased sensitivity had appeared to have followed an increase in the number of insulin receptors on cell surface membranes.

The absorption of Metformin had been relatively slow and had sometimes extended over about 6 hours. Metformin is not metabolized, and it's primary sites of concentration had been the intestinal mucosa and the salivary glands. The plasma concentration at steady state ranges about 1 to 2 ug/ml. The additional administration of certain other drug compounds may have potentiated the effects of Metformin. Glucophage had been excreted in urine at a high renal clearance rate of approximately 450 ml/min., as the initial elimination had been rapid, with a half-life having varied between 1.7 and 3 hours. The terminal elimination phase which had accounted for about 4% to 5% of the absorbed dose had been slow, with a half-life between 9 and 17 hours.

Clinically, Glucophage had been prescribed in efforts to have controlled hyperglycemia in patients with the maturity onset type of diabetes (Type II), which could not have been controlled by proper dietary management, exercise, weight reduction, or insulin therapy. Glucophage had been occasionally warranted for the treatment of obese diabetic patients.

A few athletes had utilized the compound of Glucophage in attempts to have mimicked the oral insulin compound. Glucophage had appeared to have been the "safer" compound to have administered, as it had been less potent than Debeone, therefore, the risks of self-administration had also been somewhat lessened.

Usual Clinical Recommendation:

In some diabetic subjects, short-term administration of the Glucophage may have been sufficient during periods of transient loss of blood sugar control. The usual dose had been 850 mgs (1 tablet) administered 2 or 3 times a day. Maximal dose had not exceeded 2.5 grams a day.

Usual starting dose - in general, clinical significant responses had not been seen at doses that had been greater than 1500 mg/day. However, a lower recommended starting dose and a gradual increased dosage had been advised in efforts to have had minimized gastrointestinal symptoms. The usual starting dose had been 1 x 850 mg tablet daily, taken with the morning meal. This dosage had increased in increments of 850 mg (1 tablet) every other week, in divided doses, up to a maximum of 2550 mg/day.

The usual maintenance dose had been 850 mg (1 tablet) taken twice daily with the morning and evening meals. If it had been necessary, patients had been given 850 mgs (1 tablet) taken 3 times daily with meals.

Adventitious Dosage and Administration:

Glucophage tablets had been intended for oral administration, which had implied that they should have been swallowed by mouth. Many athletes had claimed that these tablets had produced the best results, when they had been consumed with water, and always with meals, in efforts to have minimized gastric intolerance such as nausea and vomiting. They did not require to have been crushed or chewed. A common dosage regime of some athletes, has been discussed in the following:

Several athletes also had chosen to have risked the usage of this compound in efforts to have achieved a pump, and vascularity due to the mimicked insulin effect. Some nondiabetic athletes had generally claimed that a dosage of 1,700 mg (2 x 850 mg tablets) of Glucophage a day had been effective. A few athletes had further divided this dosage into equally divided amounts, which had been consumed 6 times a day prior to meals. A few athletes who had not utilized steroidal compounds had expressed that Glucophage combined with Creatine Monhydrate, with 30 to 50 grams of glucose, administered three times a day (on an empty stomach), immediately having followed exercise, had mimicked the insulin effects quite satisfactorily.

Side Effects:

Some of the most frequently reported adverse reactions which had been experienced both clinically and in athletic application, had been a metallic taste in the mouth, epigastric discomfort, nausea and vomiting, flatulence, but rarely, diarrhea and anorexia. Impairment of Vitamin B12 and Folic acid absorption had been reported in some patients. Most of these reactions had been transient and had been easily brought under control by having reduced the dosage or by having had discontinued the therapy.

However, if vomiting had occurred, Glucophage had been temporarily discontinued in attempts to having had ruled out the possibility of lactic acidosis. Particular attention had also been paid to short and long ranges every 6 months while having had administered Metformin.

Lactic acidosis refers to a metabolic irregularity which had resulted in a mortality rate of 50% to 75%, and has still been under investigation for cause and effect. It is a serious and often fatal metabolic complication observed, among other conditions, in diabetic patients, often characterized by acidosis (decreased blood pH); electrolyte disturbances with an increased anion gap and an increased lactate level with altered lactate-pyruvate ratio; azotemia may also have been present. It had been very important for an individual who had engaged in the administration of Glucophage, to have recognized the symptoms which could have signaled the onset of lactic acidosis.

WARNING:

The administration of Glucophage should have only been considered as a treatment in addition to proper dietary regimen, and not as a substitute for diet. If acidosis of any kind had developed, Glucophage had been discontinued immediately. The risk of lactic acidosis had increased with the degree of renal dysfunction, impairment of creatinine clearance and the age of the individual. Individuals who had serum creatinine levels above the upper limit of the normal range, or a pre-existing contraindication, had not administered Glucophage.

Certain pharmaceutical compounds may have also had potentiated the effect of Metformin, and other drugs had tended to have produced hyperglycemia, which had sometimes led to the loss of blood sugar control. These compounds had included diuretics (thiazides, Furosemide), corticosteroids, oral contraceptives (Estrogen plus Progesterone) and nicotinic acid in pharmacologic doses.

It had been extremely important for the individual to have adhered to dietary instructions, regular exercise and regular testing of blood glucose, glycosylated hemoglobin, renal function and hematologic parameters.

Rating:

Based on a 1 to 5 star scale, with 1 considered low, and 5 considered high, a -- symbol is indicative of no value. This compound of Phenformin Hydrochloride has rated as the following:

	MALES	FEMALES
Fat Burner	****	****
Contest Preparation	***	***
Side Effects	***	***
Cost Efficiency	*	*

(HCG: HUMAN CHORIONIC GONADOTROPIN)

Chemical Name: Chorionic Gonadotropin.

Common Generic Name: HCG.

Other Trade Names Found in Mexico:
Gonadotropyl.
Gonakor.
Pregnyl (N.L.M).
Profasi.

Manufacturers:

Gonadotropyl "C"	- Hoechs.
Gonakor	- Sanfer.
Profasi	- Serono.

Dosage Form:	Gonadotropyl "C"	- 5000 I.U. ampule.
	Gonakor	- injectable 10 ml bottle.
	Profasi	- 500 I.U., 1000 I.U., - 2000 I.U., 5000 I.U., 10,000 I.U. ampules.

Storage: The dry product should be stored at controlled room temperature, 15 to 30 degrees C, or 59 to 86 degrees F. After reconstitution, refrigerate the product at 2 to 8 degrees C, or 36 to 46 degrees F. Do not freeze.

Price Range:	Gonadotropyl "C "	- approx. $ 90.60 pesos for 5000 I.U. ampule.
	Gonakor	- approx. $ 86.50 pesos for injectable 10 ml bottle.
	Profasi	- approx. $ 22.55 pesos for 500 I.U.
		- approx. $ 37.90 pesos for 1000 I.U.
		- approx. $ 55.60 pesos for 2000 I.U.
		- approx. $ 63.35 pesos for 5000 I.U.
		- approx. $113.95 pesos for 10000 I.U.

Type of Drug: Mimics the Natural Luteinizing Hormone.

Ingredient: 2500 Units of Chorionic Gonadotropin, 300 mcg of hidroxocobolamin.

Drug Identification:

Gonadotrophyl "C" - is available in two separate containers, one, an ampule of sterile water, and the other a light brown, multi-injection bottle with the dry product. Gonadotrophyl "C" is on a white and blue label, along with the manufacturer. The ampule has a light blue line around the neck, which indicates where to break the ampule. The light brown bottle with the dry white substance has a silver tear-off aluminum wrap around the lids, which requires to be torn off and discarded after entry. The accompanying package is basically white, with the products' entities written in black ink. The Lot # is AG5006. There is also a light blue box displaying the company's name of Roussel and their logo. There is also a smaller stripe of navy blue just above this box. There is also a red stripe on the top of the package.

Gonakor- is available in two injectable 10 ml bottles, one with the dry white, product, and the other contains sterile water. These two bottles are cradled within plastic moldings. The Lot # is 116AR1225. Both also have silver tear-off aluminum wrap around the multiple entry lids, which requires to be torn off and discarded after initial entry. Gonakor is on the white and blue label, along with the manufacturer. The box has the same color of blue and white as the bottles do, as well as a red "tab". Prior to and after injections, to prevent contaminations of the combined contents after multiple repeated insertions, the septum of the vial should be wiped with an antiseptic solution. Also, the use of sterile, disposable needles and syringes is definitely imperative.

Profasi - is available in two clear ampules, one with the dry product, and the other contains the sterile water. The dry product has a white substance within, and the ampule has a white sticker label around it with the Profasi name, manufacturer, the I.U., amount, and the other ampule containing the sterile water is labeled in black ink directly onto the ampule itself. The Lot # is M24F009, and the 5000 I.U. version has the Reg. # of 76-20. Profasi is manufactured by Serono which can also be found on the ampule labels. The box has four stripes of light green to dark green on the front, along with the Profasi, I.U., amount, chemical name, and the manufacturer, Serono.

*****Please refer to photographs of Gonadotropyl-C, Gonakor, and Profasi for full color references.***

Drug Description: ****Gonadotropyl "C', Gonakor, and Profasi have been commonly referred to as HCG for simplicity measures in the following text.***

HCG is available in a variety of different dosages, ranging from 500 I.U. ampules, increasing up to 10,000 I.U. ampules, all containing vitamin B12. HCG should not have been confused with steroids, as it is actually a natural protein hormone which had been secreted by the human placenta, and then purified from the urine of pregnant women. It is a natural hormone which had mimicked the LH (luteinizing hormone), almost identically.

Clinically, HCG had been usually prescribed in efforts to have treated prepubertal cryptorchisim (undesended testicles), delayed adolescence, and hypogonadotropic hypogonadism. Male athletes often had utilized the compound of HCG usually after a long steroid term, in efforts to have increased the body's own natural production of Testosterone. Male users also had administered HCG in attempts to have prevented testicular atrophy, which had often resulted when high dosages of steroidal compounds had been used. High dosages of steroids had generally caused a false signal to have been transmitted to the hypothalamus, which had resulted in a depressed signal to the testicles. Over a period of several weeks, this often had damaged the testicle's ability to have responded to preventative testicular atrophy signals. When initially administered by intramuscular injection, serum Testosterone levels had been increased very quickly, usually first having appeared in approximately two hours. A second peak had been frequently experienced within two to four days later. Not only had HCG therapy been found to have been effective in the prevention of testicular atrophy, but it had also been proven to have been beneficial in raising the body's own biochemical stimulating mechanisms in order to have increased plasma Testosterone levels during training.

Several male athletes had claimed that administering HCG directly after a steroid cycle had assisted in having reduced the effect of considerable strength and muscle mass loss, which had been usually experienced in the transition phase. The administration of HCG had also helped to quickly bring back the testes to their original size, when testicular atrophy had been experienced due to extremely high steroidal dosages which had been taken for prolonged periods of time.

Unfortunately, not only could the administration of HCG have increased the androgen levels up to 400 %, but could have also raised levels of Estrogen as well. This of course, primarily had resulted in feminization effects such as gynecomastia and in feminine fat distribution.

HCG had not only been utilized by male athletes who had wished to have avoided potential hazards when they had abruptly ended a steroid cycle, but it had been also administered in efforts to have kept androgen levels high, especially before a drug tested competition. Consequently, HCG had been currently undetectable on steroid testing methods.

Most athletes had been cautious to have visually inspected parenteral drug products such as HCG, for particulate matter and discoloration before they had engaged in the administration; whenever the solution and container had permitted. The commercial HCG which had been currently available, had been sold as a dry substance, that had required reconstitution before it had been ready for administration.

Usual Clinical Recommendation:

The dosage regimen in each case, had depended upon the indication for use, the age, and weight of the patient, and the physician preference.

The selected cases of hypogonadotropic hypogondism in males:

1. 500 - 1,000, USP I.U.'s x 3 times a week, for 3 weeks, followed by the same dose twice a week, for 3 weeks.

2. 4,000 USP I.U.'s 3 times weekly for 6 to 9 months, following which the dosage may have been reduced to 2,000 USP I.U.'s 3 times a week, up to an additional 3 months.

Adventitious Dosage and Administration:

Before HCG had been administered, it had required to have been reconstituted. Initially, the sterile air had to have been withdrawn from the lyophilized vial and injected into diluent vial. Then, up to 10 ml of diluent had been removed, and added to the lypohilized vial, shaken gently, and the solution had become complete. It had been imperative that this reconstituted solution had been used within 30 days. Dry HCG had a life span of approximately ten weeks. Therefore, athletes had paid particular attention to the product's expiration dates, to have ensured that the product had not expired.

Once this had been obtained, the solution had been intended for deep intramuscular injection. HCG had not been administered orally, as it had been destroyed in the gastrointestinal tract. Therefore, the best site for this type of injection had primarily been in the gluteus medius muscle area, which had been the upper outer portion of the buttock, approximately 2 to 3 inches below the hip bone (iliac crest). Most athletes had frequently alternated injections from one side to the other, (first injection on the left side, the second time injection administered on the right, or vice versa) in efforts to have alleviated pain somewhat, which had also allowed the area to have slightly "healed". This practice had also often prevented a thick scar tissue from having had potentially formed. However, the more injections that had been administered, the greater possibility of scar tissue had also increased. A common dosage regime of some athletes, has been discussed in the following:

Females:

Female athletes had not usually engaged in the administration of HCG, as this compound had been ineffective as an athletic or bodybuilding enhancer when it had been administered to the female system. HCG had been primarily utilized clinically to have triggered ovulation, and to have produced Estrogens and yellow bodies in female patients.

Males:

Male athletes often had kept their cycles on HCG down to approximately three weeks at any one given time, with a rest interval of abstinence for at least a month between cycles. Also, male athletes often had practiced previously to having contemplated HCG, that their steroidal regimes had been slowly and evenly reduced.

Several male athletes had generally entertained a regime of HCG, which often had involved initially having "kick started" the system with approximately 2,000 - 4,000 I.U.'s every third day, following any steroid cycle. This then had been maintained at approximately 1000 mgs per week, for two to three weeks. HCG had also been used for two to three weeks in the middle of a steroid cycle, in efforts to have avoided testicular atrophy.

Cycles had been ideally kept down to a 2 or 3 week maximum, and maintained at approximately 1,000 I.U.'s. This had been administered once every 2 to 3 months, in efforts to have given the body's natural Testosterone levels a boost. However, as previously indicated, short cycles of HCG had often been primarily utilized by most male athletes, due to potential feminization side effects, and the possibility that the prolonged use of HCG could have permanently repressed the body's own production of gonadotropins.

Side Effects:

Some of the more common side effects which had been experienced by male athletes who had administered the compound of HCG had included nausea and vomiting, mood alterations, increased sex drive, headaches, high blood pressure, water retention and gynecomastia. However, other effects may have been associated with this compound which have been experienced by men, but not documented, due to the possibility that they had not been recognized in association to administration of this compound.

WARNING:

If Testosterone levels had become too elevated from high doses of HCG, severe incidences of gynecomastia had frequently resulted. There had been no reported cases of overdose complications with the parental use of HCG. Also, there had been no associated carcinomas, liver or renal impairments documented.

Rating:

Based on a 1 to 5 star scale, with 1 considered low, and 5 considered high, a -- symbol is indicative of no value. This compound of Chorionic Gonadotropin has rated as the following:

	MALES	FEMALES
Testosterone Stimulant	****	--
Side Effects	**	--
Cost Efficiency	**	**

HUMAN GROWTH HORMONE

Chemical Name: Somatropin.

Common Generic Name: Human Growth Hormone.

Other Trade Names Found in Mexico:
Biotropin (made for institutional use).
Genotropin.
Humatrope.
Nanorm (N.L.M.).
Norditropin.
Saizen.

Manufacturers:
Biotropin - Biotec Labs.
Genotropin - Pharma.
Humatrope - Lilly.
Norditropin - PISA.
Saizen - Serono.

Dosage Form:
Biotropin - 4 I.U. 1 ml ampule.
Genotropin - 4 I.U. 1 ml ampule.

Humatrope	- 5 mg. ampule.
Norditropin	- 12 I.U. ampule.
	- 4 I.U. ampule.
Saizen	- c/10 I.U.
	- c/4 I.U.

Storage: Before and after reconstitution with Bacteriostatic water for injection, USP, this must be stored at 2 to 8 degrees C (36 to 46 degrees F) in the refrigerator. With the exception of Saizen, the biological activity of Growth Hormone is usually not impaired when storing the dry substance at 15 to 30 degrees C (59 to 86 degrees F). However, refrigeration temperature as discussed above is preferable. Reconstituted vials should be used within 7 days after reconstitution. Expiration dates are stated on the product's labels. Do not freeze.

Price Range:

Biotropin	- currently, only available for institutional use.
Genotropin	- approx. $ 729.30 pesos for 4 U.I. 1 ml ampule.
Humatrope	- approx. $1,200.00 pesos for 5 mg ampule.
Norditropin	- approx. $ 416.92 pesos for 4 U.I. ampule.
	- approx. $1,063.15 pesos for 12 U.I. ampule.
Saizen	- approx. $1,350.00 pesos for c/10 U.I.
	- approx. $ 597.00 pesos for c/4 U.I.

Type of Drug: Synthetic DNA Growth Hormone.

Ingredient: 5 mgs Somatropin.

Drug Identification:

Humatrope - available as an injectable solution, is available in two separate containers, one bottle of sterile water, and the other a clear glass, multi-injection bottle with the dry product. Humatrope is on a white label, with the product's entities written in black, along with the manufacturer and I.U. amount displayed in red. The bottle has a silver tear-off aluminum wrap around the lid which requires to be torn off and discarded after entry which reveals a multiple injection type lid underneath. The accompanying package looks identical to the bottle's label. No. 7346. Clave # 5155.

Saizen - available as an injectable solution, is available in two separate containers, one bottle of sterile water, and the other a clear glass multi-injection bottle with the dry product. The accompanying package is white with the products entities displayed in gray, blue and black ink. Reg. # 208MM8. Clave #5155.

Unfortunately, not all of the Human Growth Hormone products had been obtained for illustrational and identification purposes, however, they are all available in most farmacias.

Please refer to the photographs of Humatrope and Saizen for full color references.

Drug Description:

Initially, biological active forms of Growth Hormone had been extracted from the pituitary glands of cadavers, and formally used in both clinical and athletic applications. However, these versions had been quickly abandoned and had been removed from the market due to it's association with a rare brain virus known as Creutzveldt Jacob Disease. Although this virus reportedly had only affected a minute minority of clinical patients, it nevertheless, had developed symptoms very quickly and had proved to have been fatal within six months of the onset of the disease.

Consequently, synthetic recombinant versions of Growth Hormone (which had been genetically produced either from E-coli, or from the transformed mouse cell lines), had replaced the original biological active forms, and have been widely available and so far, safely utilized today.

Somatropin and Somatrem are polypeptide hormones which have been purified, and are of recombinant DNA origin. In Mexico alone, the synthetic versions of Somatropin have included those by the trade names of Biotropin, Genotropin, Humatrope, Nanorm, Norditropin, and Saizen; all of which have contained an amino acid chain of 191 amino acids. Another synthetic form of Growth Hormone, had been slightly chemically different, as it had contained an additional amino acid, for a total of 192. This synthetic form had been referred to as Somatrem, which had been more easily recognized by the trade name of Protropin.

Growth Hormone is an endogenous hormone, which is produced by the pituitary gland; and had reached particularly high levels during puberty. This duration primarily had been when the growth of all tissues, muscles, and bones had been especially significant. Since Growth Hormone had been necessary for having had increased muscle, it had a direct therapeutic effect on body composition, and increased bone density had also been theorized to have occurred. Growth Hormone also had promoted the deposition of protein and the breakdown of fat, for the body to have used as a source of energy. However, as puberty had ended and the body had reached full maturity, these endogenous levels had significantly diminished, but had continued on a limited basis to have aided in protein synthesis, RNA and DNA reactions, and in having converted bodyfat into sources of energy. Unfortunately, this performance generally had often progressed at a much lower level, which had often expressed the finishing sensation of a vast growth period, as levels in the elderly, when compared to levels in young males, had been markedly reduced. Also, Growth Hormone levels did not attain the same peak values after exercise in the elderly as they had in young, healthy males.

Growth Hormone is produced in the hypophysis, and if stimuli such as proper sleep intervals, stress, low blood sugar levels, and efficient training methods had been provided, then it had inadvertently been released to have been advantageous to the system. Interestingly, the body had released this Growth Hormone specifically at two different times; approximately 15 to 30 minutes after intense exercise, and during REM sleep. Theoretically, it would have been definitely beneficial to have provided the body with the proper macronutrient ratio to have ensured maximum release of Growth Hormone during these durations.

Clinically, the administration of Growth Hormone had been intended for the long-term treatment of children who had experienced growth failure, which had often been due to an inadequate secretion of normal endogenous Growth Hormone. The application of Growth Hormone in these patients had often resulted in the increase of linear, tissue, skeletal and cell growth, as well as an improvement in protein, carbohydrate, and lipid metabolism. However, mineral metabolism had not been significantly altered by the use of these compounds.

Peculiarly, athletes often had entertained the administration of the Somatropin versions of Growth Hormone which had contained the 191 amino acid chain, as this had allegedly been more effective than it's contender of 192 amino acids, Protropin. Since Human Growth Hormone is a master hormone, exogenous administration had acted as a messenger which had ultimately resulted in the endocrine system having returned to the natural biological harmony.

Synthetic Growth Hormone had a strong anabolic effect that had caused an increased protein synthesis which had led to an increase, and an enlargement of the muscle cells. The ability of muscular hyperplasia, had made the synthetic Growth Hormone unique, as this property had been unattainable by steroidal compound intake alone. The administration of synthetic Growth Hormone had also strengthened the connective tissues, tendons and cartilages that had often been responsible for strength increases, which had often prevented potential injuries.

Consequently, several athletes had claimed that the exclusive use of synthetic Growth Hormone although anabolic, had very little anti-catabolic activity, and had not produced any beneficial gains by itself. However, the addition of anabolic steroids (characteristic of preventing catabolism), had produced a tremendous degree of synergism, which inevitably had often promoted a very much desired, significant increase in lean tissue.

In fact, many athletes had claimed that an injectable synthetic Growth Hormone, along with the required combination of Humulin (insulin), and Cynomel (a LT-3 thyroid hormone) had not only allowed for the maximum anabolic effect, but also had enabled the liver to have produced and have released the maximum amounts of Somatomedin and insulin-like growth factors. These growth factors had been the ones which had caused various effects in the body. This effect had been however, somewhat restricted, as the liver had only been capable of having produced a limited amount of these substances.

Some athletes also had frequently engaged in the administration of exogenous synthetic Growth Hormone, for the added desired entity of having burned bodyfat for energy, which distinguishably had often led to a pronounced fat reduction, even on a high caloric intake. In fact, if this compound had been utilized when calories had been restricted, the body had generally counteracted by having reduced the release of insulin and the L-T3 thyroid hormone. This in turn, had reduced the anabolic effect. Miraculously, many athletes had also reported that a reasonable increase in proper calories had not resulted in the accumulation of fat. However, if this compound had been utilized by athletes only for the lipolysis properties, then the thyroid hormone levels had also been required to have been increased during the synthetic Growth Hormone treatment. Most athletes had generally easily accomplished this by having consumed a complete meal every three hours.

Consequently, many athletes had claimed that the effects of Growth Hormone had not been advantageous (particularly when dieting), when they also had combined an anti-catabolic compound such as Spiropent. This combination had actually reduced the body's own natural release of insulin and L-T3. On an average of 6 to 8 months, most athletes had encountered an increase in lean muscle tissue of approximately 8.8%, and 14% reduction in bodyfat.

Unfortunately, several athletes had been unsuccessful in having attempted the utilization of exogenous synthetic Growth Hormones, therefore, had often rendered this compound's efficacy worthless. Accordingly, there had generally been many probable reasons for these warranted accusations; which had argumentatively not supported these theories.

All of the current synthetic versions of Somatropin had been expensive, and for the most part, several self-administering athletes simply could not have afforded the required dosages which would have produced the desired results. Unless a possible cycle had been affordable or obtainable, most athletes had not ventured to have wasted both money and effort in an amount that would have been insufficient to have produced a positive outcome. A full dosage taken regularly over a extended enough duration, had been necessary for this compound to have been effective.

Other common problems which some athletes had sometimes encountered had been that the body also had required more thyroid hormones, insulin, corticosteroids, gonadotropins, Estrogen, androgens, and anabolics, in addition to the administration of synthetic Growth Hormone. If these substances had been absent, or if the synthetic Growth Hormone had been singularly taken, it had usually resulted in considerably lessened effects, if any had been experienced at all. Therefore, if athletes had also entertained the additional combination of steroidal compounds, thyroid hormones, and in particular, insulin, they had often been able to have had produced potential optimal anabolic results.

In fact, in the administration of a particular amount of IGF-1 and/or Growth Hormone, only a tiny fraction of these substances had caused the system to shutdown. However, the body had a tendency to have generated a new LH pulse more rapidly, which had reinitiated the system's production of Testosterone. As the new LH pulse usually had occurred before the body's own Testosterone had been totally eliminated from the system, the total sum amount of Testosterone frequently had been raised. Possibly, this interaction may have had explained the reason why Growth Hormone had seemed to have worked so efficiently with anabolic injections combined with the administration of Growth Hormone (in average individuals, this had generally caused the pituitary output of Growth Hormone to have become short circuited as a consequence). Generally, the sole administration of anabolic steroids had resulted in the body primarily having shut down the production of Testosterone, which in turn, had caused the testes to have become atrophied. Consequently, the administration of Growth Hormone with a cycle of anabolic steroids had not allowed the system's own production of Testosterone to have shut down, therefore, the testes had remained unaffected, and levels of Testosterone had also been increased, which had resulted in great gains by many athletes.

However, in a few very rare cases, the athlete's body had actually reacted against the synthetic Growth Hormone compound; that had made it ineffective, due to the development of antibodies which had destroyed it.

Although the 191 amino acid sequence versions (Somatropin) had been proven to have produced less of an antibody reaction, they still had not been able to have produced consistent results. However, many athletes who had been able to afford the high price of this compound, had often been willing to have taken this risk, in attempts to have achieved the possible wondrous effects, which had been generally associated with the administration of Somatropin.

Some athletes had generally reported that the major drawbacks to Growth Hormone administration had been that it not only had required to have been injected frequently (daily to several times a week), but had been tremendously expensive. This treatment also allegedly, had not produced as an appealing overall result which had usually been experienced with anabolic steroid supplementation. Therefore, many athletes often had administered Growth Hormone for a short term treatment, concurrently with anabolics, in efforts to have kept cost factors to a minimum, and results at a maximum.

Presently, methods have not been available to have detected the use of the synthetic Growth Hormone compound in athletic utilization, but this compound had been banned by most athletic committees and federations. Synthetic Growth Hormone had also, currently not been added to the Controlled Substance List; unlike most of the other athletic enhancement compounds which had been found in Mexico.

Usual Clinical Recommendation:

This recommended dosage had been recommended up to 0.06 mg/kg (0.16 I.U./kg) of bodyweight administered three times a week by either subcutaneous or intramuscular injection. The dosage and administration had been usually individualized for each patient, and had depended on the circumstance.

Some studies which had been performed on the administration of synthetic Growth Hormone had been shown to have had enhanced the efficacy of parenteral (IV) and enteral (oral) feedings. A dose of approximately 25 u/kg/day had been required to have provided an overall anabolic effect in the elderly, (this had been most beneficial when it had been administered at night, in attempts to have approximated the natural circadian rhythmic release).

Adventitious Dosage and Administration:

Athletes precisely had reconstituted the 5 mgs of Somatropin, with 1.5 to 5 ml of diluent. The diluent had been carefully injected into the vial of the dry substance, by having aimed the stream of liquid against the glass wall. Following the reconstitution, the vial had been swirled gently in a circular motion until all of the contents had been completely dissolved. This mixture had been NEVER SHAKEN. The resulting solution had to have been clear, without particulate matter. If the solution had been cloudy or contained particulate matter, the **contents had never been injected.** There had been approximately 13.3 I.U's of synthetic Growth Hormone in a bottle (the conversion had been .375 mg = 1 I.U.). Therefore, if the usual 4 I.U.'s had been utilized each time, then 3 cc's of diluent had been put into the powder; and the injection of one cc each time had been administered, so that the bottle had generally lasted one week (4 I.U.'s three times a week).

Before and after an injection, cautious athletes always had wiped the septum of the vial with rubbing alcohol or an alcoholic antiseptic solution, which had prevented potential contamination of the contents, that could have been often caused by repeated needle insertions. Sterile disposable syringes and needles had always been used. The volume of the syringe had been small enough so that the desired dose could have been withdrawn from the vial with reasonable accuracy.

Female & Males:

Many athletes had claimed that the utilization of small regular dosages had seemed to have been the most effective, as the administered synthetic Growth Hormone effect had been almost immediate due to the rapid increase of the serum concentration in the blood. The administration of synthetic Growth Hormone had also stimulated the liver which in turn, had produced and released somatomedins and insulin-like growth factors. This effect had generally transpired into desired results in the athlete's body. Consequently, since the liver had been only able to have produced a limited amount of these substances, and had reacted more favorably to smaller dosages, it had not proven to have been advantageous to have increased the administered injection, in further attempts to have acquired larger quantities of somatomedins and insulin-like growth factors.

Several athletes had claimed that if the synthetic Growth Hormone had been administered subcutaneously (beneath the skin) at the same point of injection, for a repeated amount of times, that a loss of fat tissue had been frequently experienced. Evidently, in order to have avoided lipoatrophy (localized fat tissue loss), many athletes had generally alternated the injection sites from one side of the body to the other. Commonly, daily subcutaneous injections had been preferred (when financially permitted), at dosages of usually 8 I.U.'s per day.

Top athletes had claimed to have injected the synthetic form of Growth Hormone anywhere in the range of 4 to 16 I.U.'s a day. Since this compound had a half-life time of less than one hour, many athletes had often further divided their daily dose into 3 or 4 subcutaneous injections of 2 to 4 I.U.'s each. However, the effect of synthetic Growth Hormone had largely been dosage-dependent. Sometimes, a typical 200 lbs (91 kg) bodybuilder had often administered approximately 5.5 mg (or approximately 15 I.U.'s) daily, which had been slightly more than the 5 mg amount in the bottle.

Consequently, a female athlete had generally entertained dosages that had similarly been in relation to her bodyweight. For example, if a female athlete had weighed 130 lbs (59 kg), the administration of approximately 2 to 3 mgs (or 5 to 8 I.U's) of synthetic Growth Hormone may have had been utilized, in divided daily dosages.

Most athletes had often administered minimal dosages at 4 I.U.'s a day, which had allegedly provided effective results, especially when it had been administered for a duration of at least six weeks, to several months. Several athletes had reported that the effect of this compound such as newly acquired muscle and strength gains had not appeared to have terminated after a few weeks after discontinuation, which had usually allowed for continued improvements at a steady dosage.

To further exacerbate the results of the administered synthetic Growth Hormone compounds, many athletes had also utilized other anabolic and androgenic steroids. These additional substances had allegedly produced phenomenal results which many athletes had claimed could not have been acquired by the sole administration of synthetic Growth Hormone alone.

Humulin (insulin) had even sometimes had been administered, even though it had posed an increased threat when utilized by non-diabetic individuals, and had frequently counteracted when used incorrectly, which had resulted in actually making an individual fat, instead of lean. Evidently, too much insulin had generally activated particular enzymes which had converted glucose into glycerol; then triglycerides. An insufficient amount of insulin which had generally been apparent when a restriction in calories had been present, had reduced the anabolic effect of the synthetic compound of Growth Hormone. In efforts to have avoided an improper insulin status, most athletes had wisely monitored their glucose levels by means of a glucometer, and had adjusted the administration of insulin accordingly.

Most athletes who had engaged in the administration of synthetic Growth Hormone while they had been in their build-up phase, usually had not required the injection of exogenous insulin. Instead, most often these athletes had consumed a complete meal every three hours, which had generally resulted in 6 daily meals. This practice had often caused the body to have continuously released insulin, so that the blood sugar level had not fallen too low.

The utilization of Cynomel (LT-3 thyroid hormone) in the build-up phase, had also been entertained by a few athletes, who periodically had a physician check the thyroid hormone levels to have ensured normalities. The application of a thyroid hormone, in particular, LT-3, in addition to injected insulin, had not been clearly determined.

Some athletes had successfully stacked the synthetic compound of Growth Hormone with Orimeten (currently, not available in Mexico). The aminoglutethimide had provided the anabolic qualities of Growth

Hormone, and the anti-catabolic activity of Orimeten, (which also had been able to have inhibited the conversion of androgens to Estrogens, by effecting the aromatizing enzyme system). This combination had also allegedly been successful in having passed any drug test known.

Side Effects:

Although the media had often sensationalized many of the side effects that had been feasible with the compound of synthetic Growth Hormone, they had often neglected to have indicated that these adverse effects had affected primarily pre-pubescent individuals. Side effects such as Gigantism, Acromegaly, increased heart muscle and kidney size, fatigue, weakness, diabetes, heart conditions, and early death, had not usually been experienced by adult athletes.

Technically, however, even though the possibility had been rare, Acromegaly specifically involving the elongation of the feet, forehead, and hands, or overgrowth of the elbows and jaw, thickening of the skin, carpal tunnel, thyroid insufficiency, heart muscle hypertrophy, enlargement of the kidneys, hypertension, exacerbation of glucose intolerance, (hypoglycemia) leading to diabetes, and an increased incidence of neoplasm (but only in high and long-term doses) had sometimes been experienced by a few unconservative dosing, long-term administering adult athletes. In some cases antibodies had developed against Growth Hormones, but had been clinically irrelevant.

Consequently, some athletes had reported incidences of headaches, nausea, vomiting, and visual disturbances during the first few weeks of initial intake, which had generally subsided and disappeared in most cases, even with continued utilization. However, most athletes had frequently experienced a slight retention of fluid for the first three months of the administration of synthetic Growth Hormone, as the body's hormonal system had to rebalance. Incidentally, athletes who had utilized conservative measures of synthetic Growth Hormone, had not often experienced negative side effects. The most common problem had occurred, when synthetic Growth Hormone had been combined with the injection of Humulin (insulin).

Therefore, synthetic Growth Hormone had not presented the typical side effects of most other anabolic and androgenic steroids. Studies had indicated that there had also been no causal relation between treatment with Somatropin and a possible higher risk of leukemia.

Rating:

Based on a 1 to 5 star scale, with 1 considered low, and 5 considered high, this compound of Somatropin had rated as the following:

	MALES	**FEMALES**
Strength Increase	****	****
Mass & Weight Increase	****	****
Fat Burner	*****	*****
Contest Preparation	*****	*****
Side Effects	**	**
Cost Efficiency	*****	*****

HUMULIN

Chemical Name: Human Biosynthetic Insulin.

Common Generic Name: Insulin.

Other Trade Names Found in Mexico:
Beriglobina* P.
Humulin.
Seroglubin.

Manufacturer:
Beriglobina* P - Quimica Hoechst de Mexico.
Humulin - Lilly.
Seroglubin - PROBIF.

Dosage Form:
Beriglobina* P - 2 ml ampule.
Humulin 10/90 injectable solution, 100 I.U.
Humulin 20/80 injectable solution, 100 I.U.
Humulin 30/70 - 100 I.U.
Humulin L Lenta - ampule 10 ml.
Humulin N NPH - ampule 10 ml.
Humulin N NPH - ampule c/5 cart.
Humulin R REG - ampule c/5cart
Humulin R REGULAR - ampule 10 ml.
Humulin NPH - 100 I.U. 30/70.
Seroglubin - 2 ml bottle.

Storage: Humulin must be stored in a cold place, preferably in a refrigerator, but not in a freezer. Do not let it freeze or leave it in direct sunlight. The vial in use can be kept at room temperature (below 25 degrees C or 77 degrees F) for no longer than one month. The cartridge in use may be kept at a temperature below 30 degrees C (86 degrees F) for up to 21 days.

Price Range: Humulin - all dosages are approx. $93.60 pesos.
Beriglobina* P - approx. $46.30 pesos for 2 ml ampule.
Seroglubin - approx. $61.30 pesos for 2 ml bottle.

Type of Drug: Antidiabetic Agent. Recombinant DNA origin.

Ingredient:

Humulin 10/90	- Each ml contains 10 units of NPH insulin.
Humulin 20/80	- Each ml contains 20 units of Regular insulin and 80 units of NPH.
Humulin 30/70	- Each ml contains 30 units Regular insulin and 70 units of NPH insulin.
Humulin L	- Each ml contains 100 units of Lente insulin.
Humulin N	- Each ml contains 100 units of Lente insulin.
Humulin R	- Each ml contains 100 units of Regular insulin.
Humulin NPH	- Each ml contains 100 units of Insulin Isophane.

Drug Identification:

Beriglobina* P - For injectable administration, it is available in a clear glass ampule, with two green stripes near the top of the ampule tip. It is in a 2 ml ampule. The label is a white sticker with the product's entities displayed in green ink. There is also a red and green box on the top right corner of the sticker. The Lot # is 102011. The solution itself is clear and colorless. The accompanying box is identical to the ampule, as it is also white, with green print.

Humulin L - Available for injectable administration, the substance itself is a suspension, which has a milky-white water appearance. The glass bottle is clear with a white sticker label displaying the product's entities. The company Lilly is displayed in red outlined by a black border, within a light gray stripe across the top of the label. The "L" and all other printing is in black ink. Lot # 51448WC. The multi-injectable lid is enclosed by a silver, tear-off aluminum cap. The accompanying box is identical to the bottle, with a red tab on the top.

Humulin N - Available for injectable administration, is exact in appearance to Humulin L, with the exception of a "N" appearing on the label printed in a very light gray color, with a black ink border. Lot # 51448WC.

All forms of Humulin Insulins have a milky-white water appearance, with the exception of the short-acting Insulin Humulin-R, Regular. Humulin-R is a clear, colorless solution.

Seroglubin - Is also available for injectable administration, and is presented in a clear glass bottle. It is a 2 ml x 330 mg bottle. The Lot # is MEA212. The label is a white sticker, with the colors of green blue, and red ink displaying various entities of this product. There is a silver aluminum tear-off lid, which conceals a multiple-injection type lid underneath. The solution itself is clear and colorless. The accompanying box is white with a navy blue triangle in the left top corner, with a red tab, and a red and green stripe through the middle of the box. The products entities are displayed in both red and navy blue ink.

*****Please refer to the photographs of Humulin L & N, Beriglobina* P, Seroglubin for full color references.***

Drug Description:

*** All brands of Insulin have been commonly referred to as Humulin for simplicity measures in the following text.*

The substance of Humulin is a polypeptide hormone which consists of a 21 amino acid A-chain, and a 30 amino acid B-chain that is linked by two disulfide bonds. Humulin had been found to be "chemically, physically, biologically, and immunologically equivalent to human insulin" which is created by the pancreas. Insulin can be considered to have been somewhat of a nutrient storage hormone; as it had escorted amino acids (protein) and glucose (carbohydrates), into various cells of the body, where it had either been used for energy or stored. Insulin also had aided amino acids and glucose to have been absorbed by the muscle cells which had facilitated anabolism, and possibly had helped to have prevented the breakdown of muscle tissue, in attempts to have avoided anti-catabolism.

Clinically, suitable doses of insulin had been intended for the administration in patients who had been diagnosed with diabetes mellitus. Injectable insulin such as Humulin, had been administered for many years by diabetics, who had this disease which had prevented the body from making enough insulin (Type I diabetes), or had a defect which had caused the cells not to have recognized insulin (Type II diabetes). Insulin, such as Humulin, combined with a controlled diet and exercise, had temporarily been able to have restored the ability to have metabolized carbohydrates, fats and proteins; to store glycogen in the liver; and also to have converted glucose to fat. When insulin had been administered in suitable doses at regular intervals to an individual who had been diagnosed with diabetes mellitus, the blood sugar had usually been maintained within a reasonable range, the urine had remained relatively free of sugar and ketone bodies, and diabetic acidosis and coma had usually been prevented.

There are three main types of insulin; long acting, intermediate acting, and short-acting. Short-acting insulin usually had remained in the body for about six to eight hours after injection; peak hours within 2.5 to 5 hours, and the onset of action had generally been approximately 0.5 hours after administration.

Intermediate acting insulin usually had a duration in the body ranging from 18 to 24 hours after administration; peak hours within 4 to 15 hours, and the onset of action had usually been in 1.5 to 3 hours.

Long acting insulin generally had remained in the body anywhere from 24 to 36 hours, peaking anywhere from 8 to 30 hours, with the onset of action within 4 to 6 hours after injection.

There had also been different sources of insulin which have included standard and purified animal insulins, as well as human insulins. The main difference between standard and purified insulins had been in their degree of purification and content of non-insulin material. These insulins had also been derived from different sources, such as beef, pork, or a mixture of both. Consequently, human insulin had been identical in structure to the insulin that had been produced by the human pancreas, and had been only slightly different from the animal insulin. Changes in refinement, purity, strength, brand, type and/or method of manufacture (recombinant DNA versus animal source insulin) had often required a change in dosage.

Similarly, several professional bodybuilders had indicated that if they had switched from animal to human insulin (or vice versa), they frequently had noticed a different reaction from the same dosage. Therefore, an adjustment frequently had been made either with the first dose, or over a period of several weeks. Professional bodybuilders who had made a change of insulin, cautiously had done so, as this should only have been attempted with medical supervision.

Biosynthetic human insulin (produced by recombinant DNA technology), had been less likely to have produced immunogenicity problems than with the administration of insulin which had been derived from animal origin. Consequently, Biosynthetic human insulin had not contained protein contaminants of pancreatic origin, which had normally been present in trace amounts in all insulins which had originated from the pancreas.

Professional bodybuilders who had systemic allergies to either pork or beef insulins, had also often reacted to the administration of human insulin. Clinically, patients who sometimes had encountered these problems had undergone appropriate procedures such as intradermal testing and even desensitization, before therapeutic doses of human insulin had been administered. Several cautious professional bodybuilders had either similarly undergone these procedures, or, had abandoned the concept of using insulin altogether. For the most part, the use of administering animal insulins had lowered significantly, almost to the point of extinction in both clinical and athletic application. Novo-Toronto and Humulin-T insulin had been examples of animal insulins (which are currently, not available in Mexico).

Formulations of Humulin had appeared to have produced a slightly faster onset and slightly shorter duration of action than the corresponding forms of animal-source insulins. Humulin-L and Humulin-U had generally resulted in the reduction of the quick-acting effect of regular insulin.

Insulin preparations had been different in onset, peak and duration of action. The addition of Protamine to insulin, and the presence of Zinc, had been able to have produced a stable complex due to it's slow dissolution, which had been less intense; with a more prolonged action.

The following insulins have all been biosynthetic human insulins, and the differences between them have been listed as follows:

Humulin-R, Regular, Insulin Injection Beriglobina* P:	Are fast-acting insulins that have a relatively short duration of activity which lasts for 6 to 8 hours.
Humulin-N, NPH, Insulin Isophane, Humulin-L, Lente, Insulin Zinc Suspension Medium:	Are intermediate-acting insulins which have a a longer duration of activity of up to 24 hours, but have a slower onset of action than Regular insulins.
Humulin-U, Ultalente, Insulin Zinc Suspension Prolonged, Seroglubin:	Are long-acting insulins with a longer duration of activity of at least 24 hours or more, but have a slower onset of action than Regular insulins.
Humulin Mixtures (10/90, 20/80, 30/70, 40/60, and 50/50 Insulin Injection, Human Biosynthetic and Insulin Isophane	Are intermediate-acting insulins which have a more rapid onset of action than NPH alone, and also have a duration of activity of up to 24 hours.
***Humulin-N, Humulin-L, Humulin-U*:**	May be mixed with Humulin-R to treat individual metabolic requirements. This should be determined by a physician.

Some professional bodybuilders had incorporated the administration of insulin into their enhancement regimes, in attempts to have increased definition and muscle fullness. However, if an inactive individual had attempted to have applied this method in efforts to have obtained the same results, a very different outcome had transpired, as the self-administration of insulin had also prevented the breakdown of bodyfat, which actually had increased the bodyfat storage in these sedentary individuals. Apparently, too much insulin had generally activated particular enzymes which had converted glucose into glycerol; then triglycerides. It had been evident that if an extreme physical demand had been placed upon the body such as performing intense weight training, (without the consumption of an excessive caloric intake), the insulin had selected to transport the nutrients to the muscle cells, instead of to the fat cells.

Within the last few years, the self-administration of insulin had appeared to have had a major impact in the athletic environment; particularly in bodybuilding. A few professional or top amateur bodybuilders have engaged in the administration of insulin, often combined with Growth Hormone, steroidal compounds, including Testosterones, thyroid drugs, such as Eutirox or Tiroidine, and Cynomel, and/or IGF-1 (currently, only experimental in Mexico). These "top" bodybuilders had claimed that the additionally utilization of insulin had been even more effective, as it allegedly could have induced the Growth Hormone and IGF-1 to have become more potent muscle builders and fat burners, than the sole utilization of these other enhancement entities alone.

Of course, the self-administration of prescription pharmaceutical drugs had always been dangerous, however, the self-use of insulin had been so jeopardizing, that in fact, **immediate death had resulted if it had been misused.** In efforts to have avoided an improper insulin status, most athletes had wisely monitored their glucose levels by means of a glucometer, and had adjusted the administration of insulin accordingly.

Insulin administration had only been utilized by a few competitive bodybuilders in the top professional ranks, and even then, many had not ventured the effects of this very risky substance; as frequently, most had felt that the gains had not outweighed the risks associated with this substance. If death had not occurred with the misuse, then other possible serious health problems had sometimes become apparent, such as sometimes having acquired the diabetes disease itself, which had required the administration of insulin for life; in addition to other potential problems such as possible blindness etc.

In attempts to have dissuaded athletes from these dangers, the invention of "drug-free" substances which had been able to have mimicked the results that had allegedly been obtained by professional bodybuilders from the administration of insulin, had been undertaken. These compounds also had been able to have safely produced the anabolic and anti-catabolic effects of insulin. The manufacturers of Creatinine Monohydrate have been designing a product which has worked very similarly to insulin injections, and will have been able to have assisted with the building of muscle, but, will not be so powerful that it will have caused hypoglycemia or other health concerns. Currently, however, many athletes have safely perused the compound of Vanadyl Sulfate, which also has a "drug-free" insulin mimicking ability.

Usual Clinical Recommendation:

Dosages of Humulin should have been determined by a physician according to the requirements of the patient. Therefore, there had been no "general" guidelines to a possible starting dosage, and to a possible overdosage. These factors had been extremely dependent upon the individual's blood sugar level, and the dosages had therefore, been concluded from these results.

Patients who had received insulin for the first time, had usually started on Humulin in the same manner as they would have been on an animal-source insulin.

Patients who had been transferred from an animal-source insulin to the administration of Humulin, usually had continued to have utilized the same dose and dosage schedule. However, close monitoring had been practiced during the adjustment period, as some patients who had been transferred to Humulin, sometimes had required a change in dosage from that used previously with the animal-source insulin. If an adjustment had been required, it had been either obtained with the first dose, or over a period of several weeks.

Changes in total dosage, the number of injections per day, and/or timing of injections had often been necessary in order to have achieved maximum glycemic control. When a patient on high doses of animal insulin had been switched to Humulin, it had been sometimes appropriate to also have reduced the starting dosage and to have continued to have monitored the patient carefully. Usually, the most satisfactory injection time had been before breakfast.

Adventitious Dosage and Administration:

The use of insulin had been intended for subcutaneous injection. The best site for this type of injection had primarily been in the upper arms, thighs, buttocks, or abdomen. The few professional bodybuilders who had engaged in insulin administration had rotated injection sites so that the same site had not been used more than approximately once a month. Of course, extreme caution had been taken to have ensured that a blood vessel had not been entered, and also that the area had not been massaged after the injection. Professional bodybuilders had not administered the Humulin-N, Humulin-L, Humulin-U, or Humulin Mixtures when floating lumps or substances which had stuck to the sides of the vial had been visible; or if the contents of the vial had been clear and had remained clear after the bottle had been shaken or rotated. *(The contents of the vial of Humulin-R should be clear, and consequently had not been administered if it had been cloudy).* Humulin-R is a clear, colorless solution which had been usually administered subcutaneously, but clinically, could have been administered also by intramuscular, or intravenous injections. Humulin-N, Humulin Mixtures, Humulin-L and Humulin-U are suspensions compounds which professional bodybuilders had administered by subcutaneous injection only. One cc had been equivalent to 100 units. A common dosage regime of these few professional bodybuilders, has been discussed in the following:

Insulin had primarily been utilized for precontest preparation by a few professional and top amateur bodybuilders. These bodybuilders had claimed that it had appeared that when the body had been depleted of glycogen, the administration of insulin during the "carbing up" phase, had been able to allegedly have produced dramatic effects in the swelling of the muscles. One of the most common complication that most bodybuilders had generally encountered had been in the stage of reintroducing carbohydrates back into the system ("carbing up"). If the muscles had been depleted of glycogen, the muscle's appearance often had presented to have been small and flat. This had been most apparent when the consumption of a low-carbohydrate diet (approximately 100 grams or less daily), had been followed for 3 to 5 days, combined with intense training.

However, with the reintroduction of high quantities of carbohydrates, the muscles had appeared to somewhat over-compensate, and had consumed more carbohydrates then they would have normally. Consequently, this practice had been extremely difficult to perfect. If the professional bodybuilder had not consumed enough carbohydrates, the muscles had appeared to have been small and flat; and if the consumption of too many carbohydrates had transpired, this had usually resulted in subcutaneous water retention; which had caused the muscles to have appeared larger, however, still flat.

Consequently, these life-gambling bodybuilders had reported that the administration of insulin during the phase of having reintroduced carbohydrates back into the system, had produced very desired, dramatic results, which had often allowed for the necessary peak with maximal muscle fullness, and definition. This of course, had been the primary objective of having engaged in a variation of a high and low carbohydrate consumption; however, the administration of insulin allegedly had allowed for somewhat of a guarantee of these optimal results.

Females
& Males:

As previously indicated, the administration of insulin had been very individualized as the dosage and duration had been largely dependent upon the blood sugar levels. This had been closely monitored by an instrument called a glucometer, which would have rendered blood sugar level readings for an individual at their convenience. However, a few professional bodybuilders who did not have abnormal readings in their blood sugar levels, had reportedly administered insulin in efforts to have obtained the above mentioned results by having consumed approximately 10 grams of simple carbohydrates (glucose, per Unit of insulin) approximately 20 to 30 minutes after the administration of insulin. Therefore, when these bodybuilders had administered for example, 10 units of insulin before breakfast, the consumption of approximately 100 grams of simple carbohydrates within 20 to 30 minutes later had been generally followed. The dosage of insulin had generally remained between the ranges of 20 to 40 units per day, and the simple carbohydrate consumption had been adjusted accordingly.

Some professional bodybuilders had not administered an insulin injection before breakfast, in order to have avoided having to have consumed any extra *simple* carbohydrates, but instead, had consumed a meal with only *complex* carbohydrates. Other professional bodybuilders sometimes had engaged in short-acting insulins requiring 2 or 3 daily injections, with a 6 hour duration between each injection. Short-acting insulins had been easier to manage and predict. A few professional bodybuilders, had even chosen to have administered insulin which had both short and long-acting characteristics. This had required very careful monitoring of the diet regimes in efforts to have eaten precisely every three hours, being extremely cautious to have included proportioned servings of protein and carbohydrates.

As the longer-acting insulin could have remained in the system for approximately 24 to 36 hours, it could have peaked several times throughout the day. This characteristic had often made it much more difficult for some professional bodybuilders to have predicted and managed. A few professional bodybuilders had been able to have overcome this dilemma by having eaten properly, and by having consumed a sufficient amount of carbohydrates throughout the day; which at the same interval, also had somewhat reduced the risk of hypoglycemia. If hypoglycemia had been experienced, and the professional bodybuilder had been unable to have consumed a soluble carbohydrate or fruit juice orally, hypoglycemia had then usually been treated with 10 to 20 grams of Dextrose intravenously, or by the administration of Glucagon, either subcutaneously or intramuscularly. Of course, the latter two treatments had been under the immediate medical supervision.

Another alleged advantage of the long-acting form of insulin when it had been administered by professional bodybuilders, had been since it had remained in the system throughout the day, when the blood glucose levels had been increased, the extra insulin had permitted the glucose and available amino acids to have been consumed by the muscle cells.

Another example which had been perused by some professional bodybuilders, had included the administration of a long-acting insulin such as Humulin-U at 15 units, with the additional 5 units of the short-acting insulin Humulin-R first thing in the morning, before breakfast. This had been followed by the administration of another 10 units of the short-acting insulin Humulin-R approximately 6 hours later, and another 10 I.U.'s of Humulin-R after another 6 hours, for a total of 40 units of insulin a day. These professional bodybuilders had been very careful in not having administered the last dose of insulin before they had went to sleep, as the symptoms of hypoglycemia had not been easily detected, or treatable, while asleep.

Some professional bodybuilders had even tried to have cycled the administration of insulin primarily by having had entertained an insulin cycle for a 6 to 8 week period, then had practiced abstinence for the same time duration. However, this practice had not generally been followed, as insulin had been a very dangerous substance to have engaged in self-administration to begin with; therefore, professional bodybuilders who had attempted the alleged effects of insulin, generally had preferred to have utilized it's properties primarily prior to a competition. This practice had lessened the dangers somewhat, as it had allowed for a minimization of possible long-term insulin administration side effects, which might have included a disruption in the body's ability to have produced certain neurotransmitters in response to low blood sugar levels.

Side Effects:

The self-administration of insulin such as Humulin had posed to have been very dangerous when an individual had been administering this substance in efforts of athletic enhancement. Some milder side effects which had been experienced by a few professional bodybuilders, had included local inflammatory responses, which had frequently resulted from several incidences such as improper cleansing of the skin, contamination of the injection site with alcohol, the use of an antiseptic which had contained impurities; or even accidental intracutaneous rather than subcutaneous injections. Local reactions which often had resulted in skin sensitivity phenomena, usually had subsided spontaneously. However, more extreme, dangerous side effects had also been experienced if too much insulin had been administered along with an insufficient quantity of carbohydrates, hypoglcemia (low blood glucose, also referred to as "insulin reaction") and/or a comatose state had frequently occurred.

Hypoglycemia had also often occurred if a professional bodybuilder had administered too much insulin, missed meals, or had an infection or had become ill (especially with diarrhea or vomiting), or if the body's requirement for insulin had changed for other various reasons. Hypoglycemia had frequently been manifested by hunger, nervousness, warmth and sweating, and palpitations. Additional symptoms had also included headaches, confusion, drowsiness, fatigue, anxiety, blurred vision, diplopia, or numbness of the lips, nose or fingers. Consequently, the clinical manifestations of hypoglycemia had often been masked by the commitant administration of Propranolol or other beta-adrenergic blockers.

A few professional bodybuilders who had experienced hypoglycemic reactions after being transferred to Humulin, had reported that the early warning symptoms such as nervousness, sweating and palpitations, had appeared to have been less pronounced, than they had been with an animal source insulin.

Symptoms had often appeared when the blood sugar concentration had fallen below 2.2 mmol/L (40 mg/100 ml), but had also often occurred with a sudden drop in blood glucose; even when the value had remained above 2.2 mmol/L (40 mg/100ml).

Primarily, if insulin had been intentionally or unintentionally misused, it had undeniably resulted in a rapid death. Insulin lipohypertrophy had also been reported with the administration of Humulin. This complication had been usually accredited to the local pharmacologic effects of the subcutaneous injection of insulin. A few clinical cases of lipoatrophy and serum sickness had also been reported.

WARNING:

The self medicine of the utilization of insulin had been very risky, and should have been left to the supervision of the medical profession. This practice should never have been entertained by amateur or novice athletes or bodybuilders. It ideally, should not even have been attempted by those had been in the professional ranks.

Under no circumstances had any professional bodybuilder administered any Humulin Mixture intravenously, nor had they engaged in the mixture of Humulin with glandular insulins.

Rating:

Based on a 1 to 5 star scale, with 1 considered low, and 5 considered high; a -- symbol is indicative of no value. This compound of Human Biosynthetic Insulin had rated as the following:

	MALES	FEMALES
Fat Burner	****	****
Contest Preparation	****	****
Side Effects	*****	*****
Cost Efficiency	*	*

LASIX

Chemical Name: Furosemide.

Common Generic Name: Lasix.

Other Trade Names Found in Mexico: Currently, just Lasix.

Manufacturer: Lasix - Quimica Hoechst Mexico

Dosage Form: Lasix - 2 ml ampule.
- 20 and 40 mgs tablets.

Storage: Furosemide tablets should be stored at room temperature in a tightly closed light-resistant container. The oral solution should also be stored in a tightly, closed, light-resistant container but should be refrigerated at 2 to 8 degrees C (36 to 46 degrees F). This medication should never be frozen.

Price Range: Lasix - approx. $17.30 pesos for 5 x 2 ml ampule.
- approx. $13.90 pesos for 36 x 20 mgs tablets.
- approx. $20.10 pesos for 24 x 40 mgs tablets.

Type of Drug: Strong Diuretic and Antihypertensive.

Ingredient: Furosemide.

Drug Identification:

Lasix - is available as an oral administration tablet, in 2 packages of 12 tablets, for a total of 24 tablets per box. The tablets are packaged individually in in a total dark green front, with a silver foil punch-through backing. On the back, Lasix, Furosemida Tabletas 20, Lot # 96G0734, or

40 mgs, Lot # 96H0834, the Quimica Hoechst company label, and the Reg. #, can be found written throughout the back, in yellow. The packing itself is white, with the product's entities written in black ink. The company's logo is displayed in the top right hand corner, overtop of three yellow vertical lines.

The ampule version of Lasix are available in five per box, 2 ml ampules, totaling 10 mls. These ampules are glass, and are a golden color with the break-off type top. All five of these ampules are cradled within a plastic molding. There is a light blue line around the neck of the ampule, indicating where the ampule should be broken. The product's entities are written in black ink upon a white sticker label on each individual ampule. There are three yellow lines identical to accompanying package itself, and on the other side, the Lot # 96C0241 and the expiration date are indicated.

*****Please refer to the photographs of Lasix for full color references.***

Drug Description:

Lasix belongs to the loop-agent diuretic family, which has indicated that it is one of the strongest types of diuretics. These diuretics have been able to have incurred incredible changes to have taken place within the body. Lasix's effects had been usually noticeable within minutes after administration, and often had concluded within an hour's time. The Furosemide compound however, had not only been powerful, but had been fast-acting, and could have been administered orally, intramuscular injection, or intravenously. The administration of Lasix had not only had increased the elimination of water excretion, but also had caused the body to have lost sodium, chloride, calcium, and potassium as well, through the kidneys. It had also been utilized to have reduced fluid accumulation in the body, and in efforts to have lowered high blood pressure (hypertension).

Athletes had often utilized the compound of Lasix in the past in attempts to have diluted urine samples, so that traces of banned substances had not been detected. However, Lasix, and other diuretics had been since added to the list of banned substances of the U.S. Olympics, and most other competitions and organizations. At one time, Lasix had proven to had been a very effective method of masking steroid cycles, therefore, had been no longer allowed. Unprepared athletes frequently still have administered Lasix in untested competitions, as a last alternative in the attempts of having shed subcutaneous water to uncover their peak physiques, or in efforts to have made a weight class. However, the use of this diuretic compound had not only been controversial, but had occasionally proved to have been extremely dangerous if it had not been used properly. Some athletes have died from the miscalculation, and misuse of this diuretic product.

Usual Clinical Recommendation:

The usual initial dose of Lasix had been 20 to 80 mgs, when administered as a single dose. This would ordinarily have caused prompt diuresis. If required, the same dose had been administered 6 to 8 hours later, or the dosage had been increased to 20 or 40 mgs. Lasix should not have been administered any sooner than the previous dose; until the desired diuretic effect had been achieved.

Adventitious Dosage and Administration:

Lasix tablets had been intended for oral administration, which had implied that they had been designed to have been swallowed by mouth. These tablets had provided the best results when they had been ingested with a bit of water. They had not require to have been crushed or chewed. The use of Lasix injectables had been intended for deep intramuscular injection. The best site for this type of injection had been in the gluteus medius muscle area, which had been the upper outer portion of the buttock, approximately 2 to 3 inches below the hip bone (iliac crest). Athletes often had alternated injections from one side to the other, (first injection on the left side, the second time injection administered on the right, or vice versa) in efforts to have alleviated pain somewhat, and in attempts to have allowed the area to slightly "heal". This practice had often prevented a thick scar tissue from potentially forming. However, the more injections that had been administered, the greater possibility of scar tissue had resulted. Finally, most athletes had not entertained the use of Lasix as an intravenous administration, as this had not been a method which had been ultimately practiced. Consequently, some professional bodybuilders had perused the intravenous administration of Lasix, with very high levels of risks involved. A common dosage regime of some athletes, has been discussed in the following:

Females
& Males:

Most female and male athletes only had resorted to the utilization of diuretics such as Lasix, when they had been ill-prepared. Both females and male athletes had preferred the oral compound of Furosemide, but the injectable had provided much more effective results. Depending upon the amount of subcutaneous water held within the body's shape; the amount, duration, and dosage of diuretic had been varied. However, usually a half or a whole 40 mgs tablet had initially been taken, and then the body had been monitored for results. Depending upon the outcome, this procedure had been repeated once or twice usually within a few hours. The injectable version of Lasix had worked very quickly, usually within 15 minutes, and had been easier to have controlled, than the oral administration.

Beginning the evening prior to the competition, usually 10 mgs intravenously had been initially attempted by some athletes. The maximum dosage had never been higher than 40 mgs. If the desired results had not been achieved with this dosage, athletes had realized that they probably had not been going to have been obtained with the administration of the Lasix compound. If this occurred, athletes had generally attempted to have switched to a thiazide or potassium-sparing diuretic (however, usually these compounds had been much more effective if they had been taken 4 to 6 days prior to competition). All in all, most athletes had agreed that proper calculation would had totally have eliminated the considered requirement of a diuretic in the last few days or hours previous to a competition.

Side Effects:

Lasix had been one of the strongest diuretic, and therefore, had been considered to have been the most dangerous compound in an athlete's regime. Clinically, and in athletic application, some of the known side effects which had been caused by loop-agent diuretics such as Lasix had been, constipation, blurred vision, dizziness, headaches, cramping, diarrhea, itching, rash, loss of appetite, nausea, sore mouth, dry mouth, sore throat, increased thirst, dehydration, stomach upset, severe abdominal pain, vomiting and weakness, confusion, difficulty breathing, fainting, joint pain, muscle spasms, muscle cramping, mood changes, palpitations, ringing in the ears, tingling in the fingers or toes, numbness of the arms and hands, unusual bleeding or bruising, or even yellowing of the eyes or skin. The administration of Lasix had also caused increased sensitivity to sunlight. Cardiac arrest and death have also resulted from use of this compound. Of course, other side effects may have had been experienced which had not been recognized by the athlete, therefore, had not been documented.

WARNING:

Another common practice amongst bodybuilders especially, had been to have also administered Slow-K, which had been a prescription strength potassium supplement, in the attempts of having replaced some of the removed potassium, in efforts to have reversed the adverse effects. However, this had not been as easily accomplished, and had only been periodically successful. This practice only had allowed for the probability of having obtained damaging side effects; even to the extent of cardiac arrest.

Occasionally, the utilization of Lasix in the injectable or intravenous form the night or morning previous to the competition, had produced the opposite effect; which had caused the muscles to have become small and flat, with the loss of vascularity, and loss of "pump" during the warm-up interval. Having removed water out of the skin, also had depleted muscle tissue, due to too much water and minerals having been excreted through the urine. However, some professional, experienced athletes had been sometimes able to have corrected this by having injected glucose intravenously, in efforts to have had increased the blood volume once again. Novice athletes had not attempted this practice, at any measure, as Loop-agents had not been experimental compounds, and mistakes had proven to have been fatal.

Excessive diuresis may also have caused dehydration and blood volume reduction with circulatory collapse; and possible vascular thrombosis and embolism (blocking of blood vessels by blood clots). Electrolyte depletion also had occurred, especially when a high dosage of Lasix had been administered while on a restricted salt intake. Treatment of having overdosed had generally consisted of replacement of excessive fluid and electrolyte loss.

The concentration of Furosemide associated with toxicity or death had been unknown. In athletic application, Lasix had been considered to be a "hit or miss" compound, and had not left room for trial and error. Therefore, all athletes had claimed that it had been much wiser to have prepared for a competition well in advance, so that drastic measures such as the administration of diuretics did not have to be considered as a last resort.

Rating:

Based on a 1 to 5 star scale, with 1 considered low, and 5 considered high, a -- symbol is indicative of no value. This compound of Furosemide had rated as the following:

	MALES	FEMALES
Contest Preparation	****	****
Side Effects	*****	*****
Cost Efficiency	*	*

MADECASSOL

Chemical Name: Centella Asiatica Extract.

Common Generic Name: Madecassol.

Other Trade Names Found in Mexico: Currently, just Madecassol.

Manufacturer:

Dosage Form: Madecassol "C" tablets.
Madecassol 'N' 12 tablets.
Madecassol 20 tablets
Madecassol 20 gram cream.

Storage: Anapolon tablets should be protected from light and moisture, (keep in the blisters until contents are used), and stored at controlled room temperature 15 to 30 degrees C (59 to 86 degrees F).

Price Range: Madecassol "C" - approx. $55.40 pesos for 12 tablets.
Madecassol 'N' - approx. $50/20 pesos for 12 tablets.
Madecassol - approx. $46.00 pesos for 20 tablets.
Madecassol - approx. $43.00 pesos for 20 gram cream tube.

Type of Drug: Cicatrising Agent.

Ingredient: 10 mg of Centella Asiatica Extract.

Drug Identification:

Madecassol - the different availability of forms of Madecassol, had not been obtained for illustration and identification purposes. Although these compounds are readily produced and obtainable in Mexico, Madecassol may still be extremely difficult to acquire, and may have to be specially ordered by a farmacia in order to obtain this product.

Drug Description:

The compound of Madecassol is not a steroidal compound, or any other related athletic enhancement pharmaceutical item. Instead, it is actually a titrated extract of Centella asiatica, which also contains triterpenes asiaticoside, asiatic acid, and madecassic acid; which had been able to have stabilized the production of collagen fibers when they had been disturbed; such as experienced in the formation of scar tissue. The administration of Madecassol had been able to have acted upon the connective tissue which in turn, had slowed hypertrophic and possible keloidal reactions by having reduced; or even totally had eliminated the reaction. This characteristic in some cases, could often have had converted the problematic lesion, into that of a mature scar.

The oral administration or topical application of Madecassol had generally resulted in symptomatic relief of itching, reduction of pain, and an improvement of the physical appearance of the affected scar area. A reduction in size, induration and redness had also been frequently experienced by several individuals.

Clinically, the application of Madecassol had been prescribed for the treatment of keloids, hypertrophic scars, and in capsular contractures which had been in the active stage. Scar tissue which had shown only chronic inflammatory reactions had been modified by the utilization of Madecassol. Madecassol however, had an insignificant effect upon the acute inflammatory process, that had generally accompanied the normal healing of wounds; and also had little effect on the scar connective tissue which had been common in long-established asymptomatic contractures.

As the practice of breast, pectoral, calf and other associated types of implants have recently become popular amongst many athletes, particularly, bodybuilders, the application of Madecassol had often been warranted in attempts to have relieved pain, which had often been associated to capsular contracture. Capsular contracture had usually been the result of a buildup of scar tissue around the inserted foreign implant. Basically, a scar contracture had been somewhat of a defense mechanism in which the body had produced in an effort to have voided an unknown substance, such as that of an implanted device. All foreign objects which had been embedded surgically or otherwise, have had some extent of a scar contracture built up around it. This capsular contracture could have been unilateral, or bilateral, and had been frequently presented as a firmness, which had sometimes resulted in somewhat of a distorted abnormal appearance, with occasional associated pain.

Depending upon the degree of the contracture, I, II, or III, had classified the amount of scar tissue buildup. With the Type I classification, sometimes the medical attempt of physically having "broken" the scar contracture had often offered relief of the symptoms. However, many athletes who had developed either a Class I or Class II degree of capsular contracture, had often acquired relief from the utilization of Madecassol. The Class III classification had been the most serious, and the most disfiguring; therefore, the only relief from this occurrence had been with the capsulotomy or capsulectomy, scar contracture release surgical intervention.

However, surgically, it had been very difficult to have established which individual had a greater potential to have suffered from a high degree of scar contracture; as opposed to those who would have not been bothered by a slight contracture, which would not have produced any symptomatology. Consequently, subsequent surgical intervention would not have guaranteed permanent relief from the continued occurrence of the capsular contractures.

Sometimes, complete removal of the implant had to have been undergone, in attempts to have acquired physical relief from pain and disfigurement. However, many physicians had opted to have prescribed the compound of Madecassol, which had prevented the buildup of the scar tissue in several patients. Not only had this substance aided in scar contractions related to implant surgery, but it had also helped with other disfiguring, even painful scars such as keloids (thickened red scars obtained by accidental laceration, or by surgical incision/excision), and had also reduced the swelling and often associated redness.

Currently, Madecassol is of course, obtainable by prescription in Mexico. However, this could also have been acquired through a physician in Canada (currently, it has not been available in the United States), as it had not been considered to be a controlled substance, such as many other featured pharmaceutical entities. Consequently, occasionally Madecassol had been difficult to find, as not all farmacias, or pharmacies frequently had it in stock. Therefore, most athletes had often sought this prescription early in their visit within the country of Mexico, if they had wished to have utilized it's entities.

Usual Clinical Recommendation:

The usual clinical dosage in adult individuals had generally been 1 to 2 10 mgs tablets administered three times daily with meals. If no sign of improvement had been apparent after 20 days, then this medication had been discontinued; as this had been an indication that Madecassol would not have been efficacious as a treatment for this particular suffered symptomatology.

If the administration of Madecassol had proven to have been effective, then the treatment had been continued for an average of 3 to 6 months, according to the response. However, the duration of treatment had often been dependent upon the degree of capsular contracture, thickness of the keloid, intensity of the hypertrophic scar, and clear signs of maturation of the scar, or total disappearance of all the signs of inflammatory reactions.

Adventitious Dosage and Administration:

Madecassol tablets had been intended for oral administration, which had meant that they had been designed to have been swallowed by the mouth. These tablets had produced the best results, when they had been also consumed with water and meals. They did not require to have been crushed or chewed. The cream had been applied directly to the bothersome area, usually twice a day. A common regime of some athletes, has been discussed in the following:

Since Madecassol had recently been introduced to the athletic environment, not only had it not been misused or abused, but efforts of doing so would undeniably have proven to have been ineffective. As stated in the clinical application, if the above mentioned dosage had not been effective with the administration of 1 to 2 x 10 mgs tablets taken three times daily for a period of 20 days, then it would not have been, no matter what the dosage or duration had been increased to.

Females:

A large number of female athletes, and other individuals often had been victims of capsular contractures due to the popular breast implant surgery. It had been estimated that approximately 6 out of every 10 women have undergone breast augmentation, and therefore, these individuals had been very likely to have had experienced a certain degree of scar contracture surrounding the breast implant. However, the above mentioned suggestions had sometimes helped tremendously in the relief from the sometimes disfiguring and painful symptomatology, without the requirement of having to undergo corrective surgery.

Males:

Only a few male athletes had been affected by scar contractures (primarily, those who had engaged in the implantation of pectoral, calf and other possible enhancement implants). However, the administration of Madecassol had not only proven to have been effective in these incidences, but also had aided in reducing the symptomatology of keloids and other acquired scars which again, had sometimes been acquired from previous lacerations or surgical incision/excision. Accordingly, the clinical recommendation had been effectively followed by several male athletes.

Side Effects:

Some of the side effects which had been associated to the oral administration of Madecassol had included gastrointestinal intolerance such as transient anorexia, heartburn, nausea, feeling of heaviness, and sometimes, the occasional feeling of vertigo, allergic skin reactions such as contact dermatitis and urticaria had sometimes become apparent with the topical cream application of Madecassol.

Clinically, adverse effects which had become evident due to an overdosage of Madecassol, had been treated symptomatically. Of course, other problems could have occurred if this substance had been misused or abused by athletes who had chosen to self-administer this compound.

Consequently, there had been no need for the practice of self-medicine in regards to the application of Madecassol, as a physician would have readily written a prescription for it, if symptomatology had been warranted.

WARNING:

Madecassol does not possess antiseptic or antibiotic properties, therefore, antibiotic treatment and/or prophylaxis must additionally have been utilized when indicated.

Rating:

This compound of the Centella Asiatica Extract had been rated as an excellent alternative in efforts to have reduced the disfigurement, and sometimes associated pain of scar contractures.

MAXIBOL

Chemical Name: Co-enzyme B12.

Common Generic Name: Co-enzyme of Vitamin B12.

Other Trade Names Found in Mexico: Maxibol.

Manufacturer: Maxibol - Hoechs.

Dosage Form: Maxibol - 16 x 1000 mg capsules.

Storage: Maxibol capsules should be protected from light, (keep in the carton until contents are used), and stored at controlled room temperature 15 to 30 degrees C (59 to 86 degrees F), away from heat and moisture. Do not freeze.

Price Range: Maxibol - approx. $27.20 pesos for 16 x 1000 mg capsules.

Type of Drug: Co-enzyme B12/dibencozide.

Ingredient: Dimethyl Benzimidazole Cobamine Co-enzyme.

Drug Identification:

Maxibol - is available in oral administration, black capsules. There are two, 8 capsules per sheet, for a total of 16 capsules in each box. These are individually packaged in a plastic see-through blister, with a silver aluminum foil punch-through backing. The back of the packaging states Maxibol Capsulas, Roussel and the company logo, 1000 mcgs,and the Reg. #68199 and the Lot # AM6001 is written throughout, in navy blue. The accompanying package is white in color, with the product's entities written in black ink. There is a light blue box on the right hand corner, which contains the company's name Roussel, and logo. Above this box is a smaller navy blue stripe. There is also a red tab on the top of the package.

****Please refer to the photographs of Maxibol for full color references.***

Drug Description:

Similar to Neurofor, Maxibol (Co-enzyme B12) had also been essential to growth, as it had regenerated red blood cells, maintained a healthy nervous system, and had increased energy levels to have provided a general sensation of well being. It had also increased appetite levels which had been appreciated particularly when weight and size increases had been desired. The administration of Maxibol had also been able to have utilized fats, carbohydrates and proteins properly, which had aided in the necessity of proper utilization of macronutrients.

Maxibol had appeared to have benefited many athletes and bodybuilders in several ways, as it had seemed to have aided in DNA and RNA production lines, at a cellular level. Maxibol seemed to have worked much the same way as Neurofor, and had been as effective. Cyanocobalamin had not been as effective as an oral entity, as it had not been well assimilated in the stomach. However, Maxibol had been a potent 1000 mg capsule. The Vitamin B12 injections had been generally preferred over the Maxibol tablets, however, the Maxibol tablets had been more effective and longer lasting in the system; although the oral form had not been as dependable as the the parenteral injection of Vitamin B12. The administration of Maxibol had often prolonged the sense of appetite and energy stimulation in most athletes who had administered this compound.

Usual Clinical Recommendation:

The usual dosage had been 1 to 2 x 1000 mcg capsule taken by mouth daily.

Adventitious Dosage and Administration:

Maxibol capsules had been intended for oral administration, which had implied that they had been designed to have been swallowed by mouth. Many athletes had claimed that these tablets had produced the best results, when they had been consumed with water. A common dosage regime of some athletes, has been discussed in the following:

Female & Male:
Both female and male athletes had often engaged in the oral administration of the Maxibol compound. A range from 5000 to 10,000 mcg (or 5 to 10 capsules) in divided doses spread evenly throughout the day, had usually been successful in allowing the athlete to have achieved a state of well-being, increased energy, and increased appetite levels.

Side Effects:

Some of the more common side effects that some athletes had associated with the oral administration of Maxibol had included those of pulmonary edema, congestive heart failure early in treatment, peripheral vascular thrombosis, diarrhea, itching, and a swelling sensation of the entire body.

WARNING:

Many athletes had first investigated clinically, if there had been a sensitivity to this compound, before they had self-administered it. This test had usually been obtained by a competent physician through an intradermal testing dose.

Rating:

Based on a 1 to 5 star scale, with 1 considered low, and 5 considered high, a -- symbol is indicative of no value. This compound of Cyanocobalamin had rated as the following:

	MALES	FEMALES
Strength Increase	*	*
Mass & Weight Increase	*	*
Fat Burner	*	*
Contest Preparation	*	*
Appetite Stimulant	*****	*****
Side Effects	**	**
Cost Efficiency	**	**

NAXEN

Chemical Name: Naproxen.

Common Generic Name: Naprosyn.

Other Trade Names Found in Mexico: Currently, just Naxen.

Manufacturer: Naxen - Syntex.

Dosage Form: Naxen
- 24 x 1 gram tablets.
- 45 x 250 mg tablets.
- 45 x 500 mg tablets.

- 2 x 5 ml 500 mg ampule.
- 100 ml suspension.
- 40 gram gel tube.

Storage: Naxen tablets and gel tube, suspension and ampules, should be protected from light and moisture, (keep in the blisters until contents are used), and stored at controlled room temperature 15 to 30 degrees C (59 to 86 degrees F). Store at controlled room temperature 15 to 30 degrees C (59 to 86 degrees F). Do not permit to freeze.

Price Range: Naxen
- approx. $106.20 pesos for 24 x 1 gram tablets.
- approx. $68.70 pesos for 45 x 250 mg tablets.
- approx. $114.30 pesos for 45 x 500 mg tablets.
- approx. $23.80 pesos for 2 x 5 ml 500 mg ampule.
- approx. $34.80 pesos for 100 ml suspension.
- approx. $42.60 pesos for 40 gram gel tube.

Type of Drug: Nonsteroidal. Anti-inflammatory with Analgesic and Antiphyretic properties.

Ingredient: Naproxen.

Drug Identification:

Naxen - is available as an oral administration tablet, each containing 250, 500 mgs or 1 gram of Naproxen. It is available in 3 packages of 15 tablets, for a total of 45 tablets of either 250, or 500 mgs, or in 4 packages of 6's, for a total of 24 tablets, of 1 gram Naproxen. The tablets are individually packaged in a see-through plastic blister, with a silver aluminum foil punch through backing. However, the 1 gram tablet is oblong, with

SYNTEX impressed on one side, with the other side scored. On the back, 250, 500 mgs or 1 gram, Naxen Tabletas, Reg. #38245, Lot # (actually there had not been one indicated), and Syntex with the company logo, is printed throughout in black. The 250 and 500 mgs Naxen tablets are uncoated, white, and have the Syntex company logo debossed across one side, and the other side is plain. The accompanying carton is white, with a block of light blue on top, and in the bottom block, contains the product's entities and manufacturer, Syntex, along with the logo, written in black.

Naxen - is also available in 2 x 5 ml 500 mg ampule, for injection, and 100 ml suspension bottle, intended for oral administration. These bottles are dark brown in color, with a white sticker label with a medium colored blue box on the front top of the label with the product's entities displayed in black ink. The twist-off white lid is intended for multiple entries, and should be screwed back on after utilization. There is also a plastic safety-seal covering the lid. The accompanying carton is white, with a block of light blue on top, and in the bottom block, contains the product's entities and manufacturer, Syntex, along with the logo, written in black.

Naxen - is also available in a topical gel tube of 40 grams. This is an aluminum type type covered in a white paint, which is identical to the all the other Naxen product accompanying packages. It has a twist-off white lid which is also intended for multiple entries, and should be screwed back on after utilization. The tube itself is similar to that of "toothpaste".

Please refer to the photographs of Naxen, for full color references.

Drug Description:

Clinically, Naxen had been utilized in efforts to have treated a condition referred to as Rheumatoid Arthritis, as the administration of this product had been able to have reduced joint swelling, stiffness, and discomfort, which often had accompanied this disease. The compound of Naxen, is nonsteroidal, nonthyroidal and nonhormonal. In fact, the only reason why it had been featured within this text, had been due to it's application as an anti-inflammatory, which had been commonly utilized by many athletes in efforts to have treated tendonitis, and injuries that had been often sustained from training. Anti-inflammatories had even occasionally been required to have alleviated pain from injuries, which had been sometimes experienced from overtraining a particular bodypart.

The muscles had tended to have tensed around the injured or sore area, which often had caused extreme discomfort when exertion had been emphasized in activity. Anti-inflammatory agents such as Naxen had often aided in relaxing the swelling around the area, which in turn, had lead to relief from pain. This compound had worked by having prevented the production of hormones referred to as prostaglandins, and consequently, had not been degenerative. The use of anti-inflammatories such as Naxen had frequently sped up recovery time, and had even masked pain to a certain extent, which had allowed activity to have somewhat resumed.

Usual Clinical Recommendation:

The usual total daily dosage for osteoarthritis, rheumatoid arthritis, and ankylosing spondylitis had been 500 mg (20 ml) daily, in divided doses. Depending upon the patient's response, it had been increased gradually to 750 to 1000 mgs, or decreased. Naxen tablets had always been taken with meals, or milk.

Adventitious Dosage and Administration:

Naxen tablets had been intended for oral administration, which had meant that they had been designed to have been swallowed by mouth. These tablets had been most effective when they had been ingested with either water or milk, and taken with meals. They did not require to have been crushed or chewed. The use of Naxen as an injectable, had been intended for deep intramuscular injection. The best site for this type of injection had been in the gluteus medius muscle area, which had been the upper outer portion of the buttock, approximately 2 to 3 inches below the hip bone (iliac crest). Many athletes had alternated injections from one side to the other, (first injection on the left side, the second time injection administered on the right, or vice versa) in attempts to somewhat have alleviated associated pain, and in efforts to have also allowed the area to have slightly "healed". This practice had occasionally prevented a thick scar tissue from having formed. However, the more injections that had been administered, the greater possibility of scar tissue had resulted. Naxen, in the form of a gel, had been designed to have been applied directly onto the problematic area. A common dosage regime of some athletes, has been discussed in the following:

Several athletes had indicated that Naxen, as an anti-inflammatory had worked relatively well, having provided the proper dosage had been obtained. The administration of Naxen had usually been initiated with a low dosage, then gradually had been increased until relief from pain had been obtained. This relief amount usually had indicated which dosage seemed to have provided results for each individual. However, clinically, it had been recommended that the Naxen's dosage of 1000 mgs not be exceeded. However, as with many compounds athletes had self-administered, this amount had been frequently surpassed. Consequently, as with most compounds, the higher the dosage, the more side effects had generally resulted.

Females
& Males:

Female and male athletes had usually initiated the administration of Naxen with 650 mgs (for simplicity measures, a 250 mgs tablet version is equivalent to 2 1/2 tablets) a day, divided up evenly over the day's extent, or in other words, had been taken 3 times a day. This amount had usually been experimented with for approximately 3 days. If no alleviation had been obtained, then this amount had been increased to a dosage of 750 mgs (3 x 250 mgs tablets) a day for 3 days, and so forth until a dose had appeared to have offered some relief.

A common dose had been approximately 600 mgs (approximately 2 1/4 x 250 mgs tablets) administered twice a day. Naxen had usually been administered p.r.n., which had meant that it had been taken whenever it had been necessary, in efforts to have alleviated joint pain due to inflammation.

Side Effects:

Some of documented side effects which had been associated clinically, and in athletic application, with the use of Naxen had included peptic ulcers, heartburn, constipation, nausea, diarrhea, headaches, dizziness, fatigue, depression, alopecia, skin eruptions and rashes, apnea, palpitations, congestive heart failure and vasculitis, hearing and visual disturbances, thirst, fever and chills, and muscle weakness. Of course, other side effects may have had been experienced which had not been recognized by the athlete, (especially when dosages had been increased to high amounts), therefore, had not been documented.

WARNING:

Having utilized the compound of Naproxen had been known to have induced peptic ulceration, perforation and gastrointestinal bleeding, which sometimes had been severe, and occasionally had proved to have been fatal. If any type of a stomach ulcer had ever previously been experienced by an athlete, the use of Naxen had been avoided and not used.

Rating:

Based on a 1 to 5 star scale, with 1 considered low, and 5 considered high, a -- symbol is indicative of no value. This compound of Naproxen had rated as the following:

	MALES	FEMALES
Anti-inflammatory	****	****
Side Effects	***	***
Cost Efficiency	*	*

NEUROFOR

Chemical Name: Cyanocobalamin.

Common Generic Name: Vitamin B12.

Other Trade Names Found in Mexico: Neurofor.

Manufacturers: Neurofor - Hoechs
- Roussel.

Dosage Form: Neurofor - 50,000 mcg ampule.

Storage: Cyanocobalamin injectables should be protected from light, (keep in the carton until contents are used), and stored at controlled room temperature 15 to 30 degrees C (59 to 86 degrees F). Do not freeze.

Price Range: Neurofor - approx. $39.00 pesos for 50,000 mcg ampule.

Type of Drug: Vitamin.

Ingredient: 100 or 1000 mcg Cyanocobalamin.

Drug Identification:

Neurofor - is available in an injectable of 50,000 mcg per each 10 ml, in a dark brown bottle for multiple injections. The company name of Roussel is labeled on the front of on a blue and white sticker, along with the same colors as the bottle. The multiple-entry lid is covered by a tear-off silver aluminum wrap. The box is plain, with the product's entities written in black. Prior to and after injections, to prevent contaminations of the combined contents after multiple repeated insertions, the septum of the vial should be wiped with an antiseptic solution. Also, the use of sterile, disposable needles and syringes is also a prerequisite.

Neurofor - is also available in a clear glass ampule with a breakoff tip, containing Neurofor 50,000 10 ml, with it's entities written in black. The accompanying box is white and blue, again with the product's inscription also written in black. Once the ampule tip has been broken off, the contents are withdrawn into the syringe for sterile storage. However, it is important to have a new, sterile needle with each and every injection.

*****Please refer to the photograph of Neurofor for full color references.***

Drug Description:

Vitamin B12 appears as dark red crystals or crystalline red powder. It has been essential to growth, regeneration of red blood cells, maintenance of a healthy nervous system; and had been known to have had provided a general well feeling, due to it's ability to have increased energy levels. Vitamin B12 also had been able to have had utilized fats, carbohydrates and proteins properly. Some other known values of Vitamin B12 had also included the improvement of concentration, memory and balance, relief from irritability, and the ability to have been able to have increased appetite levels.

The administration of Vitamin B12 had been quantitatively, as it had been absorbed into the system very quickly from either intramuscular, or deep subcutaneous injections. However, it had not been well assimilated through the stomach. Usually within one hour from administration, the plasma level of the compound had reached it's peak level. Within two days, up to 98% of the injected dose of Vitamin B12 had frequently surfaced in the urine, and the majority of it had been excreted within the first eight hours after it had been injected. The average diet usually had been usually able to have supplied approximately 5 to 15 mcgs a day of Vitamin B12, which had been available for absorption after normal digestion.

Vitamin B12 had been found only in foods of animal origin, therefore, it had not been present in plants. Strict vegetarians often have suffered from deficiencies of this vitamin, which inevitably had led to *Pernicious Anemia.* Clinically, Vitamin B12 had been utilized in efforts to have treated Pernicious Anemia, pregnant and nursing women who had required the additional vitamins, and other related conditions which had often resulted in malabsorption of Vitamin B12.

Athletes frequently had administered Vitamin B12 due to it's abilities of having been able to have increased appetite and energy levels. The ability of having increased the appetite usually had helped most athletes to have consumed numerous amounts of calories, which had often been required for most gains in strength and weight. Steroid cycles also had depended on proper and abundant caloric intakes of protein, carbohydrates and fats. Increased energy levels had also aided in daily functioning, and training regiments.

Usual Clinical Recommendation:

Patients who had been diagnosed with Pernicious Anemia, had been required to have administered Vitamin B12 injections for the remaining part of their lives. Parenteral injections had been recommended as the oral form had not been dependable. The intravenous method usually had resulted in virtually all of the vitamin having been lost in the urine.

An usual dose of 100 mcg daily x 6 to 7 days, frequently had been administered intramuscularly, or deep subcutaneously to most patients. If an improvement had resulted, then the same amount had been administered on alternate days x seven doses, then every 3 to 4 days for another two weeks. This regimen had often then maintained by 100 mcg monthly, for life.

Adventitious Dosage and Administration:

The use of Neurofor had been intended for intramuscular or deep subcutaneous injection. The best site for this type of intramuscular injection, had been in the gluteus medius muscle area, which had been the upper outer portion of the buttock, approximately 2 to 3 inches below the hip bone (iliac crest). Most athletes had also alternated the injections from one side to the other, (first injection on the left side, the second time injection administered on the right, or vice versa) in attempts of having alleviated pain somewhat, and also in efforts to have let the area to have slightly "healed". This practice had sometimes allotted for the prevention of a thick scar tissue from potentially forming. However, the more injections that athletes had administered, the greater possibility of scar tissue had often resulted. Subcutaneous injections, which had been just underneath the layer of skin, had usually been best administered in the outer surface of the arms and forearms. Some athletes had often easily accomplished this by having gathered the skin in a pinch-like fashion, then having injected the substance within this grasped area. A common dosage regime of some athletes, has been discussed in the following:

Females
& Males:

Most female and male athletes usually had administered one injection of 10,000 mcgs every second day (2 cc's) x one week on, one week off, for three dosing sessions, which had been used to have increased both appetite and energy levels.

Side Effects:

Some of the more common side effects both female and male athletes had associated with the parenteral administration of Vitamin B12 had included those of pulmonary edema, congestive heart failure early in treatment, peripheral vascular thrombosis, diarrhea, itching, and a swelling sensation of the entire body.

WARNING:

No overdosage had been reported with Vitamin B12. However, clinically, Anaphylactic shock and death had been reported after parenteral Vitamin B12 administration.

Many athletes had first investigated clinically, if there had been a sensitivity to this compound, before they had self-administered it. This test had usually been obtained by a competent physician through an intradermal testing dose.

Rating:

Based on a 1 to 5 star scale, with 1 considered low, and 5 considered high, a -- symbol is indicative of no value. This compound of Cyanocobalamin had rated as the following:

	MALES	FEMALES
Strength Increase	*	*
Mass & Weight Increase	*	*
Fat Burner	*	*
Contest Preparation	*	*
Appetite Stimulant	*****	*****
Side Effects	**	**
Cost Efficiency	**	**

NOLVADEX

Chemical Name: Tamoxifen Citrate.

Common Generic Name: Nolvadex.

Other Trade Names Found in Mexico: Currently, just Nolvadex.

Manufacturers:

Nolvadex - ICI-Farma.
Crioxifeno - Cryo Pharma Mexico (N.L.M).
Tamoxan - Tecnimed PL; Kener Mexico (N.L.M).
Taxus - Andromaco Mexico (N.L.M).
Tecnofen - Tecnofarma Mexico (N.L.M).

Dosages: Nolvadex - 10 and 20 mgs tablets.

Storage: Nolvadex tablets should be protected from light and moisture, (keep in the container until contents are used), and stored at controlled room temperature 15 to 30 degrees C (59 to 86 degrees F).

Price Range: Nolvadex - approx. $161.00 pesos for 30 x 10 mg tablets.
- approx. $157.50 pesos for 14 x 20 mg tablets.

Type of Drug: Nonsteroidal. Anti-estrogen and Anti-neoplastic (anticancer).

Ingredient: 10 or 20 mgs of Tamoxifen.

Drug Identification:

Nolvadex - as oral administration tablets are round, binconvex, film coated, and white. The tablets are individually welded within a silver "meshed" strip, with the product's entities written on one side in blue ink. Nolvadex is available in boxes of either 14 tablets at 20 mg strength, Reg. # 90749, Lot # 429-OK, or 30 tablets at the 10 mg strength. The accompanying package is white and blue containing the product's entities, along with the Lot #429-OK, and expiration date. There is also a large UPC code located on the front of the package.

***Please refer to the photographs of Nolvadex for full color references.*

Drug Description:

Nolvadex is a nonsteriodal anti-Estrogen drug, which had been primarily clinically utilized in the treatment of advanced breast cancer in postmenopausal women. As an anti-Estrogen, Nolvadex had worked against this by having inhibited a bonding of Estrogens and receptors, by having blocked the Estrogen. Nolvadex also had stimulated FSH and LH production. It had not prevented Testosterone and it's synthetic steroids from having converted into Estrogens, but actually had competed with them for the Estrogen receptors. Therefore, the administration of the compound of Nolvadex had often aided in having prevented edema, gynecomastia, and female fat distribution, which had often occurred when a male's Estrogen level had become too elevated.

Nolvadex had worked as an anti-Estrogen by having blocked the Estrogen receptors of the effected body tissue, which had limited the bonding of the Estrogens and receptors. It also had worked as an Estrogen antagonist, but had not prevented Testosterone and steroids from having converted into Estrogens. Instead, as previously mentioned, it actually had competed with them for the Estrogen receptors. For many male athletes, this had often been a disadvantage when having completed the use of Nolvadex, as a backfire effect had occasionally occurred; as the suddenly released Estrogen receptors had now been able to have assimilated the Estrogen which had existed in the blood. Many male athletes had claimed that the additional use of Proviron combined with the administration of Nolvadex had often prevented this from having transpired.

Another venture of many male athletes with the utilization of Nolvadex compound, had been that it had a direct influence on the hypothalamus, which had increased the release of gonadotropins, therefore, had stimulated the Testosterone production in the testes. This had not been immensely, but had been a moderate amount of increase of the body's own Testosterone level. Unfortunately, this had not been adequate enough to have significantly increased the Testosterone production which had often been reduced by the administration of anabolic and androgenic steroidal compounds. Nolvadex not only had reduced the Estrogen level, but also had weakened the anabolic effect of some steroids. Certain steroids, particularly the various Testosterone compounds, had only accomplished their full anabolic effect if the Estrogen level had been sufficiently high. Tremendous results had been obtained from Nolvadex when it had been stacked with powerful compounds such as Anapolon and Metandiabol or Reforvit B (veterinarian products). However, when stacked with weaker steroids such as Primobolan or Deca-Durabolin, unsatisfactory results had often occurred, since Nolvadex already had a moderate anabolic effect, which had caused an additional loss of effect. In some instances, Nolvadex had actually increased the Estrogen levels instead of having lowered it. If this had occurred, slight increases in the serum Estrogen concentration had been required to have overcome the anti-Estrogen effects.

Nolvadex had also been administered for it's possible fat burning entities, even though this had not been a direct enterprise. Instead, it's anti-Estrogenic effect had been able to have contributed to the maintenance of the lowest Estrogen level possible. Athletes who already had a low body fat percentage, had been able to have acquired observable muscle hardness with the use of Nolvadex.

Most male athletes had generally initiated the administration of Nolvadex at the end of a steroid cycle, primarily to have increased their body's own Testosterone production, and at the same time, counteract potential side effects which may have been caused by Estrogens. The androgen level had usually been low compared to the Estrogen level, in which case, Estrogen became the dominant hormone, that had often lead to side effects of feminization problems.

Female athletes had also used the compound of Novaldex for it's fat burning qualities. For some reason, Nolvadex had worked wondrously on having eliminated bodyfat and water retention in females. Consequently, at the same time, because Tamoxifen had been developed to have treated certain types of breast cancer in women, it had also been known to actually have prevented it in otherwise healthy women. Adverse reactions from taking Nolvadex, had been recognized to have caused uterine cancer. Studies performed on mice had also revealed that high doses of Tamoxifen had also caused ovarian tumors in females, and testicular tumors in males.

Usual Clinical Recommendation:

Nolvadex had been usually administered in approximately 20 to 40 mgs daily, either in a single dose, or 2 equally divided doses. The lowest effective dose should have always been utilized.

Adventitious Dosage and Administration:

Nolvadex tablets had been intended for oral administration, which had meant that they had been designed to have been swallowed by mouth. Most athletes had claimed these tablets had produced the best results if they had been ingested with water. They did not require to have been crushed or chewed. A common dosage regime of some athletes, has been discussed in the following:

Nolvadex is an oral compound which should have been taken with meals. An usual dosage amount had been close to the clinical application of approximately 10 to 30 mgs (if the 10 mg tablet had been used, then this had been equivalent to 1 to 3 tablets; if the 20 mg tablet had been used, this had been equivalent to 1/2 to 1 1/2 tablets) daily.

***Females*:**
Female athletes typically had administered a dose of 1 tablet of 10 mgs once a day. This had often been continued for a period of 4 weeks, with a rest interval of 2 weeks for three months. Female athletes had been careful

not to have included the utilization of Proviron while having used the compound of Nolvadex.

Males:

Many male athletes had usually involved the utilization of Nolvadex approximately 3 to 4 weeks after the initiation of an anabolic steroid cycle. Nolvadex at 20 to 30 mgs (if the 10 mgs tablet had been utilized, this had been the equivalent of 2 to 3 tablets, or if the 20 mgs tablet had been used, this had been the equivalent of 1 to 1 1/2 tablet) a day, combined with Proviron 25 to 50 mgs (1 to 2 tablets) a day. This had generally been utilized by male athletes who had a tendency to have acquired feminization effects such as gynecomastia, strong water retention, and increased fat deposits. This had also been generally utilized if Anapolon, Deca-Durabolin, Metandiabol or Reforvit B (veterinarian products) and Testosterones had also been administrated. Dosages of approximately 10 mgs (1 of 10 mgs tablet version, or 1/2 of the 20 mgs tablet version) daily had usually been sufficient for Estrogenic side effect prevention. Athletes had been careful in not having administered high dosages of Tamoxifen, and had generally limited the Nolvadex cycle to 6 to 12 weeks.

Some studies had indicated that muscle growth had been often inhibited by the use of Nolvadex, and many athletes allegedly had acquired better mass gains without it. Nolvadex had been, as previously mentioned, beneficial as an anti-Estrogen. The decision of having administered Nolvadex had been greatly dependent on which entity had been of greater importance to the athlete, the lessening of feminization effects, or the building of muscle mass.

Side Effects:

Nolvadex had been nontoxic, and consequently, had not shown any side effects when it had been used in low dosages as an anti-Estrogen. However, the following adverse side effects had been associated with the use of Tamoxifen in both clinical and athletic application had been; a distaste for food, dizziness, headache, light-headedness, nausea, vomiting, visual disturbances such as blurring, corneal changes, cataracts, and Retinopathy, fever, chills, depression, rapid weight gain, sore throats, rash, unusual weakness, and hepatocellular carcinomas.

Side effects which had been particularly associated with females had been menopausal symptoms such as hotflashes, menstrual irregularities, disturbances of menstrual function including oligomenorrhea, and amenorrhea, endometrial cancer, uterine cancer, hyperplasia, polyps, abnormal vaginal bleeding, and vaginal itching.

Of course, other side effects may have been experienced which had not been recognized by the athlete, therefore, had not been documented.

WARNING:

Female athletes always had exercised caution in not having combined the use of Nolvadex when they had also been taking birth control pills for contraceptive measures. The compound of Nolvadex as an anti-Estrogen, and the birth control pills as an Estrogen, had counteracted, therefore, had generally canceled the effect of birth control as a pregnancy preventative.

Also, if extreme gynecomastia had been present in males, high dosages of Nolvadex had not reduced this condition. If the gynecomastia had been too pronounced, surgery had often been warranted.

Rating:

Based on a 1 to 5 star scale, with 1 considered low, and 5 considered high; a -- symbol is indicative of no value. This compound of Tamoxifen had rated as the following:

	MALES	FEMALES
Fat Burner	***	***
Anti-Estrogen	***	*
Side Effects	***	***
Cost Efficiency	**	**

NUBAIN

Chemical Name: Nalbuphine Hydrochloride.

Common Generic Name: Nubain.

Other Trade Names Found in Mexico: Currently, just Nubain.

Manufacturer: Nubain - Rhone.

Dosage Form: Nubain - 5 x 1 ml ampule.
- 10 ml injectable solution bottle.

Storage: Store at controlled room temperature 15 to 30 degrees C (59 to 86 degrees F). Do not permit to freeze. Protect from light. It is advisable to keep in packaging until use.

Price Range: Nubain - approx. $ 71.35 pesos for 5 x 1 ml ampule.
- approx. $100.90 pesos for 10 ml injectable solution bottle.

Type of Drug: Synthetic, Narcotic Agonist-Antagonist Analgesic.

Ingredient: Nalbuphine HCI.

Drug Identification:

Nubain - As a clear injectable solution administration. It is bottled within a clear, glass bottle, with the product's entities displayed in red ink. Lot # MKA507A imprinted in black ink, which has been added to the bottle at a latter date. The solution itself is clear, and colorless. The multiple-entry lid has a bluish-green flip-off cap, which is to be discarded after initial entry. The product's accompanying package is white with the product's entities written in black ink. There are two dark navy blue stripes joining a navy blue box containing a white figure. There is also a red tab displayed on the front right corner of the package.

****Please refer to the photograph of Nubain for full color references.***

Drug Description:

Nubain is a potent analgesic which had been equivalent to that of morphine on a milligram basis. It had been utilized by some athletes in attempts to have alleviated moderate to severe pain. It had also been clinically utilized as a supplement to have balanced anesthesia for before and after analgesia, and also for labor and delivery. Clinically, Nubain had been stated as having had a low abuse potential, although psychological and physical dependence tolerance had often followed abuse or misuse. However, several athletes who had overly indulged in this compound, often had proven, that Nubain frequently had become addictive if it had been administered regularly. Once an addiction had been established, larger and more frequent dosages had been required to have achieved previous obtained states of relief.

Athletes had often referred to Nubain as "Nopain", which had clearly indicated the product's potential potency. Many athletes had stated that the utilization of Nubain had permitted exercising and training without the experience of pain from sustained injuries, or soreness experienced from previous workouts. This practice in the long run, not only had proven to have been unwise due to the addiction probability, but also due to the fact that the injury itself had often not received adequate recuperation time to have healed properly. Most intelligent athletes had not engaged in the administration of Nubain.

Usual Clinical Recommendation:

The recommended clinically dosage had usually been 10 mg/70 kg administered subcutaneously, intramuscularly, or intravenously, for adults.

This may have been repeated again every 3 to 6 hours, as required. Dosages should have been adjusted to the severity of the pain, physical status of the patient, and to other medications which the patient may have been taking.

Adventitious Dosage and Administration:

Although, most or even all of the compounds and the adventitious dosages which have been found within this text have been controversial when administered for athletic enhancement purposes; Nalbuphine Hydrochloride had definitely not been one compound which many athletes had chosen to have experimented with. Therefore, a possible citing of adventitious dosage or administration had not been provided. There had been numerous other compounds which athletes had been able to have obtained relief from soreness and injury, without having to had additionally inflict the possibility of addiction. The compound of Nubain should definitely have been strictly left to that of the clinical community.

Females & Males:

Intelligent, cautious female and male athletes had avoided having engaged in the administration of Nubain, due to the extreme possible addiction probabilities involved, especially which had frequently been apparent with the self-administration of this potent, addictive compound.

Side Effects:

Some of the more common side effects known to have occurred in individuals who had taken the Nalbuphine HCI compound have included, sweaty or clammy skin, nausea, vomiting, dizziness, dry mouth, bitter taste in the mouth, speech difficulty, headaches, nervousness, crying, depression, unusual dreams, numbness, high or low blood pressure, cramps, itching, disturbances in vision such as blurring, and a possible flushing or warming sensation.

Abrupt discontinuation of Nubain which had followed prolonged use, had often been followed by symptoms of narcotic withdrawal. These symptoms had included abdominal cramping, nausea, vomiting, rhinorrhea, lacrimation, restlessness, anxiety, elevated temperature and "goosebumps".

Of course, other side effects may have been experienced which had not been recognized by the self-administering athlete, therefore, had not been documented.

WARNING:

As previously mentioned, the administration of the compound Nubain had been addictive, therefore drug tolerance had always developed very quickly. Rapid withdrawal had often resulted in the same type of symptoms experienced by those associated to other narcotic forms such as crack cocaine. Of course, these symptoms had been very dramatic, and a type of detoxifying system had often been required to have established a normal state once again.

Rating:

Based on a 1 to 5 star scale, with 1 considered low, and 5 considered high, a -- symbol is indicative of no value. This compound of Nalbuphine Hydrochloride had rated as the following:

	MALES	FEMALES
Potent "Pain-killer"	*****	*****
Side Effects	*****	*****
Cost Efficiency	**	**

PRIMOBOLAN DEPOT

Chemical Name:	Methenolone Enanthate.
Common Generic Name:	Primobolan.
Other Trade Names Found in Mexico:	Currently, just Primobolan Depot.
Manufacturer:	Primobolan Depot - Schering.
Dosage Form:	Primobolan Depot - 1 x 50 mg (c) ampule.
Storage:	Primobolan Depot injectables should be protected from light, (keep in the carton until contents are used), and stored at controlled room temperature 15 to 30 degrees C (59 to 86 degrees F).
Price Range:	Primobolan Depot - approx. $79.00 pesos for 1 x 50 mg (c) ampule.
Type of Drug:	Anabolic Steroid.
Ingredient:	50 mgs Metenolone Enanthate.

Drug Identification:

Primobolan Depot - Each ml of sterile, colorless to pale yellow solution which contains 50 mgs of Methenolone Enanthate in sesame oil, with 5 mgs of Chlorobutanol as a perservative. Primoteston Depot is written on the glass vial itself. It is available in a singular brown, 50 mg ampule, and has blue printing on the vial. There is also a blue ring around the neck of the ampule. The ampule is individually enclosed within a silver aluminum package, cradled in plastic, with a clear plastic front, so that the ampule can be visually seen. The back is silver, with Schering and the company's logo, written throughout in black ink. The accompanying package is white, with a greenish-gold stripe bar close to the bottom of the package, with the product's entities written in black ink.

*****Please refer to the photograph of Primobolan Depot for full color references.***

Drug Description:

Clinically, Primobolan Depot had been utilized in efforts to have treated conditions such as breast cancer, osteoporosis, geriatric protein deficiencies, primarily in postmenopausal females, and to have treated prostate cancer in males.

Several athletes had claimed that Primobolan Depot as an intramuscular oil-based injectable, had not caused liver damage, and had not aromatized, which had allowed it to have been considered one of the more safer injectable compounds that had currently been available in Mexico. Most athletes had reported that the administration of Primobolan Depot had appeared to have had very strong anti-catabolic and fat-burning entities, which had permitted increases in lean body mass. These acquired gains had generally appeared to have been almost of a permanent nature. Most of the time, results of 10 to 15 lbs weight increases had often been obtained within 6 to 8 weeks; without the potential threat of having lost these accomplishments once Primobolan Depot had been discontinued. These desired, positive effects had also been achieved on a low caloric diet regime.

Several athletes often had chosen Primobolan Depot (Methenolone Enanthate) as opposed to Primobolan tablets, (Metheonolone Acetate), as the injections had not only been faster-acting, but this compound had also been considered to have been a good, basic anabolic steroid, with the least minimal amount of possible side effects. The administration of Primobolan Depot also had not negatively affected water and electrolyte balances, (water retention) therefore, had not caused hypertension, and had allowed the blood lipids to have remained unchanged. These properties of course, had been widely highly regarded by all athletes. Primobolan Depot had often been utilized weeks prior, in preparation for competition especially, by many female and male bodybuilders.

Usual Clinical Recommendation:

The usual dosage had been 1 x 50 mg ampule intramuscularly once every two to three weeks.

Adventitious Dosage and Administration:

The use of Primobolan Depot, had been intended for deep intramuscular injection. The best site for this type of injection had been in the gluteus medius muscle area, which had been the upper outer portion of the buttock, approximately 2 to 3 inches below the hip bone (iliac crest). Many athletes had often alternated injections from one side to the other, (first injection on the left side, the second time injection administered on the right, or vice versa) in attempts to have alleviated pain, and to possibly have allowed the area to have slightly "healed". This practice allegedly had prevented a thick scar tissue from having potentially formed. However, the more injections that athletes had administered, the greater possibility of scar tissue had resulted. A common dosage regime of some athletes, has been discussed in the following:

The administration of Primobolan Depot had been very flexible, which had enabled it to have been easily stacked with many other androgens in efforts to have produced significant results; which had been permanent. Both female and male bodybuilders had very commonly used Primobolan Depot in precontest preparations as well.

***Females*:**
Although most female athletes had preferred the Primobolan tablets (Acetate) to the injectable, Primobolan Depot (Enanthate), many still had chosen to have utilized the Primobolan Depot, due to the low possibility of virilization side effects (if it had been properly used, and in low dosages).

Many female athletes had additional stacked Primobolan Depot, 100 mgs (2 x 50 mg ampules) with 50 mgs of Winstrol Depot (currently, not available in Mexico) per week, which had allegedly produced productive results for most women. However, dosages had often exceeded these amounts, and sometimes had reached up to 100 to 200 mgs (2 to 4 x 50 mg ampules) per week, which had been dependent on the individual goal, and benefit/risk ratio, the female had wished to have chanced. To have lessened the risks of virilization and other potential side effects, cautious female athletes had not injected Primobolan Depot earlier than every 3 to 4 days.

***Males*:**

Since Primobolan Depot had a long duration (it had been able to have remained in the system for a long period of time), many male athletes had utilized approximately one injection per week of 100 mgs, (2 x 50 mg ampules), up to 300 mgs (6 x 50 mg ampules). These dosages had appeared to have had sufficed most male individuals. However, this had been often increased far beyond this dosage, up to a 100 mgs (2 x 50 mg ampules) a day, by some more adventitious male pro-bodybuilders.

Consequently, a low water retention had been established, while strength and muscle size had been gained, if Primobolan Depot had been taken in an average dosage of 200 mgs (4 x 50 mg ampules) per week. This often had worked well for male athletes who had initiated a steroid cycle; and for those who had wanted to especially have avoided the unwanted side effects. Novice male athletes had often generally experienced an increase in lean body mass while having used 100 mgs (2 x 50 mg ampules) every ten days. Primobolan Depot had been frequently stacked with Stanozolol, Durabolin or Winstrol (all three compounds are currently not available in Mexico), for bulking cycles.

Having achieved mass size quickly, had been obtained by Primobolan Depot, stacked with Sustanon 250, Parabolan (currently, not available in Mexico) and Metandiabol or Reforvit-B (veterinarian products). Another possible stack which had also been used by novices, or by those who had wanted to avoid potential side effects, had been Primobolan Depot 100 to 200 mg (2 to 4 x 50 mg ampules) a week, stacked with Deca-Durabolin 200 to 400 mgs (4 to 8 x 50 mg redi-ject ampules) per week.

A common stack which had been commonly used by several bodybuilders prior to a competition had included Durabolin (currently, not available in Mexico) x 8 ampules, with 12 to 16 tablets of Oxandrolone (currently, not available in Mexico), with 6 to 8 capules of Restandol (also currently not available in Mexico), a day.

Side Effects:

Although Primobolan Depot had generally been considered to have been one of the most safest injectable steroids that had been available, there had been some minimal potential side effects, which had been associated with the administration of this compound. Some of these had included a slight experience of acne, and virilization for women such as deepening of the voice, increase of body hair growth, and increased sex drive. Particularly, in males, the Primobolan Depot injectable solution also had somewhat of a small influence on the hypothalamohypophysial testicular axis when very high dosages had been taken over a prolonged period of time. Therefore, this often had reduced the body's own natural Testosterone production.

Of course, other side effects may have been experienced which had not been recognized by the athlete, therefore, had not been documented.

WARNING:

The utilization of Primobolan Depot had been associated to the development of prostate cancer in males.

Rating:

Based on a 1 to 5 star scale, with 1 considered low, and 5 considered high, a -- symbol is indicative of no value. This compound of Methenolone Enanthate had rated as the following:

	MALES	FEMALES
Strength Increase	***	****
Mass & Weight Increase	***	***
Contest Preparation	*****	*****
Side Effects	**	**
Cost Efficiency	**	**

PRIMOBOLAN TABLETS

Chemical Name: Methenolone Acetate.

Common Generic Name: Primobolan.

Other Trade Names Found in Mexico: Currently, just Primobolan.

Manufacturer: Primobolan Tablets - Schering.

Dosage Range: Primobolan Tablets 30 x 5 mg tablets.

Storage: Primobolan Tablets should be protected from light and moisture, (keep the blisters in the carton until all the tablets are used), and stored at controlled room temperature 15 to 30 degrees C (59 to 86 degrees F).

Price Range: Primobolan Tablets are approx. $54.50 pesos for 30 x 5 mg tablets.

Type of Drug: Anabolic Steroid.

Ingredient: 5 mg Methenolone Acetate.

Drug Identification:

Primobolan Tablets - available as oral administration tablets. These tablets have been individually welded into a silver aluminum blisters. There are 3 strips of 10 tablets each in each package, for a total of 30 tablets. Primobolan Tabletas, Schering Mexico and the Reg. # 58504 is displayed throughout the silver strip, in black ink. The accompanying packaging and the tablet itself had not been obtained for identification and illustrational purposes.

*****Please refer to the photograph of Primobolan Tablets for full color references.***

Drug Description:

Primobolan Tablets are very low in androgens, are highly anabolic, and although it is a very powerful form of oral Primobolan, it had been considered to have been a relatively safe steroid compound. However, Primobolan Acetate had not typically promoted dramatic size or strength increases, as it had only a limited effect in having built up muscle mass and strength; there had been reports that quality muscle gains had been achieved while having utilized this product. Interestingly, Primobolans had been one of very few anabolic steroidal compounds, which had demonstrated any effectiveness on caloric restrictions.

Several athletes had often administered Primobolan over a prolonged period of time, as it had provided only a slow, but high-quality muscle gains, which mostly had remained after it had been discontinued. Consequently, it had been one of the very few steroids which female athletes had also felt comfortable using. Primobolan Tablets had most frequently been utilized in a pre-contest situation by bodybuilders, as this compound had been eliminated from the system very quickly. Several athletes had indicated that Primobolan Tablets had been frequently administered successfully, up to three weeks prior to a drug-tested competition.

The administration of Primobolan tablets had proven to have been advantageous, as it had also actively helped to burn bodyfat, as a source of energy. However, it had been extremely important that Primobolan tablets had never been exclusively taken during a restricted caloric intake, due to it's extremely low androgenic effect. This effect had often resulted in a significant loss in muscle and strength, and also had increased the possibility of overtraining.

Usual Clinical Recommendation:

The usual recommended dosage had usually been 1 to 1.5 mg per pound of body weight/day, which had been equivalent to 20 to 30 tablets for each 100 lbs of bodyweight.

(So, for an average 200 lb athlete, this would have been approximately 40 to 60 x 5 mgs tablets a day. Even though this may have appeared to have been excessive, it had displayed the high quantity which had been required for this compound to have been effective. Through oral consumption, Primobolan tablets had been atrociously deactivated in the liver, leaving only a small portion to have been distributed into the bloodstream).

Adventitious Dosage and Administration:.

Primobolan Acetate tablets are not 17-alpha alkylated, therefore they are passed through the gastrointestinal tract, then into the liver, where a large part of the substance had been destroyed and ultimately deactivated, having only left a much smaller portion of the substance to get into the blood.

Due to the fact that the Primobolan tablets had an effect on fat burning, but, consequently, had been mostly deactivated in the liver; many athletes had most efficiently applied this compound directly to the problematic areas. This practice had permitted for the penetration of the substance to have been absorbed directly into the blood through the skin, in areas where undesired fat deposits had existed. This had also been conceivable by the assistance of the DMSO compound. Dimethyl sulfoxide (DMSO) had been one of few substances which had been fully absorbed through the skin, which had allowed the skin to have become permeable to other substances which could have been distributed through the body.

One possible way in which many athletes had applied this compound topically, had been by finely having grounded up 5 x 5 mg Primobolan tablets, by having them placed on the back of a hard surface with a piece of paper or foil cover, and then having applied pressure with the back of a spoon (much like crushing an aspirin tablet). Then, it had been mixed with a half a teaspoon of DMSO gel, a thin layer had then been applied to the skin, and finally, the selected area had been covered with a piece of "Saran" plastic wrap. This had allowed for a "warming" of this mixture, which had further enabled for quicker absorption into the system. It had been important that it had been applied, and NOT rubbed into the skin. One or two applications had usually sufficed. Athletes had generally claimed that it had been best to have applied this mixture for approximately 20 to 40 minutes in order to have achieved the full effect.

Another feasible method which many athletes also often had used to in efforts to have avoided the liver and consequent destruction of this substance, had been by having ground up the Primobolan tablets (again, approximately 4 to 5) in a mortar (which is a dish with a smooth surface), and then having swallowed this powder mixture together with heated Vitamin E oil. This method allegedly had allowed the Primobolan tablets combined with the Vitamin E mixture, to have reached the blood through the lymph system, which had prevented the solution from having reached the liver through the portal vessel.

Yet, another more difficult approach which had also been utilized by a few athletes, had been by ultimately having grounded a few Primobolan tablets approximately 4 or 5 into a fine powder, then having added a half teaspoon of DMSO (nondiluted), and gently having swirled this mixture in a rotary fashion, until the solution had practically dissolved (this had only been partially obtainable due to the insolubility of the acetate tablet binders). After this had been achieved, this solution had been diluted with water in efforts to have made it half of the strength; 50/50 in nature. This mixture now had been ready to have been applied directly to the skin, in the desired problematic areas. It had also been important that it had been applied, and NOT rubbed into the skin. Again, the practice of covering the area with "Saran" plastic wrap had helped to intensify this compound's action. This mixture had frequently been applied directly to the skin for approximately 20 to 40 minutes, in attempts to have achieved the full effect.

Females:

The Primobolan steroid had been the only compound which when it had been administered strictly by itself, had successfully led to strength and muscle gains in both females and beginners.

Steroid novices and the less advanced users, had also achieved valuable strength and muscle gains by having administered 50 to 100 mgs (10 to 20 x 5 mg tablets) of Primobolan tablets daily, stacked with 150 mgs of Winstrol Depot (this is currently not available in Mexico), taken once a week without having retained water. Some female athletes had frequently combined other steroidal compounds which had been moderately to highly androgenic (but did not aromatize or retain water), with Primobolan tablets, in efforts to have greatly optimized it's effects.

Other suitable possible steriodal compounds utilized by many female athletes had also included Masteron, Parabolan, Winstrol (these are not currently available in Mexico), and Equi-Gan, Maxigan, or Crecibol (Equipoise). Most female athletes generally had not experienced an enormous strength increase, but usually had been capable of having acquired 2 to 4 pounds of muscle in 6 to 8 weeks, accompanied by a visibly harder, and tighter appearance.

Female bodybuilders who had been willing to take a higher risk, had often ventured to combine 75 mgs (15 tablets) daily of Primobolan, with 50 mgs of Winstrol (this is currently not available in Mexico) weekly, and 50 mgs of Testosterona 25 or 50. Clenbuterol 80 to 100 mcgs daily, on a two day on, two day off pattern, Oxandrolone 2 to 3 tablets, and the 2 mgs Winstrol tablets (the latter two compounds are also not currently available in Mexico), had also often been taken together with the application of Primobolan.

Steroid novices and the less advanced athletes had also achieved good strength and muscle gains by having administered 50 to 100 mgs (10 to 20 x 5 mg tablets) of Primobolan daily, and 150 mgs of Winstrol Depot (currently, not available in Mexico) weekly, safely without the possibility of water retention. Having combined Primobolan with one of these compounds had been further exacerbated with the additional intake of Oxandrolone (also, currently not available in Mexico).

Several athletes had claimed that all of these possible combinations had been also further advantageous by also having restricted caloric intake and proper diet regiments, especially prior to competition. Even competing female athletes had acquired good quality gains with continuously harder muscles, by having applied 150 mgs (30 tablets) of Primobolan daily, combined with 50 mgs of Winstrol Depot (currently, not available in Mexico) every two days, as well as 76 mgs of Parabolan (currently, not available in Mexico), every two days.

Males:

The average dosage for most male athletes had been approximately 100 to 200 mgs, (20 to 40 tablets) daily. Again, this dosage had been dependent upon the individual's weight, and had been adjusted accordingly.

An effective daily dose observed in most male athletes had been in the range of 50 to 200 mgs (10 to 40 tablets). Obviously, the 25 mg tablets had been preferred to the 5 mg tablets. Unfortunately, the 5 mg tablet had been the only form currently available in Mexico, and for that matter, most other countries.

Side Effects:

Since the Primobolan tablets are not 17-alpha alkylated, but had a 17-beta hydroxy group, they had been almost non-toxic to the liver. However, in high dosages, they had been able to have influenced the liver values, which had resulted in higher bilirubin, GPT, GOT, and alkaline phosphatase. Since Primobolan usually had not aromatized, it had not caused any significant side effects such as water retention. It had been also only slightly androgenic. However, it had been a precursor of dihydrotestosterone, which had allowed it to have accelerated hair loss if such a predisposition had existed. Blood pressure, liver values, cholesterol levels, HDL and LDL values usually had remained unaffected, which often had permitted Primobolan to have been well tolerated.

In female athletes, dosages around 50 to 100 mgs daily, had generally very rarely experienced virilization effects. The acetate form of Primobolan also did not aromatize into Estrogens, therefore, it had not caused water retention.

Of course, other side effects may have been experienced by topical application of Primobolan Acetate, which had not been recognized by the athlete, therefore, had not been documented.

WARNING:

The administration of this compound may have upset a female's normal hormonal system. In males, it may have caused hepatic tumors.

Rating:

Based on a 1 to 5 star scale, with 1 considered low, and 5 considered high, a -- symbol is indicative of no value. This compound of Methenolone Acetate had rated as the following:

	MALES	FEMALES
Strength Increase	**	****
Mass & Weight Increase	**	***
Contest Preparation	****	****
Side Effects	**	**
Cost Efficiency	**	**

PRIMOTESTON DEPOT

Chemical Name: Testosterone Enanthate.

Common Generic Name: Primoteston Depot.

Other Trade Names Found in Mexico: Primoteston Depot.
Testosterona 200.

Manufacturer: Primoteston Depot - Schering.

Dosage Form: Primoteston Depot - 1 x 250 mg ampule.

Storage: Primoteston Depot injectables should be protected from light, (keep in the carton until contents are used), and stored at controlled room temperature 15 to 30 degrees C (59 to 86 degrees F). Do not freeze.

Price Range: Primoteston Depot - approx. $28.00 pesos for 1 x 250 mg ampule.

Type of Drug: Strong Anabolic and Androgenic Steroid.

Ingredient: 200 mgs of Primoteston Depot.

Drug Identification:

Primoteston Depot - Is available as an oil-based injectable solution, in two 1 ml, medium brown ampules. One ampule has the product's entities written in blue ink, while the other accompanying ampule is similarly written in green ink. Both ampules are cradled within a plastic mold, with a silver push-through backing with the product's entities displayed across in navy blue ink. Reg. # 47334 SSA. The accompanying package is basically white, with a navy blue box close to the bottom, and the product's entities are also written in black ink.

*****Please refer to the photograph of Primoteston Depot for a full color reference.***

Drug Description:

Primoteston Depot is a synthetic version of the naturally occurring androgen, Testosterone. Clinically, it had been responsible for the normal development of the male sex characteristics, and had been normally used in efforts to have treated hypogonadism which had resulted from androgen deficiency and anemia. Primoteston Depot is a long acting injectable Testosterone, which had been commonly utilized amongst athletes for it's alleged mass building characteristics. However, similar to all Testosterones, Primoteston Depot also had aromatized easily, and had been moderately toxic to the liver.

Many athletes had claimed that a distinct advantage of Primoteston Depot, had been that it had a very strong androgenic effect combined with an intense anabolic component. This entity had generally resulted in an increased amount of strength and mass, within a short time interval.

Consequently, the rapid and strong weight and mass increase had frequently been associated with distinct water retention, as a withholding of electrolytes and water usually had often occurred. Many athletes had generally achieved mass and an increase of strength with the administration of Primoteston Depot, however, only a very few had been able to have retained their size after having discontinued the compound. This had been a common reason why some athletes unfortunately, had often refused to have taken a break from a Primoteston Depot cycle, which undoubtedly, had increased the potential of risks that had often been associated with steriodal abuse.

Other advantages of the water retention had included temporary relief for athletes who had frequently experienced problems with knee, elbow and shoulder joint pain, and intervertibral disk erosion. Ordinarily, after a few weeks of having administered Primoteston Depot, a flat, puffy appearance had often been displayed by the muscles. Another common problem which had also been commonly experienced by some athletes had been that the conversion rate to Estrogen had been very high, which had allowed the body to have stored more fat, or had developed other feminization symptoms such as gynecomastia. Again the athlete's predisposition usually had determined whether these side effects would have posed to have become problematic. If they had, many athletes had often counteracted these effects by the additional combination of Nolvadex and Proviron, which had generally been entertained at a dosage level of approximately 500 mgs or greater per week.

The administration of Primoteston Depot had also demonstrated a strong influence on the hypothalamohypophysial testicular axis. The hypophysis had been inhibited by a positive feedback, which had lead to a negative influence on the endogenic Testosterone production. Therefore, high dosages of Primoteston Depot which had been taken over a prolonged time interval, had often resulted in a reversible interruption or even a reduction of the sperm count in the testes. Inevitably, the testes had also been reduced to a smaller size. Again, many athletes had been able to have avoided these potential occurrences, by having had administered Gonadotropyl-C, Gonakor, or Profasi (HCG) for an interval of every 6 to 8 weeks, at 5000 I.U.'s every fifth day, over a period of 10 days (a total of 3 injections), which had greatly minimized this problem.

Primoteston Depot had allegedly produced results for every athlete who had administered it, as it strongly had promoted the regeneration process, which in turn, had encouraged an increased feeling of well-being, and increased energy levels. For some athletes, this had often been the explanation of the additional increased intense training and exercise allotment, that had frequently been accompanied by the increase of strength and mass; without the usual associated lethargy. A few athletes had indicated that it had been common to have experienced an exorbitant, strong pump during training. Increased blood volume combined with a high oxygen supply, and a high quantity of red blood cells had been particularly responsible for this acquired feeling of a "steroid pump". The administration of extremely large doses of Primoteston Depot had usually resulted in a tremendous pump sensation. Several athletes had claimed that this had mostly been experienced in the both the upper thigh and calf regions, and had often been provoked from the slightest activity, such as having climbed a flight of stairs or having ridden a stationary bike.

Primoteston Depot along with Testosterone Cypionate, (not available as a sole entity currently in Mexico) and Sostenon 250, had appeared to have been the primary choice for many steroid-practicing athletes. Primoteston Depot had been long-acting and therefore, had been able to have remained in the system for one to two weeks, which had been dependent upon the body's metabolism and initial hormone level. This characteristic had also enabled for a longer interval between injections, and consequently, could therefore have been injected anywhere from once a week, to once every two weeks, and still had been able to have remained very effective. Several athletes had professed that the administration of Primoteston Depot had been able to have provided a much more convenient, less expensive, and considerably more comfortable injection cycle.

Usual Clinical Recommendation:

The usual recommendations had been dependent upon etiology. To treat hypogonadism and impotency in males had been 150 mg intramuscularly every 3 to 6 weeks. In efforts to have treated breast carcinomas in postmenopausal women, the recommended dosage had been intramuscularly 250 mg every 2 weeks.

Adventitious Dosage and Administration:

Primoteston Depot had been intended for deep intramuscular injection. The best site for this type of injection had been in the gluteus medius muscle area, which had been the upper outer portion of the buttock, approximately 2 to 3 inches below the hip bone (iliac crest). Many athletes often had alternated injections from one side to the other, (first injection on the left side, the second time injection administered on the right, or vice versa) which had somewhat alleviated the associated pain, and also had permitted the area to have slightly "healed", in attempts to have prevented a thick scar tissue from potentially forming. However, the more injections that athletes had administered, the greater possibility of scar tissue had resulted. A common dosage regime of some athletes, has been discussed in the following:

Athletes who had been steroid novices usually had always avoided all Testosterone compounds, and instead, had utilized milder steriodal substances to initiate their ventures. Once these compounds had become somewhat ineffective, the entertainment of a stronger anabolic such as Primoteston Depot had then possibly been considered.

Females:
Most female athletes had not engaged in the administration of Testosterone steriodal compounds, as it had generally been not well tolerated, as severe side effects of virilization had often occurred. However, for those females who had been willing to have neglected the risk/benefit ratio, and had indulged in this compound anyways, a maximum of 1 ampule of Primoteston Depot every 7 to 10 days had been used. If higher and more frequent injections had been entertained, then the greater potential of having acquired male characteristics had greatly prevailed.

Males:
Male athletes had been able to have had tolerated this compound rather easily, and often had encouraged it's effects of increased strength, mass, aggressiveness and stamina. For the more advanced male athlete, Primoteston Depot had been either taken alone, or in combination with other steriodal compounds.

Singularly, there had been a wide range of dose administration which had ranged from 2 ampules of Primoteston Depot, all the way up to 6 ampules of Primoteston Depot per day! However, the latter dosage had been somewhat extreme and unnecessary, as Primoteston Depot had a plasma half-life time in the blood of a week, which had generally remained in the system for approximately 7 to 10 days.

Generally, most athletes had utilized the range between 1 to 4 x 250 ampules, or 1 to 4 cc's a week. If the dosage had been at a minimum of 1 to 2 x 250 ampules, or 1 to 2 cc's, it had been usually administered all at once, often once a week or once every ten days. Dosages that had been higher than this range, had often been equally divided into two injection intervals per week, or every ten days.

In having had determined the proper amount of required dose, most athletes often had considered the following variables such as age, goals, steriodal stack, temperament, and of course, financial situation. The latter had frequently been considered primarily due to the quantity of Primoteston Depot which had usually been required to have been administered, had often caused this steriodal compound to have become very expensive.

Primoteston Depot had primarily been combined with several other steriodal compounds in order to have gained size and mass. As Primoteston Depot was an androgen, it had somewhat of a synergetic effect with the anabolic steriodal compounds, which had resulted in the bonding with several receptors.

Many athletes had claimed that Primoteston Depot had stacked remarkably well with Anapolon, Metandiabol or Reforvit-B, (veterinary products) Deca-Durabolin or Norandren 50 (veterinary product), and Parabolan (currently, not found in Mexico). Another possible stack which had often also been utilized, had consisted of Anapolon 100 mgs (2 x 50 mg tablets) a day, Deca-Durabolin or Norandren 50 (veterinary product) at 200 mgs (2 x 1 ml redi-jects) a week, along with Primoteston Depot 2 x 250 mg ampules a week. Also, Metandiabol or Reforvit-B (veterinary product) at 40 mgs (approximately 1 1/2 to 3/4 cc's) daily, had usually replaced the Anapolon dosage after approximately six weeks.

Another feasible combination which many male athletes had utilized, had included Primoteston Depot at 2 x 250 mgs ampules, or 2 cc's weekly, with Metandiabol or Reforvit-B (veterinary product) at approximately 1 1/2 to 3/4 cc's per week, or Anapolon 2 tablets daily, which often had kept water retention at a minimum. Reportedly, Primoteston Depot combined with Oxandrolone or Winstrol (both are currently not found in Mexico), had permitted the increase of strength and mass, without the associated bodyweight increase.

At the conclusion of a Primoteston Depot cycle, the administration of Testosterone-stimulating compounds such as Gonadotropyl, Gonakor, or

Profasi, (HCG), Omifin, or Serofene (Clomid), Nolvadex and anti-catabolic substances such as Novegam or Spiropent (Clenbuterol), or Ephedrine (currently not available in Mexico), or even Human Growth Hormone (Biotropin, Genotropin, Humatrope, Nanorm, Norditropin, Saizen or Protropin) had also been necessarily entertained. The administration of these compounds often had aided in the absorption of the catabolic phase; which had helped in the elevation of the endogenic Testosterone level. Consequently, these compounds had also reduced the potential strength and mass loss, which usually had been inevitable. Allegedly, slowly having tapered down the dosages of Primoteston Depot had not unfortunately, helped to have maintained the strength and mass increases. Another preventative measure which had also been entertained by some athletes had involved the possibility of having had switched to milder steriodal compounds such as Deca-Durabolin or Norandren 50 (veterinary product), Primobolan Depot, or Winstrol (currently, not available in Mexico). The discontinuation of these compounds usually had permitted the acquired gains to have remained.

Side Effects:

The side effects that had been experienced by some athletes which had been associated with the use of Primoteston Depot had primarily been the distinct androgenic effects, and increased water retention. Other side effects had included acne, which had been predominantly harsher on the chest, back, arms, and shoulder areas, than on the face. This had often been a recognizable indication to other athletes that a particular individual had administrated Testosterones, including Primoteston Depot. However, sometimes a type of rebound effect had occurred, and these side effects had sometimes not appeared until after discontinuation of the Testosterone.

Primoteston Depot had only slightly been toxic when it had been administered in conservative quantities. Although Primoteston Depot had been broken down through the liver, the liver values changes had not occurred as often as they had with the oral 17-alpha alkylated steriodal compounds. Male athletes had especially experienced feminization effects such as gynecomastia, testicular atrophy, reduced spermatogenesis and increased aggressiveness. Some athletes had also experienced hair loss and further deepening of the voice.

Female athletes generally had avoided Testosterone steriodal compounds such as Primoteston Depot, due to potential masculizational traits. These androgen-linked side effects of virilization which had often been encountered included acne vulgaris, increased facial and body hair growth, male pattern baldness, a hoarseness or deepening of the voice, menstrual irregularities, increased clitoral size, and a great increase in sex drive. Some of these side effects had been somewhat irreversible, such as the increased facial and body hair growth, increased libido, male pattern baldness, however, often once the damage had occurred to the voice and clitoris, it had been generally that of a permanent nature. Depending on the quantity of Testosterone which had been administered, and if the cycle had been completely terminated before these effects had become evident, had sometimes resulted in a lessening effect of these associated problems.

WARNING:

If hypertension had become elevated at the initiation of Primoteston Depot, or athletes who had a predisposition for high blood pressure, often routinely had it monitored by a competent physician, or had learned to have taken blood pressure readings themselves. *(Usually, any pharmacy or Clinic had offered to have taught these instructions, or had devices which had rendered a free Blood Pressure reading for an individual*). An antihypertensive compound such as Catapresan (available in Mexico), had also been warranted to some athletes in efforts to have helped kept the blood pressure within normal limits.

Rating:

Based on a 1 to 5 star scale, with 1 considered low, and 5 considered high, a -- symbol is indicative of no value. This compound of Testosterone Enanthate had rated as the following:

	MALES	FEMALES
Strength Increase	*****	**
Mass & Weight Increase	*****	**
Side Effects	**	*****
Cost Efficiency	*****	*****

PROTROPIN

Chemical Name: Somatrem.

Common Generic Name: Protropin (Human Growth Hormone).

Other Trade Names Found in Mexico: Currently, just Protropin.

Manufacturers: Protropin - Lilly.

Dosage Form: Protropin - 10 I.U. per 10 ml.

Storage: Before and after reconstitution with Bacteriostatic water for injection, USP, this must be stored at 2 to 8 degrees C (36 to 46 degrees F) in the refrigerator. With the exception of Saizen, the biological activity of Growth Hormone is usually not impaired when storing the dry substance at 15 to 30 degrees C (59 to 86 degrees F). However, refrigeration temperature as discussed above is preferable. Reconstituted vials should be used within 7 days after reconstitution. Expiration dates are stated on the product's labels. Do not freeze.

Price Range: Protropin - not known.

Type of Drug: Synthetic DNA Growth Hormone.

Ingredient: 5 mgs Somatropin.

Drug Identification:

Protropin - Protropin is not manufactured in Mexico, and is very difficult to acquire, therefore, it had not been obtained for illustrational and identification purposes. However, this product had been very similiar in appearance to the other synthetic Human Growth Hormones of Somatropin. It may possibly be obtainable in a few select farmacias.

Drug Description:

Protropin Growth Hormone is a sterile, white, lyophilized powder, which had been intended for intramuscular or subcutaneous injection, after reconstitution with Bacteriostatic water. Protropin has 192 amino acids residues, and a molecular weight of approximately 22,000 daltons. The product contains the identical sequence of 191 amino acids constituting pituitary derived human growth hormone, with an additional amino acid, Methionine, on the N-Terminus of the molecule. Somatrem is also a polypeptide hormone which had been purified, and is recombinant of DNA origin. Somatrem amino acid sequence had been identical to that of Human Growth Hormone of pituitary origin.

Some athletes had utilized the synthetic compound of Protropin in efforts to have had enhanced the anabolic effects of their steroid regimes. It had also been reported to have had superior fat-burning entities, and thus, had been very popular amongst many female athletes. Protropin, similarly to the other forms of 191 amino acid synthetic versions of Growth Hormone, had also been expensive, and rather difficult to have attained.

It had been a common phenomenon that Protropin had been primarily used by those in the professional ranks of bodybuilding. Consequently, many novice athletes had a tendency to have shyed away from Protropin;

not only because of the cost, difficulty in obtaining, but also because sometimes due to ignorance in application, administration, and of possible fear of the rumored potential side effects. Some athletes had often disputed the fact that this compound's application had not been as spectacular as it had been rumored; as many administrators sometimes had appeared not to have benefited from Protropin's utilization.

Unfortunately, this may have resulted from several reasons such as improper dosing, improper reconstitution, improper storage, and the possibility that the compound had been counterfeit. Sometimes, a few athletes even had experienced a possible immune reaction, which had rendered the compound ineffective. Clinically, it had been reported that approximately 30% to 40% of all patients who had engaged in the administration of the compound of synthetic Protropin, had developed persistent antibodies. In patients who had been previously treated with Protropin (a pituitary-derived Growth Hormone), one of 22 subjects had developed persistent antibodies. Another study had stated that one of 84 subjects who had been treated for 6 to 36 months had developed antibodies that had been associated with high binding capacities, and therefore, had failed to have responded.

However, many athletes had positive experiences with this compound of Protropin, and had reported that the administration had been successful in the maintainence of the gains, which had been acquired from anabolic steroids; as well as having had exceptional fat-burning capabilities.

Usual Clinical Recommendation:

The Protropin dosage had been individualized for each patient. A common dosage of up to 0.1 mg/kg (0.26 I.U./kg) bodyweight, administered three times per week, by either intramuscular or subcutaneous injection had been recommended.

Adventitious Dosage and Administration:

After the desired dosage had been determined, it had been reconstituted by having had chosen between either a 5 mg vial, in which case, it had been reconstituted with 1 to 5 ml of Bacteriostatic Water for injection, USP (Benzyl alcohol preserved), or each 10 mg vial with 1 to 10 ml of the Bacteriostatic Water for injection, USP (Benzyl alcohol preserved) only. The Protropin solution had been prepared by having had injected the Bacteriostatic Water for injection USP (Benzyl alcohol preserved), into the vial which had contained the Protropin Growth Hormone, by having aimed the stream of liquid against the glass wall. Immediately having followed this, it had been gently swirled in a circular motion, until the combined contents had been completely dissolved. It had never been SHAKEN.

Protropin Growth Hormone is a protein, therefore, having shaken the solution had resulted in a somewhat cloudy solution usually immediately after reconstitution. The small, colorless particles of protein may have been present in the Protropin solution, which was not considered to have been unusual for this kind of protein. But, if the solution had been cloudy immediately after it had been reconstituted or refrigerated, the contents had not been injected.

Prior to and after injections, to have prevented contaminations of the combined contents after multiple repeated insertions, the septum of the vial had been always wiped with an antiseptic solution. Athletes had perused a needle of sufficient length, which had be more than 1 inch, to have ensured that the injection had reached the muscle layer. Also, the use of sterile, disposable needles and syringes had definitely been always undertaken. The 5 mg bottle had been equivalent to 13 I.U.'s, and the 10 mg bottle had been equivalent to 26 I.U.'s.

The administration of synthetic Protropin appeared to have been more effective when it had been included with a stack of anabolic steroids. It had also been important not to have exceeded more than the dosages of 4 I.U's in any one given day. A common dosage regime of some athletes, has been discussed in the following:

Females

Female athletes had claimed that effective dosages usually had been approximately 1 I.U. daily, or every other day, administered anywhere for 2 to 8 months, and sometimes even longer if it had been so desired.

Males

Male athletes usually benefited from 2 I.U.'s daily, or every other day, also had been administered anywhere from 2 to 8 months or longer.

Side Effects:

The side effects of Protropin, such as Acromegaly had been uncommon, but had occasionally occurred in dosages that had been higher than 4 I.U.'s. Other side effects, which had sometimes rarely been experienced by adult athletes who had administered unconservative, long duration dosages, had included overgrowth of the elbows and jaw, thickening of the skin, carpal tunnel syndrome, thyroid insufficiency, heart muscle hypertrophy, enlargement of the kidneys, hypertension, exacerbation of glucose intolerance, (hypoglycemia) which had generally lead to diabetes, and an increased incidence of neoplasm (but only in high and long-term doses). In some cases, antibodies had developed against Protropin, (which the incidence had been higher with this compound than the other synthetic versions of Growth Hormone).

Some athletes had also reported headaches, nausea, vomiting, and visual disturbances during the first few weeks of initial intake, which had generally subsided and had disappeared in most cases, even with continued administration. Most athletes had also experienced a slight water retention for the first three months of administration. However, athletes who had utilized conservative dosages of synthetic Protropin, had not often had experienced negative side effects.

WARNING:

An acute overdosage of Protropin may have lead initially to hypoglycemia, and subsequently to hyperglycemia. Long-term overdosage may have also resulted in signs and symptoms of Gigantism, or Acromegaly, which had been consistent with the known effects of excess Human Growth Hormone.

Rating:

Based on a 1 to 5 star scale, with 1 considered low, and 5 considered high, this compound of Somatrem had rated as the following:

	MALES	FEMALES
Strength Increase	****	****
Mass & Weight Increase	****	****
Fat Burner	*****	*****
Contest Preparation	*****	*****
Side Effects	**	**
Cost Efficiency	*****	*****

PROVIRON

Chemical Name: Mesterolone.

Common Generic Name: Proviron.

Other Trade Names Found in Mexico: Currently, just Proviron.

Manufacturer: Proviron - Schering.

Dosage Form: Proviron - 10 x 25 mg tablets.

Storage: Proviron tablets should be protected from light and moisture, (keep in the carton until contents are used), and stored at controlled room temperature 15 to 30 degrees C (59 to 86 degrees F).

Price Range: Proviron - approx. $59.90 pesos for 10 x 25 mg tablets.

Type of Drug: Androgenic Steroid. Estrogen Antagonist.

Ingredient: 25 mgs of Mesterolone.

Drug Identification:

Proviron - Is available as an oral administration tablet. These tablets are round, white in color and have been scored on one side, and plain on the other. They are individually separated into one package of 10, in blisters with a push-through silver meshed backing. On the back, the product's entities have been displayed throughout written in navy blue ink. The accompanying package is basically white with a navy blue box near the right side, with the product's entities written in black ink.

*****Please refer to the photographs of Proviron for full color references.***

Drug Description:

Many male athletes had frequently administered Proviron at the end of a steroid treatment; in attempts to have increased their own reduced Testosterone production. This oral androgenic steroid had been commonly utilized as an Estrogen antagonist. Once the substance of Proviron had entered the blood, it had competed with Estrogen at the receptor sites, which sometimes had resulted in cessation of aromatizing effects of other steroids. However, it had no effect on the body's own Testosterone production, as it actually only had reduced, or even completely had canceled the dysfunctions which had been caused by the Testosterone deficiency.

These deficiencies specifically had referred to impotence, that had mostly been caused by an androgen deficiency (which had often resulted after the discontinuance of steroids). The second, had referred to infertility, which had exhibited itself in either a reduced sperm count or in a reduced sperm quality. These had been the primary clinical reasons for having had utilized the compound of Proviron. Also for these reasons, Proviron had been frequently preventatively entertained either during steroid administration, or after the discontinuance of the steroids.

Unlike the anti-Estrogen Nolvadex, which only had blocked the Estrogen receptors, Proviron had already prevented the aromatization of steroids. Also, since Proviron strongly had suppressed the constituting of Estrogens, no rebound effect had occurred after discontinuation of it's use. This had often been apparent with the utilization of the compound of Nolvadex, as the aromatization of steroids had not been preventable.

The main difference between Proviron and Nolvadex had been that Proviron actually had "cured" the problem of aromatization at it's source, while Nolvadex simply had only been able to have alleviated the symptoms. Unfortunately, Proviron had not contributed to the maintenance of strength and muscle mass after the abstinence of a steroidal treatment. More valuable compounds which had allegedly featured this characteristic had been Gonadotropyl-C, Gonakor, and Profasi (HCG), Omifin or Serofene (Clomid) or Teslac (Teslac is not currently found in Mexico). For this entity alone, Proviron had been considered by many athletes, to have been a valueless and unessential compound.

However, Proviron itself, had not only not aromatized, but it had also been only moderately toxic to the liver, which had frequently resulted in successfully having blocked gynecomastia and increased water retention. Obviously, for this purpose, most male athletes had preferred the application of Proviron, as opposed to Nolvadex.

Usual Clinical Recommendation:

The usual recommendation in efforts to have treated hypogonadism in males had been: Initial starting dosage at 75 to 100 mg per day, while the maintenance dosage had been at 50 to 75 mg per day. In attempts to have treated infertility problems in males, the recommended dosage had been 100 mg per day.

Adventitious Dosage and Administration:

Proviron tablets had been intended for oral administration, which had implied that they had been designed to have been swallowed by mouth. These tablets had provided the best results when they had been ingested with water, prior to meals. They did not require to have been crushed or chewed. A common dosage regime of some athletes, has been discussed in the following:

Proviron had often primarily been used in contest preparation, and also by those athletes who had wished to have achieved a hard appearance to their muscles.

Females:

Some female athletes who already naturally had a higher Estrogen level, often had supplemented their steriodal regimes by having included Proviron. This had permitted for an enhancement to their androgen levels, which had further permitted for a much harder look to their muscles. Generally, Proviron had often been stacked with the other steriodal compounds, at a common daily dose of 1 x 25 mg tablet administered over several weeks, or several months. However, the compound of Spiropent (Clenbuterol) had recently gained popularity due to it's entities of both lower virilization symptoms, and for the fact that it could have been taken for longer periods of time; up to a year, without having imposed harmful ill effects.

One to two tablets had frequently sufficed most female athletes, however, those who had experienced no problems with Proviron, had obtained desirable results with 25 mgs (1 tablet) of Proviron daily, with 20 mgs (2 x 10 mgs tablets, or 1 x 20 mgs tablet) of Nolvadex daily. This combination often had included a controlled caloric intake, which had further achieved an accelerated fat breakdown, and continuously harder muscles.

Males:

Since Proviron had been very effective, most male athletes had usually required only 50 mgs (2 tablets) a day. For Proviron's full potential, it had generally been administered as 1 x 25 mg tablet in the morning and another 25 mg tablet in the evening. In some instances, some male athletes had utilized the regime of one 25 mg tablet per day, however an average dose had usually been between 50 to 100 mgs (2 to 4 tablets) a day.

The administration of Proviron at 50 mgs (2 tablets) daily combined with Nolvadex at 20 mgs (2 x 10 mgs tablets, or 1 x 20 mgs tablet) daily, had provided an almost complete suppression of Estrogen. Several male athletes had claimed that more valuable results had been achieved with 50 mgs (2 tablets) daily of Proviron, combined with 500 to 1000 mgs of Teslac also taken daily (Teslac is not currently found in Mexico). However, this combination had usually not been considered by most athletes, as Teslac had usually been a very expensive compound, therefore, sometimes had been unaffordable.

Side Effects:

If most compounds had been administered in conservative dosages, few side effects had posed to have been problematic. For instance, the side effects of Proviron in male athletes had been relatively low at a dosage of 2 to 3 tablets daily, so that Proviron, taken for example, in combination with a steroid cycle, could have been used comparatively without risk over several weeks. However, if these dosages had been excessive, ill effects had often prevailed. These had included occasional retention of electrolytes and water, and edemas. Athletes who had administered less than 2 to 4 tablets daily had often not been concerned about these problems.

The most common side effect of Proviron, particularly in male athletes, had been the potential of a distinct sexual overstimulation, and the possibility of continuous penis erection (priapism). This condition had proven to have been not only painful, but also had lead to possible damage. Male athletes had either lowered the dosage, or had discontinued Proviron if this had initiated.

Female athletes had often been careful when they had utilized the compound of Proviron, due to the possible androgenic side effects which may have occurred. However, females who had still desired to have attempted the use of Proviron, had often not exceeded more than one 25 mgs tablets per day, as an increased dosage and period of intake for more than four weeks had considerably increased the risk of virilization symptoms.

These virilization side effects had included such problems as deepening or hoarseness of the voice, menstrual irregularities, clitoral enlargement, skin changes, including acne, increased hair growth on face and body, increased libido, as well as other ill effects associated with the use of Proviron. Since Proviron had been well-tolerated by the liver, liver dysfunctions had not usually occurred in the previously mentioned dosages.

WARNING:

If the compound of Proviron had been administered for long durations, it had been able to have caused prostate cancer, and in some cases, had caused a continued state of erection of the penis. If this had resulted, discontinuance of Proviron had been warranted in efforts to have retarded further damage associated with a permanent erection.

Rating:

Based on a 1 to 5 star scale, with 1 considered low, and 5 considered high, a -- symbol is indicative of no value. This compound of Mesterolone had rated as the following:

	MALES	FEMALES
Testosterone Stimulant	****	--
Side Effects	***	**
Cost Efficiency	***	***

SOSTENON 250

Chemical Name: Testosterone Propionate, Phenylpropionate, Isocaproate, Decanoate.

Common Generic Name: Sustanon.

Other Trade Names Found in Mexico: Deposterona* (veterinary).

Manufacturers: Sostenon 250 - Organon.

Dosage Form: Sostenon 250 - "250" 1 ml ampule.
- "250"- 1 cc redi-ject.

Storage: Sostenon 250 injectables should be protected from light, (keep in the carton until contents are used), and stored at controlled room temperature 15 to 30 degrees C (59 to 86 degrees F), away from heat. Do not freeze.

Price Range: Sostenon 250 - approx. $40.30 pesos for "250" 1 ml ampule or 1 cc redi-ject.

Type of Drug: Androgenic Hormone.

Ingredient: 30 mgs Testosterone Propionate, 60 mgs Testosterone Phenylpropionate, 60 mgs Testosterone Isocaproate, 100 mgs Testosterone Decanoate.

Drug Identification:

Sostenon 250 - Is available in 1 x 1 ml redi-ject syringe as an sesame-oil based pre-loaded injectable. The redi-ject itself is plastic with the product's entities written in light purple ink. It is individually cradled within clear plastic, with a silver aluminum push-through backing with the product's entities written throughout in black ink. Reg. # 50064. Lot # 9628ABR99. There is also an individual sterile capped needle, which also separately accompanies the redi-ject, for assembly. The accompanying package is white, with the product's entities also written in black ink. There is a light blue pin-stripe across the front, near the bottom of the package, and the top of the package is light blue with a red tab, outlined in white.

****Please refer to the photographs of Sostenon 250 for full color references.***

Drug Description:

Clinically, Sostenon 250 had been prescribed to patients in efforts to have treated deficiencies in external genitalia development, low libidos, eunichism, impotency, hypertrophic prostates after castration in males.

The compound of Sostenon 250 has consisted of a concoction of four Testosterones which have responded very assertively together both in continued usage, or re-establishment of a cycle. This combination of Testosterones had appeared to have been recognized by the steroid receptors for longer periods of time. For many athletes, this characteristic had been ideal, as it could have been used in lower doses, therefore, also had posed to have presented fewer potential side effects. Sostenon 250 had been fast acting and had remained active, as it had been time released. Sostenon 250 became generally effective usually after administration the first day, as it had contained Decanoates, which had frequently existed approximately three to four weeks in the system.

Sostenon 250 had both a distinct androgenic and a strong anabolic effect. Most athletes had preferred this compound, as it had been recognized to have increased bodyweight, strength, and mass, very rapidly. These characteristics had also been very desirable for those male athletes who had difficulty with elevated Estrogen levels, which had been very common of other long-acting depot Testosterones.

Most athletes had claimed that Sostenon 250 had been generally well tolerated as a basic steroid during treatment, which had stimulated the regeneration, as it also had provided a "boost" for intense training and exercising purposes.

Again, most cautious female athletes had avoided the administration of Sostenon 250, as well as most Testosterones, due to potential undesirable virilization problems. These steroidal compounds had frequently appeared to have been too harsh on the female system, regardless of desired anabolic effects. Instead, several female athletes had depended on other "milder" substances in efforts to have achieved these gains, without having to have acquired the detrimental adverse effects.

Usual Clinical Recommendation:

The usual clinical recommendation had been 1 ml injected intramuscularly once every 4 days, depending upon the clinical response of the patient.

Adventitious Dosage and Administration:

Sostenon 250 had been intended for deep intramuscular injection. The best site for this type of injection had been in the gluteus medius muscle area, which had been the upper outer portion of the buttock, approximately 2 to 3 inches below the hip bone (iliac crest). Many athletes had wisely alternated these injections from one side to the other, (first injection on the left side, the second time injection administered on the right, or vice versa) in attempts to have alleviated pain somewhat, and to also have allowed the area to have slightly "healed". This practice had often prevented a thick scar tissue from having formed. However, the more injections that athletes had administered, the greater possibility of scar tissue had resulted. A common dosage regime of some athletes, has been discussed in the following:

Females:

Most female athletes had totally avoided the administration of Sostenon 250, and other Testosterone steroids. However, some females had ventured, and had ignored the risks of virilization, and had administered 250 mgs (1 ampule, or 1 redi-ject) every 10 to 14 days, for a period of generally 6 weeks. However, these dosages and duration had never wisely been exceeded.

Males:

Male athletes usually had injected Sostenon 250 once a week, or even up to once every ten days. The usual dosage range had been anywhere from 250 to 1000 mgs (1 to 4 ampules, or 1 to 4 redi-jects) a week. Most male athletes however, had frequently obtained satisfactory results from dosages in the 500 mgs (2 ampules, or 2 redi-jects) range. If Sostenon 250 had also been combined with an oral compound, it had often been lowered to 250 mgs (1 ampule, or 1 redi-ject) once a week.

Some male athletes had claimed that in order to have achieved rapid increases in strength, Sostenon 250 in combination with Deca-Durabolin, or (Deposterona*) Metandiabol or Reforvit-B, or Norandren 50 (all veterinary products), or Anapolon had been utilized. Primobolan, Oxandrolone, Parabolan or Winstrol (the latter three are currently, not available in Mexico), had also been used by some male athletes in attempts to have gained more qualitative muscle mass.

An anti-Estrogen compound such as Nolvadex and/or Proviron, had also been frequently constituted into a cycle of Sostenon 250, in efforts to have prevented potential feminization side effects (although, Sostenon 250 had not aromatized remarkably when it had been administered in sensible dosages). Gonadotropyl-C, Gonakor, or Profasi (HCG) and Omifin or Serofene (Clomid) had been a general consideration however, at the end of a Sostenon 250 treatment due to it's characteristic of having suppressed the endogenous Testosterone production.

Side Effects:

The side effects of Sostenon 250, had been very similar to those characteristic of Testosterone Enanthate, except they had not been as numerous or severe. If the dosage of Sostenon 250 had been excessive (over the 1200 mgs range), some consequential androgenic-linked side effects had often occurred such as acne, an increased aggression, increased libido, oily skin, accelerated hair loss, mood swings, and reduced production of the body's own hormones. However, water retention and gynecomastia had not been as likely to have been problematic, having provided, that the dosage range had been kept within an reasonable range.

As mentioned previously, Sostenon 250 and other Testosterones had not been primarily utilized by female athletes, as severe virilization traits such as deepening or hoarseness of the voice, acne, increased facial and body hair growth, increased libido, enlarging of the clitoris, menstrual irregularities and changes in the skin had been known to have occurred. Most of these effects once obtained by a female, had not been reversible.

WARNING:

Liver damage, had occurred in very high dosages. However, cessation of this compound had usually resulted in the liver values having returned back to within a normal range. The administration of Primoteston Depot had also been linked to prostatic cancer.

Rating:

Based on a 1 to 5 star scale, with 1 considered low, and 5 considered high, a -- symbol is indicative of no value. This compound of Testosterone Propionate, Phenylpropionate, Isocaproate, Decanoate had rated as the following:

	MALES	FEMALES
Strength Increase	*****	**
Mass & Weight Increase	*****	**
Side Effects	**	*****
Cost Efficiency	**	**

STEN

Chemical Name: Dihydrotestosterone, Testosterone Propionate, Testosterone Cypionate.

Common Generic Name: Sten.

Other Trade Names Found in Mexico: Currently, just Sten.

Manufacturer: Sten - Atlantis.

Dosage Form: Sten - 2 x 2 ml ampules.

Storage: Sten injectables should be protected from light, (keep in the carton until contents are used), and stored at controlled room temperature 15 to 30 degrees C (59 to 86 degrees F). Do not freeze.

Price Range: Sten - approx. $8.80 pesos for 2 x 2 ml (c) ampules.

Type of Drug: Anabolic and Androgenic Steroid.

Ingredient: 20 mg Dihydrotestosterone, 25 mg Testosterone Propionate, 75 mg Testosterone Cypionate.

Drug Identification:

Sten - Each ampule of Sten consists of 2 ml of oil-base (cottonseed) Dihydrotestosterone, and Testosterones. The ampules themselves are clear glass with Sten's entities inscribed in brownish-reddish print that is burned into the glass, and can be easily felt, as it cannot be scratched off. The two ampules are packaged in a plastic mold, with a 3 ml syringe also enclosed. The box is also white with the same color of brownish-red, with the compound's entities documented.

Drug Description:

The compound of Sten can *only* be found within the country of Mexico. It is a low milligram blend of Testosterone which unfortunately, also has contained the DHT type of Testosterone. Clinically, Sten had been often prescribed in efforts to have treated hypogonadism, impotency, andropausia in males, and breast cancer and low libidos in females. This kind of Testosterone had been generally responsible for the onset of problematic acne, baldness, prostate enlargement and visceral fat accumulation. The compound of Sten had been somewhat similar to Sostenon 250, as it had also contained several Testosterone compounds. However, the substance combination of Sten and Sostenon 250 had been different, as the total amount of the Sten substance had been just slightly less than half of the amount in found in Sostenon 250. Therefore, the amount of Sten would have required to have been "doubled" in attempts to have acquired the same effects and results of having had administered Sostenon 250.

Many athletes had frequently used Sten for strength and weight gains, and to also have maintained muscle mass, while having entertained a restricted caloric intake. The results had been reported to have varied in occurrence, as athletes often had to have administered anywhere from one to three ampules a week, in order to have achieved satisfactory increases. However, along with these gains, many athletes had frequently experienced side effects such as severe aromatization and water retention.

The compound of Sten had definitely been avoided by most female athletes, due to the multiple Testosterone substances. Interestingly, it also had proved not to have been a favored compound amongst many male athletes as well. This had been primarily due to the risk/benefit ratio which could have proved to have been very detrimental to athletes administrators of both genders.

Usual Clinical Recommendation:

The usual recommended clinical dosage had been 1 ampule injected intramuscularly every 15 to 30 days, dependent upon etiology and clinical response of the patient.

Adventitious Dosage and Administration:

Sten had been intended for deep intramuscular injection. The best site for this type of injection had been in the gluteus medius muscle area, which had been the upper outer portion of the buttock, approximately 2 to 3 inches below the hip bone (iliac crest). Again, many athletes had frequently alternated injections from one side to the other, (first injection on the left side, the second time injection administered on the right, or vice versa) in attempts to have alleviated associated pain, and to also possibly have allowed the area to have slightly "healed". This practice had often prevented a thick scar tissue from having potentially formed. However, the more injections that athletes had administered, the greater possibility of scar tissue had resulted. A common dosage regime of some athletes, has been discussed in the following:

This blend of Testosterone as previously mentioned, had not been well tolerated by both female and male athletes. There had been much safer, wiser, compounds which had alternatively been used in attempts to have achieved strength and weight gains. Some athletes had chosen to have administered Sostenon 250 for example, as this compound had been much more desirable, in lower dosage amounts, with somewhat lessened associated adverse effects.

Females:

Most cautious female athletes had not entertained the administration of Sten; not even the more adventurous, risk-taking females.

Males:

Even most male athletes had often avoided the administration of this compound. However, some reckless male athletes had reportedly administered 1 to 3 ampules of Sten a week.

Side Effects:

Sten had been considered to have been somewhat of a vicious compound, as the use of it had usually resulted in many undesirable side effects. This compound had contained the DHT type of Testosterone, which had been responsible for severe associated side effects, such as those that had frequently been amplified by the media, in efforts to have shocked and dissuade the public from anabolic steroid use.

Some of the very severe side effects which most athletes who had ventured in the administration of Sten had included those of acne vulgaris, male pattern baldness, prostate enlargement, increased libido, increased aggression, mood swings, severe gynecomastia and water retention, and visceral fat accumulation.

For female athletes, this compound had been extremely androgenic, that virilization effects had occurred, no matter how low dosages had been. Some of these ill effects had included clitoral enlargement, menstrual irregularities, cessation of menstruation, hoarseness or deepening of the voice, male pattern baldness, severe facial acne, facial and body hair growth, increase in libido and aggression, and mood swings.

Of course, other side effects may have been experienced by a few athletes who had engaged in this compound, which had been possibly not recognized, therefore, had not been documented.

WARNING:

Several athletes had discovered that the potential ill effects had been too distinguished with use of this compound, as high dosages had been required to have received any anabolic or androgenic effect. High dosages of course, had greatly promoted ill effects, which in this case, most athletes had claimed definitely had not been worth the possible associated health risks.

Rating:

Based on a 1 to 5 star scale, with 1 considered low, and 5 considered high, a -- symbol is indicative of no value. This compound of Dihydrotestosterone, Testosterone Propionate, Testosterone Cypionate had rated as the following:

	MALES	FEMALES
Strength Increase	*	-
Mass & Weight Increase	*	-
Side Effects	*****	*****
Cost Efficiency	*	*

STENOX

Chemical Name: Fluoxymesterone.

Common Generic Name: Halotestin.

Other Trade Names Found in Mexico: Stenox.

Manufacturer: Stenox - Atlantis Labs.

Dosage Form: Stenox - 2.5 mg tablets.

Storage: Stenox tablets should be protected from light and moisture, (keep in the carton until contents are used), and stored at controlled room temperature 15 to 30 degrees C (59 to 86 degrees F).

Price Range: Stenox - approx. $22.80 pesos for 2.5 mg tablets.

Type of Drug: Androgenic Hormone.

Ingredient: 2.5 mgs Fluoxymesterone.

Drug Identification:

Stenox - is available as oral administration tablets which are round, white, plain on one side, and scored on the other side. There is one package of 20 tablets within each box of Stenox. These tablets are individually packaged within clear push-through blisters on a copper colored background. Lot # L631804. The backing is silver colored with the product's entities written throughout in black ink. The accompanying package is white and red.

*****Please refer to the photographs of Stenox for full color references.***

Drug Description:

Stenox is available in Mexico, in a small quantity of 2.5 mgs, which has been half the strength of the usual familiar Halotestin version of 5 mg tablets. This version of strength only had lessened the already slight presence of the anabolic component of this compound. Stenox had been however, extremely androgenic. Although it had appeared to have aromatized very poorly, it had frequently permitted for an obtainable elevated androgen level, with a low Estrogen concentration. Therefore, distinctive muscle hardness and sharpness had also been acquired when administered by athletes with a low percentage of bodyfat. Consequently, muscle diameter had not expanded, it had only actually appeared to have been more massive since the muscle density had been enhanced.

The administration of Stenox had been well known for it's characteristic of having raised aggression levels, which had been generally often welcomed by many male athletes who's energy levels had been low, which often had been due to a restricted caloric intake, or by athletes who had required an extra "boost" for intense training regimes. Male athletes generally had utilized the compound of Stenox in efforts to have maintained a specific weight within a particular weight class. Stenox had frequently enabled for an increase in strength, without the weight increase; which had usually been associated with strength gains.

Again, the steroidal substance of Stenox had not utilized by most female athletes, due to it's considerable potential virilization side effects. These adverse effects for the most part, had been irreversible once they had been obtained. Consequently, even reckless female athletes had not often been tempted by the use of this substance for possible athletic enhancement.

Next to Anapolon and Methyltestosterone (not currently available in Mexico), Stenox had been considered by many athletes, to have been the next most toxic oral steroid, with the most potential side effects associated with it's administration. Stenox had also been listed in the Controlled Substance Class, under the Anabolic Steroids Control Act. It has also of course, been assigned to the Schedule III class of drugs, which labels it as a controlled substance; narcotic.

Usual Clinical Recommendation:

The dosage had varied depending upon the individual, the condition being treated, and the severity. The total daily oral dose had been administered singularly, or in equally divided 3 or 4 doses.

To treat male hypogonadism - a daily dose of 5 to 20 mgs had usually sufficed in the majority of male patients.

Adventitious Dosage and Administration:

Stenox tablets had been intended for oral administration, which had implied that they had been designed to have been swallowed by the mouth. Many athletes had claimed that these tablets had provided the best results when they had been split into two equivalent amounts, and had been ingested once in the morning, and then again at night, with an abundance of fluids, and food. They did not require to have been crushed or chewed. A common dosage regime of some athletes, has been discussed in the following:

Stenox had been utilized almost exclusively during preparation for competition. These tablets had often been taken during meals, as they had been 17-alpha alkylated, which had enabled the compound not to have lost any of it's effect.

Females:

Female athletes mostly had avoided this substance of Stenox. As previously mentioned, even the reckless adventurous females had claimed that the benefits had not outweighed the possible risks that had been involved with the administration of Stenox.

Males:

On the other hand, many male athletes had participated in the administration of Stenox, for an average dosage total of 20 to 30 mgs (8 to 12 tablets). This dosage had usually been divided into two doses of 10 to 15 mgs or (4 to 6 tablets). Stenox had frequently been taken in a cycle of 4 to 6 weeks, but never had exceeded this duration. The dosage of 20 to 30 mgs daily had also never been exceeded by cautious male athletes.

Rapid strength increases frequently had been induced by the administration of Stenox, which had usually transpired into solid, high-qualitative muscle tissue by additionally having stacked Anadur, (currently, not available in Mexico), Deca-Durabolin, Primobolan Depot, or Equi-Gan, Maxi-Gan or Crecibol (veterinarian product). However, many male athletes had claimed that just the utilization of Stenox at 30 mgs (12 x 2.5 mg tablets), and Equi-Gan, Maxi-Gan or Crecibol (veterinarian product) at 100 mgs (4 cc's or 4 mls if the 25 mg version had been used, or 2 cc's or 2 mls, if the 50 mgs version had been used), taken on alternative days x 4 weeks, had also provided substantial results.

Doses that had been maintained at the 20 mgs (8 tablets) daily range, had limited the potential of water and salt retention in practically all male athletes who had self-administered this substance.

Side Effects:

As Stenox had been a very androgenic compound, it had also been considered to have been a very toxic steroid. Cautious administering athletes, always had limited the dosage to below 30 mgs daily, in attempts to have kept the potential side effects at a minimum. However, side effects had been known to have prevailed, even at these dosages.

Characteristic side effects associated with the administration of Stenox frequently had included those of liver damage, acne, nose bleeds, headaches, gastrointestinal pain, reduced production of the body's own hormones, irritability, and of course, increased aggressiveness. Stenox also had a notorious reputation as a cause of hair loss in chronic abusers.

Female athletes who had administered this steroidal compound had experienced harsh side effects of virilization such as acne, deepening of the voice, increased facial and body hair, enlargement of the clitoris, menstrual irregularities, male pattern baldness, and changes in skin texture. Most of these had been somewhat irreversible once they had been acquired, and had been easily obtainable, even when low dosages of Stenox had been utilized.

WARNING:

Fluoxymesterone had been known to have placed extremely high stress on the liver; which had been able to have caused liver damage. It had also caused Hypercalcemia in individuals who had been immobilized, or had breast cancer. Intelligent athletes had discontinued the use of Stenox if they had experienced any of these conditions, in efforts to have retarded further damage.

Rating:

Based on a 1 to 5 star scale, with 1 considered low, and 5 considered high, a -- symbol is indicative of no value. This compound of Fluoxymesterone had rated as the following:

	MALES	FEMALES
Strength Increase	****	*
Mass & Weight Increase	***	*
Contest Preparation	****	*
Side Effects	*****	*****
Cost Efficiency	*	*

MEXICAN VETERINARY PHARMACEUTICALS

DEPOSTERONA* *VETERINARY*

Chemical Name: Testosterone Acetate, Testosterone Valerate, Testosterone Undecanoate.

Common Generic Name: Sostenon 250.

Other Trade Names Found in Mexico: Sostenon 250 (human).
Deposterona*.

Manufacturer: Deposterona* - Syntex.

Dosage Form: Deposterona* - 60 mgs/ml, 5 ml bottle.

Storage: Store at controlled room temperature 15 to 30 degrees C (59 to 86 degrees F). Do not permit to freeze. Protect from light. It is advisable to keep in packaging until use.

Price Range: Deposterona* - approximately $60.00 pesos for 5 mls.

Type of Drug: Androgenic.

Ingredient: 12 mg Testosterone Acetate, 12 mg Testosterone Valerate, 36 mgs Testosterone Undecanoate.

Drug Identification:

Deposterona* - As an oil-based injectable solution, 60 mgs/ml is contained within 5 ml dark brown glass bottles. A black sticker label can be found on each separate bottle, with the product's entities written in white ink. There is also a white box with a dark green stripe across the bottom of the box, found at the top of the label. The multiple-injection lid is covered by a silver aluminum tear-off cap, with Syntex punch-stamped on the cap.

These bottles have most often been sold individually, but can be purchased in a package of 5. The accompanying package is identical to the product's label, and is only distributed with the purchase of 5 bottles. Otherwise, Deposterona* can be purchased in individual 5 ml bottles.

****Please refer to the photographs of Deposterona* for full color references.***

Drug Description:

Deposterona* is a veterinarian androgenic medication which had been constituted by the union of three types of Testosterone, Acetate, Valerate, and Undecanoate. This combination of Testosterone, had allowed each substance's action to have performed in a progressive series, which had generally transpired in having obtained desired hormonal concentration levels. Long therapeutic effects had been also accomplished through 8 to 9 weeks of administration.

In veterinarian utilization, this compound mixture had been usually eliminated from the system by manner of urination, at different durations. Testosterone Acetate had been eliminated by the second day after the administrated injection. However, the compound of Testosterone Valerate had been able to maintain it's effect within the system for 20 days, and then had been eliminated also from the system, within 22 days. Testosterone Undecanoate had been eliminated from the system by the 9th week after administration, and had been able to have maintained it's activity through 8 weeks.

Veterinarians had often administered Deposterona* in animals such as cattle, pigs, horses, lambs, birds and other smaller types of mammals, in efforts to have treated inhibition, geriatric (aging) conditions, and hypogonadism. It had also often been utilized to have accelerated the process of the recuperation time and the consolidation of fractures within these animals. The administration of Testosterone had also caused the anabolism of protein, which had also promoted the development of muscle tissue in the animals. This had proven to have been beneficial especially when it had been administered to horses who had matured, and had become difficult to "ride". Deposterona* had also been successful in the treatment of breast tumors and hyperfolliculism in small female animals.

Several athletes had frequently incorporated the utilization of this Testosterone compound, as it had been easily acquired without a prescription from practically any veterinarian outlet in Mexico. The cost of Deposterona* had also been less expensive than Sostenon 250. Most athletes had often considered Deposterona* as the "little brother" of the greater compound Sostenon 250. The main difference between these two compounds had primarily been that Sostenon 250 had been intended for administration in humans, and Deposterona* had been for the utilization in veterinarian medicine. Sostenon 250 had also been a much greater strength and combination of Testosterone compounds having included Testosterone Propionate, Phenylpropionate, Isocaproate, and Decanoate, for a total of 250 mg per ml. Deposterona* on the other hand, had a different combination of Testosterone at a lessened 60 mg per ml, which had displayed a milder effect when it had been utilized.

Sostenon 250 had both a distinct androgenic and a strong anabolic effect. Most athletes had preferred this compound, as it had been recognized to have had increased bodyweight, strength, and mass very rapidly. These characteristics had also been very desirable for those male athletes who had difficulty with elevated Estrogen levels, which had been very common of other long-acting depot Testosterones.

Several athletes had claimed that the administration of Deposterona* had been generally well tolerated as a basic steroid during treatment, which had (similar to the effects in animals), had generally stimulated the regeneration, as it also had provided a "boost" for intense training and exercising purposes. Deposterona* had often been considered to have been an injectable Andriol, (currently, not available in Mexico) as it had similarly contained 36 mgs of Testosterone Undecanoate and very low mgs of Testosterone Acetate and Valerate.

Several athletes had indicated that the administration of Deposterona* had provided better results than what had been experienced from the utilization of the Sostenon 250 compound. These desired results had often included increased vascularity, muscle hardness, a strength increase which had frequently been experienced by the end of the first week, without the often associated water retention.

Consequently, most female athletes had avoided the administration of Deposterona*, even though it had been considered to have been a milder compound of Testosterones, due to potential undesirable virilization problems. Testosterones, despite the amount or combination, had frequently appeared to have been too harsh on the female system, regardless of desired anabolic effects. Instead, several female athletes had depended on other "milder" substances in efforts to have achieved possible weight and strength gains, without having to have acquired the detrimental adverse effects. However, if female athletes had desired to have engaged in a Testosterone based compound anyways, Deposterona* had clearly been the preferred choice of substances.

Usual Veterinary Recommendation:

Veterinarians often had administered Deposterona* intramuscularly in the following dosages, once every three weeks:

Cattle	3 to 5 ml
Pigs	2 to 3 ml
Horses, Lambs	1 to 2 ml
Birds	1 to 1.5 ml
Small animals	0.5 to 1 ml

Adventitious Dosage and Administration:

The administration of the veterinarian compound of Deposterona* had been intended for deep intramuscular injection. The best site for this type of injection had been in the gluteus medius muscle area, which had been the upper outer portion of the buttock, approximately 2 to 3 inches below the hip bone (iliac crest). Many athletes had often alternated the injections from one side to the other, (first injection on the left side, the second time injection administered on the right, or vice versa) in efforts to somewhat have alleviated pain, and to perhaps allow the area to have slightly "healed". This practice had generally prevented a thick scar tissue from potentially forming. However, the more injections that had been administered, the greater possibility of scar tissue had often resulted. A common dosage regime of some athletes, has been discussed in the following:

Females:

Most cautious female athletes who had not wanted to have acquired masculinizing side effects which had often developed from the administration of Testosterones, had not engaged in the utilization of the Deposterona* veterinarian compound. However, female athletes who had chosen to have ventured these adverse effects, had sometimes administered 1 to 2 mls (60 to 120 mgs) every fourth or seventh day.

Males:

Many male athletes on the other hand, had often desired the androgenic effects of the Deposterona* compound, and therefore, had frequently engaged in the utilization of 4 to 5 mls (240 to 300 mgs) evenly divided over a week period. Dosages which had exceeded this amount, had occasionally had the opposite effect, and the male athlete had sometimes began to develop feminization side effects, such as gynecomastia. Therefore, most male athletes had not administered larger quantities of Deposterona*, or had increased the duration between injections intervals.

Side Effects:

The side effects of the veterinarian compound of Deposterona*, had been very similar to those characteristic of Testosterones, except they had not been as numerous or severe if utilized in conservative dosages. If the dosage of Deposterona* had been excessive (over the 320 mgs range), some consequential androgenic-linked side effects had often occurred such as acne, an increased aggression, increased libido, oily skin, accelerated hair loss, mood swings, and reduced production of the body's own hormones. Water retention and gynecomastia had been frequently experienced by some athletes, due to the compound of Deposterona* having been more readily converted into Estrogen.

As mentioned previously, Deposterona* and other Testosterones had not been primarily utilized by female athletes, as severe virilization traits such as deepening or hoarseness of the voice, acne, increased facial and body hair growth, increased libido, enlarging of the clitoris, menstrual irregularities and changes in the skin had been known to have occurred. Most of these effects once obtained by a female, had not been reversible.

In veterinarian administration of Deposterona*, side effects which had been known to have occurred in animals had included prostate cancer, and androgenic tumors. It had also resulted in defects when it had been utilized in gestational and lactating female animals.

WARNING:

Liver damage, had been known to have occurred in very high dosages. However, cessation of this compound had usually resulted in the liver values having returned back to within a normal range.

Rating:

Based on a 1 to 5 star scale, with 1 considered low, and 5 considered high, a -- symbol is indicative of no value. This compound of Testosterone Acetate, Testosterone Valerate, Testosterone Undecanoate had rated as the following:

	MALES	FEMALES
Strength Increase	****	**
Mass & Weight Increase	****	**
Side Effects	***	*****
Cost Efficiency	*	*

DIANABOL *VETERINARY*

Chemical Name: Methandrostenolone/methandienone.

Common Generic Name: Dianabol.

Other Trade Names Found in Mexico: Metandiabol.
Reforvit-B.

Manufacturer: Metandiabol - Quimber.
Reforvit-B - Oeffler.

Dosage Form: Metandiabol - 25 mg/cc 50 cc vial.
Reforvit-B - 25 mg/cc 10 cc vial.
- 25 mg/cc 50 cc vial.

Storage: Metandiabol and Reforvit-B injectables should be protected from light, (keep in the carton until contents are used), and stored at controlled room temperature 15 to 30 degrees C (59 to 86 degrees F). Do not freeze.

Price Range: Metandiabol - approx. $1375.00 pesos for 25 mg/cc 50 cc vial.
Reforvit B - not known for 25 mg/cc 10 cc vial.
- approx. $ 85.00 pesos for 25 mg/cc 50 cc vial, or approx. $639.20 pesos for a case of 50 x 25 mg/cc 50 cc vial.

Type of Drug: Strong Anabolic and Androgenic.

Ingredient: 50 mg Methandrostenolone/methandienone.

Drug Identification:

Metandiabol & Reforvit-B - Unfortunately, Metandiabol could not be obtained for illustration and identification purposes. Both Metandiabol and Reforvit-B are available at veterinarian stores, however, they are very difficult to acquire, and may require to be specially ordered by the veterinarian, as most stores do not have these products in constant stock.

*****Please refer to the photograph of Reforvit-B for full color references.***

Drug Description: *** Metandiabol and Reforvit-B have been commonly referred to as Dianabol for simple-ity measures in the following text.*

The compound of Dianabol previously had been a very desired oral tablet administration substance, that had been utilized by many, many athletes. However, it had been removed from in the market in 1982, due to the high potential of misuse that had appeared to have resulted. Consequently, there have currently been no oral tablet substances available, which had resulted in many athletes having to have perused the veterinarian versions of Dianabol; Metandiabol and Reforvit-B. However, both of these substances had been very difficult to have obtained from the veterinary stores in Mexico.

Metandiabol is a veterinarian version of Dianabol, which had not been listed in the Mexican Veterinary Desk Reference (MVDR). Several athletes had claimed that this product had been a rather unsterile item, therefore, many had been cautiously reluctant to have injected it. Instead, a few athletes had swallowed this substance and had allowed the stomach acids to have neutralized possible germs, in efforts to have obtained the Dianabol's dramatic effects.

Reforvit-B on the other hand, had appeared to have been a well manufactured product, which usually had to have been specially ordered, if an athlete had been interested in having acquired this compound from a veterinarian store. It generally had been available in cases of 50 cc x 50 bottles to a case, and had been quite inexpensive to have purchased. The compound of Reforvit-B had been red in color due to the addition of B vitamins, and one cc had been the equivalent of the 5 previously available Dianabol tablets. However, even though Metandiabol and Reforvit-B had been the only two possible versions of Dianabol that still had been somewhat obtainable in Mexico, several athletes had claimed that the usual effects of dramatic size increases had not seemed to have resulted as dramatically from these non-tablet veterinarian versions.

The former oral tablet version of Dianabol had been a derivative of Testosterone, that had exhibited strong anabolic and androgenic properties, which had generally created dramatic gains in size and strength in practically every athlete who had administered it. Athletes had claimed that there had appeared to have been no direct correlation between the increase of bodyweight, and the amount of the dosage that had been administered. An important reason why Dianabol had produced successful results in all athletes, had been that the endogenous cortisone production had been generally reduced by 50% to 70 %, which had considerably slowed down the rate at which protein had been broken down in the muscle cells. Most athletes had considered the compound of Dianabol to have been a "mass steroid", which had generally worked very rapidly and had been reliable. Many athletes had often experienced a weight increase of 2 to 4 pounds per week in the first six weeks of the administration of Dianabol. The additional body weight had consisted both of an increase in muscle tissue, and a noticeable retention of fluids.

Since the compound of Dianabol's half-life time had only been 3.2 - 4.5 hours, administration at least twice daily had often been necessary to have achieved a somewhat even concentration of the substance in the blood. Athletes who had engaged in strenuous training regimes, often had administered Dianabol three times a day, as the half-time had been even further reduced by the intense training activity. The maximum substance concentration of Dianabol had generally reached the blood after 1 to 3 hours after administration. Evidence of administration of the compound of Dianabol had not been present in the blood after the third day, however, results had differed on urine testing due to the elimination of the metabolites of the substance Methandrostenolone through the excretion of urine; had a longer duration.

Consequently, many athletes had claimed that the greatest disadvantage of the Dianabol compound had been that once it had been discontinued, a considerable loss of strength and mass had frequently resulted, primarily due to the excretion of stored water from the body. However, most athletes had stated that the utilization of Dianabol had offered several beneficial assets in addition to great increases in weight, such as a general well-feeling state, improved mood and increased appetite levels.

Usual Veterinary Recommendation:

Veterinarians often had administered Metandiabol and Reforvit-B intramuscularly in cattle, horses, pigs and sheep, once every three weeks.

Adventitious Dosage and Administration:

The use of Metandiabol and Reforvit-B had been intended for deep intramuscular injection, however, this method had been extremely painful for most humans to have endured. Nevertheless, the best site for this type of injection had been in the gluteus medius muscle area, which had been the upper outer portion of the buttock, approximately 2 to 3 inches below the hip bone (iliac crest). Many athletes had frequently alternated the injections from one side to the other, (first injection on the left side, the second time injection administered on the right, or vice versa) in efforts to have somewhat alleviated pain, and to have allowed the area to have slightly "healed". This practice had often prevented a thick scar tissue from potentially having formed. However, the more injections that had been administered, the greater possibility of scar tissue had often resulted. Some athletes had chosen to have administered the Metandiabol and Reforvit-B solution by mouth, in attempts to have avoided possible injection contamination of unsterile particles, (especially with the Metandiabol solution), and also for the fact that these two substances had produced more productive results when taken orally. This method had also eliminated the painful irritation and burning sensation which often had been experienced with the injection method. Alternatively, many athletes had simply filled two-piece gel-caps with either solution, and then had swallowed this preparation. A common dosage regime of some athletes, has been discussed in the following:

Many athletes had usually co-ordinated the dosage of Dianabol with his/her individual goals, as there had been a wide range of administered dosages; had fluctuated from 1/2 to 8 cc's daily.

Steroid novices usually had required less than a half of a cc or (15 to 20) mgs of Dianabol per day, which had been sufficient to have achieved exceptional results over a period of 8 to 10 weeks. In fact, athletes who had not been ambitious to have competed, had often acquired highly satisfying progress with the use of Dianabol. Consequently, when these athletes had begun to have experienced a decrease in these effects, (which had sometimes occurred within eight weeks), and if they had wished to have continued this treatment, the dosage of Dianabol had not been increased, but instead, the addition of an injectable steroid such as Deca-Durabolin in a dosage of 200 mg/week, or Primobolan in a dosage of 200 mg/week, to the Dianabol dose had been administered. Often, athletes even had entirely switched to either Deca-Durabolin or Primobolan, and totally had terminated the utilization of Dianabol altogether.

Many athletes had not included the administration of Dianabol in their contest preparation regimes due to Dianabol's characteristic of being able to have caused distant water retention. This had usually been experienced as a result of it's high conversion rate into Estrogen, which had often complicated the fat breakdown. However, some athletes had not experienced this problem, or had been able to have controlled it by additionally having had administered Nolvadex or Proviron; which in this phase, had utilized Dianabol together with Parabolan, Winstrol Depot, Masteron, Oxandrolone, (the latter three compounds are currently not available in Mexico) etc. This practice had allowed some athletes to have utilized Dianabol until three to four days before a competition.

Females:

Female athletes often had not engaged in the administration of Dianabol, due to it's characteristic of having contained a distinct androgenic component, in which, considerable virilization symptoms had often occurred. There had been, however, several female athletes in particular, female powerlifters, who had frequently utilized 10 to 20 mg/day of Dianabol, which had resulted in enormous progress in strength increases. Female athletes who did not have a sensitive reaction to the additional intake of androgens, or who had displayed a fear of possible masculinization symptoms, often had administered 1/4 to 3/4 cc's of Dianabol, for usually a period which had not exceeded 4 to 6 weeks. Some female athletes had claimed that higher dosages administered for longer durations of time, had generally resulted in more quantitative increases; however, the androgens often had begun to become noticeable in the female organs, which usually had resulted in the outcome of clitoromegaly. Therefore, many female athletes had avoided dosages of more than 10 mgs/day (approx. 1/4 cc), and 50 to 100 mgs of Deca-Durabolin/week, over 4 to 6 weeks, in efforts to have retained femininity, even if they had chosen to have utilized this steroidal compound.

Males:

Advanced athletes who often had competed, and athletes who had weighed more than 220 lbs, usually had not required more than approximately 1 3/4 cc (40 mg/day), and very seldom had exceeded 2 cc's (50 mg/day) of Dianabol. Many athletes had not increased the number of Dianabol injections immeasurably, as the effects that had been experienced had not doubled if the amount administered had been increased. However, these athletes often had perused a stack of Dianabol approximately just a little more than 2 cc's (20 to 30 mgs) a day, and Deca-Durabolin 4 x 50 mg 1 ml redi-jects to 8 x 50 mgs 1 ml redi-jects a day, which had allegedly produced wondrous achievements.

Many male athletes who's primary interests had been in strength, than in the increase of body mass, had often combined Dianabol with either Oxandrolone or Winstrol tablets (both of these compounds are currently not available in Mexico). These athletes had claimed that the additional intake of an injectable steroid usually had provided close to ultimate results, when they had perused the administration of the injectable form of Dianabol. Usually, in efforts to have built up mass and strength, many athletes had additionally administered Sostenon 250, 1 cc (250 mgs) or Testosterona 200 at 1 cc (200 mgs)+ per week and /or Deca-Durabolin, 4 x 1 ml redi-jects (200 mg +) per week.

Some uneducated athletes had sometimes administered dosages of Dianabol, which had exceeded more than 2 1/2 cc's (60 mg+), however, these athletes had not experienced any benefits, as the continued improper intake of steroids had often proven to have been ineffective. Also, many athletes had reported that the simultaneous intake of Dianabol and Anapolon 50 had not been beneficial either, due to the fact that these two compounds had produced similar effects.

Side Effects:

Although the administration of Dianabol had many potential side effects, they had been generally rare with small dosages of less than one cc per day. However, Dianabol had been liver toxic when it had been administrated in high dosages for long durations, as even a low dosage had been able to have increased the liver values. If liver values had become elevated, they had been able to have returned back to normal, once Dianabol had been discontinued. Also, Dianabol had generally caused a considerable strain on the liver, as it had been 17-alpha alkylated. However, 30 to 50 mgs of Dianabol had been still relatively safe while having been very effective in having produced dramatic results.

Other side effects that had been occasionally encountered had been hypertension, heart palpitations, gynecomastia, increased aggression levels, and acne vulgaris primarily having affected the face, neck, chest, back and shoulders. If athletes had a hereditary predisposition for balding, the administration of Dianabol had often accelerated hair loss, due to the high conversion of the substance into dihydrotestosterone. Also, endogenous Testosterone levels had also been reduced by 30% to 40%, when exogenous administration of Dianabol at a dosage of less than 1 cc had been administered daily for ten days, due to the distinct antigonadotropic effect which had inhibited the release of the gonadotropic FSH and LH by the hypophysis.

These substance of Metandiabol and Reforvit-B, had been intended for the use in veterinarian medicine; therefore, these pharmaceuticals had not been required to have met the same health and safety standards in which human pharmaceuticals had to surpass. The administration of Metandiabol in particular, had been very questionable by most athletes, as it had not been listed in the Mexican Veterinarian drug book, and had appeared to have been created insufficiently. Consequently, severe side effects may have occurred when applied in human self-administration.

WARNING:

The intent of this product had been indicated for use in veterinarian medicine, therefore, these pharmaceuticals had not been required to have met the same health and safety standards in which human pharmaceuticals had to surpass. Consequently, severe side effects may have occurred when applied in human self-administration. However, some other possible side effects may have been experienced which have not been recognized by the athlete, therefore, had not been documented.

Rating:

Based on a 1 to 5 star scale, with 1 considered low, and 5 considered high, a -- symbol is indicative of no value. This compound of Methandrostenolone/ methandienone has rated as the following:

	MALES	FEMALES
Strength Increase	***	***
Mass & Weight Increase	***	**
Contest Preparation	**	*
Side Effects	***	***
Cost Efficiency	*	*

(EQUIPOISE) *VETERINARY*

Chemical Name: Boldenone Undecylenate.

Common Generic Name: Equipoise.

Other Trade Names Found in Mexico:

Crecibol - Unipharm. (International) S.A.
Equi-Gan* - Laboratoios Tormie, S.A.
Maxi-Gan - Mital Pharm S.A.

Dosage Form:

Crecibol - 25 mgs/10 mls.
- 25 mgs/30 mls.
Equi-Gan* - 50 mgs/10 mls.
Maxi-Gan - 50 mgs/50 mls.

Storage: Store at controlled room temperature 15 to 30 degrees C (59 to 86 degrees F). Do not permit to freeze. Protect from light. It is advisable to keep in packaging until use.

Price Range:

Crecibol - approx. $ 36.00 pesos for 10 mls.
- approx. $300.00 pesos for 30 mls.
Equi-Gan* - approx. $140.00 pesos for 10 mls.
Maxi-Gan - approx. $475.00 pesos for 50 mls.

Type of Drug: Strong Anabolic. Moderate Androgenic Steriod.

Ingredient: 25 or 50 mg Boldenone Undecylenate.

Drug Identification:

Crecibol - Is available as an oil-based injectable, with sesame oil as the diluent which can be found within a dark-brown plastic, 10 ml bottle. Each bottle contains 25 mgs of Boldenone Undecylenate, or 25 mg/10 ml, or 25 mg/30 mls. It has a silver, aluminum, tear-off lid with a multiple-injection type lid concealed underneath. Crecibol's label is a sticker of red and yellow, with a white-colored base, with the product's entities written in black ink. The date which it was manufactured, and the expiration date can also be found on the front of the bottle's label. Unipharm's company logo is also displayed on both the bottle and box. The carton which accompanies it, looks identical to the bottle itself. A product insert is not found inside, along with the product.

Equi-Gan* - Is also available as an oil-based injectable, with sesame oil as the diluent, which can be found within a clear, glass 10 ml bottle. Lot # AG099. Each bottle contains 50 mgs of Boldenone Undecylenate, or 50 mgs/10 mls. It has a silver, aluminum, tear-off lid with a multiple-injection type lid concealed underneath. Equi-Gan*'s label is a multi-colored sticker of shades of blue and pinkish-reds, with a white-colored base. The product's entities are written in black ink. Laboratoios Tormie, S.A. company's logo is boldly displayed on the front of the bottle and carton. The carton which accompanies it, also looks identical to the bottle. A product insert written in Spanish is also found within.

Maxigan - Is available as an oil-based injectable, with sesame oil as the diluent, which can be found within a dark brown, glass 50 ml bottle. Lot # CGC08. Each bottle contains 50 mgs of Boldenone Undecylenate, or 50 mgs/50 mls. It too, has a silver, aluminum, tear-off lid with a multiple-injection type lid concealed underneath. Maxigan's label is a sticker of a dark green, with a white-colored base. The product's entities are written in both yellow and black print. Again, the carton which accompanies it, looks identical to the bottle. There is no accompanying product insert.

*****Please refer to the photos of Crecibol, Equi-Gan* and Maxigan, for full color references.***

Drug Description: ***For simplicity measures, Crecibol, Equi-Gan* and Maxi-Gan, have been referred to as Equipoise" in the following text:*

The substance of Equipoise is an oil-based veterinarian steroid, which is a derivative of Testosterone, that had been intended for the administration in horses. Equipoise is a long-acting injectable agent, that had a rapid onset of action which had proven to have been advantageous; as this characteristic had often been preferred over frequent oral dosing or repeated injections. Veterinarians had often used Equipoise as an aid for treating debilitated horses, when an improvement in weight, haircoat, or general condition had been desired. Equipoise, had been able to have increased the appetite of horses, and optimal results had been further obtained when proper diet and good management had also been applied. The application of Equipoise in horses, had frequently resulted in distinct anabolic properties, combined with a certain degree of androgenic activity, which did not have marked antigonadotrophic properties, or had produced any clear-cut effects on the endometrium of the horses (which had been commonly observed when similar substances have been used). Therefore, in veterinarian clinical trials, the administered recommended dosages of the Equipoise injectable had displayed a marked anabolic effect on debilitated horses with an improved appetite, weight gain, increased vigor, and improved musculature and haircoat.

Consequently, many athletes had frequently incorporated the administration of this compound primarily to have also enhanced their size and strength gains. Equipoise had low levels of toxicity, which had allowed it to have been non-toxic to the liver, and only had a slight aromatizing quality, therefore, aromatization effects had frequently varied for each athlete who had participated in it's application. Some athletes had often experienced a moderate aromatizing effect, while others only had only a slight encounter.

Some athletes had claimed that the administration of Equipoise, usually had not resulted in tremendous increases in strength and muscle mass within short periods of time. It had however, a very desirable effect upon the organism's nitrogen balance, which distinctly had increased protein synthesis within the muscle cell. Equipoise also had stimulated the formation of red blood cells (erythropoiesis). The consequent increase in body weight frequently had consisted of a solid quality growth of the muscles, which usually had occurred gradually and symmetrically.

Many athletes additionally had reported that the use of Equipoise also had appeared to have had an impact on having increased appetite levels, which combined together with adequately high quantity of calories and protein, had frequently resulted in increased strength, and rapid increases in quality muscles. These high quality increases, usually had resulted from the low water retention of this compound, and consequently, had become an effective drug which athletes had successively utilized in preparation for competitions. These acquired benefits, had been generally well-maintained over several weeks after the discontinuance of Equipoise substance, by many athletes.

Several athletes had compared the behavior of Equipoise similar to that of the administration of Dianabol. However, the main difference had been that Equipoise in the majority of the cases, had not resulted in as much water retention, as with the administration of Dianabol. Athletes certainly had frequently encountered an improved pump, and increased vascularity during workout sessions, while having administered this veterinarian substance.

Usual Veterinary Recommendation:

The administration of Equipoise had been intended for intramuscular use in horses only. The usual dose had consisted of 0.276-1.1 mg per kg (0.125-0.5 mg/lb) of body weight every 2 to 3 weeks. Most horses had responded with 1 or 2 treatments.

Adventitious Dosage and Administration:

The use of Equipoise, had been intended for deep intramuscular injection (in horses). However, some athletes had adapted this veterinarian pharmaceutical for their own utilization, and had reported that the best site for this type of injection had been in the gluteus medius muscle area, which had been the upper outer portion of the buttock, approximately 2 to 3 inches below the hip bone (iliac crest). Again, many athletes had often alternated the injections from one side to the other, (first injection on the left side, the second time injection administered on the right, or vice versa) in attempts to have somewhat alleviated pain, and to allow the area to have slightly "healed". This practice had often been exercised in efforts to have prevented a thick scar tissue from having potentially formed. However, the more injections that athletes had administered, the greater possibility of scar tissue had usually resulted. A common dosage regime of some athletes, has been discussed in the following:

Some bodybuilders had generally claimed that the administration of Equipoise had been very effective for "cutting", which had been of course, very beneficial prior to contest preparation. These cutting effects had often been further amplified when Equipoise had been stacked with a low androgen such as Primobolan. For this reason, bodybuilders who had also been dieting, had also frequently combined Equipoise with Winstrol Depot (currently, not available in Mexico), and still had experienced a dramatic increase in muscle hardness.

However, if Equipoise had been used in combination with Testosterone, it had generally had proven to have further enhanced the strength increases dramatically. Therefore, many athletes had reported that the administration of Equipoise had produced consistently good results, with few associated side effects.

Females:

Female athletes usually had responded well to the administration of Equipoise, at a dose of approximately 2 to 4 ml, or 2 to 4 cc's (50 to 100) mgs a week. Often, in efforts to have achieved maximum results, this dosage had been divided into multiple injections such as 1 to 2 cc's (25 to 50 mgs) every third day, which usually had provided qualitative muscle gains, with a low water retention potential. A dosage in this range had generally been well tolerated, without the harsh side effects of virilization, by most female athletes.

Males:

For most male athletes, the weekly dosage of Equipoise had generally consisted of approximately 6 to 12 ml, or 6 to 12 cc's (150 to 300 mgs) a week. If the common 25 mgs version which had been found in Mexico had been used, frequent or very voluminous injections had been necessary. Consequently, this often had resulted in inconvenience and painful injection areas due to the required multiple injections. However, for most male athletes, 2 cc's (50 mgs) a week, which had been taken every second day, for a total of approximately 6 cc's per week, appeared to have been sufficient. Advanced and ambitious athletes had often increased their dosages to approximately 2 cc's (50 mgs) daily, in efforts to have achieved dramatic results.

Side Effects:

If an overdose of Equipoise had been administered to a horse, often a prolonged androgenic effect which made the horse difficult to handle had generally resulted. If this had occurred, the treatment of Equipoise had been terminated, until all signs of androgenicity had disappeared.

Some of the associated side effects which had been associated with the veterinarian compound of Boldenone Undecylenate, when used by both female and male athletes had included; somewhat of an ill-feeling which had generally subsided within a couple of days after the initial intake. Hypertension (high blood pressure), had usually not been a problem with the administration of Equipoise, as the water and salt retention had remained relatively low.

With higher dosages of Equipoise, female athletes often especially had experienced virilization symptoms such as hoarsening or deepening of the voice, acne, increased facial and body hair, and an increased sex drive.

Male athletes however, did not seem to have experienced many problems with this compound. However, a few instances had been reported regarding acne, gynecomastia, and increased aggression.

This substance of Equipoise, had been intended for the use in veterinarian medicine; therefore, these pharmaceuticals had not been required to have met the same health and safety standards in which human pharmaceuticals had to have surpassed. Consequently, severe side effects may have occurred when applied in human self-administration. However, some other possible side effects may have been experienced which had not been recognized by the athlete, and therefore, had not been documented.

WARNING:

Equipoise had not been intended for human administration. In veterinarian medicine, the manufacturer had cautioned that this substance of Equipoise be administered in horses only. Equipoise was not to have been injected into horses which had been intended for the use of food, nor in other animals for 21 days prior to slaughter.

Rating:

Based on a 1 to 5 star scale, with 1 considered low, and 5 considered high, a -- symbol is indicative of no value. This compound of Boldenone Undecylenate had rated as the following:

	MALES	FEMALES
Strength Increase	***	***
Mass & Weight Increase	***	***
Contest Preparation	***	***
Appetite Stimulant	***	***
Side Effects	**	***
Cost Efficiency	***	***

LAURABOLIN *VETERINARY*

Chemical Name: Nandrolone Laurate.

Common Generic Name: Laurabolin.

Other Trade Names Found in Mexico:
Laurabolin 20
Laurabolin 50
Fortabol.

Manufacturers:
Laurabolin 20 - Intervet.
Laurabolin 50 - Intervet.
Fortabol - Parfarm, S.A.

Dosage Form:
Laurabolin 20 - 20 mg/10 ml bottle.
- 20 mg/50 ml bottle.
Laurabolin 50 - 50 mg/10 ml bottle.
- 50 mg/50 ml bottle.
Fortabol - 20 mg/10 ml bottle with Vitamin A.
- 20 mg/ 50 ml bottle with Vitamin A.

Storage: Store at controlled room temperature 15 to 30 degrees C (59 to 86 degrees F). Do not permit to freeze. Protect from light. It is advisable to keep in carton until use.

Price Range:
Laurabolin 20 - approx. $ 40.00 pesos for 10 ml bottle.
- approx. $145.00 pesos for 50 ml bottle.
Laurabolin 50 - approx. $ 85.00 pesos for 10 ml bottle.

		- approx. $325.00 pesos for 50 ml bottle.
	Fortabol	- approx. $ 37.00 pesos for 10 ml bottle with Vitamin A.
		- approx. $263.00 pesos for 50 ml bottle with Vitamin A.

Type of Drug: Anabolic Steriod.

Ingredient: 20 or 50 mgs of Nandrolone Laurate.
20 mgs of Nandrolone Laurate with Vitamin A.

Drug Identification:

Laurabolin 20 **-** Is available as an oil-based injectable, which can be found within a dark-brown glass, 10 ml or 50 ml bottle. Each bottle contains 20 mgs of Nandrolone Laurate, or 20 mgs/10 ml, or 20 mgs/50 mls. Both versions have a silver, aluminum, tear-off lid with a multiple-injection type lid concealed underneath. Lot # M5732. The 50 ml bottle, however, also has a yellow-swirl over the aluminum. Lot # M5745. Laurabolin 20's label is a sticker of a white-colored base, with a red and green stripe on the front, with the product's entities written in black ink. Intervet's company logo is also displayed on both the bottle and the carton. The accompanying package, look identical to the bottles themselves, with the exception of the 10 ml version, which has an additional two green stripes, for a total of three, and one red stripe. A package insert is found inside, along with the product, of course, written in Spanish.

Laurabolin 50 **-** Is also available as an oil-based injectable, which can be found within a dark-brown glass, 10 ml or 50 ml bottle. Each bottle contains 50 mgs of Nandrolone Laurate, or 50 mgs/10 ml, or 50 mgs/50 mls. Both versions have a tear-off lid with a multiple-injection type lid concealed underneath. However, the 10 ml bottle lid is silver and aluminum. Lot # M5746. The 50 ml bottle lid is somewhat of a medium brown color. Lot # M5580. Laurabolin 50's label is a sticker of a white-colored base, the 10 ml version has a thick green stripe with a somewhat smaller red stripe underneath. The 50 ml bottle looks somewhat similar to the Laurabolin 20's bottle version. The product's entities are written in black ink. Intervet's company logo is also displayed on both the bottle and package box. The accompanying packages, look identical to the bottles themselves. A package insert is found inside, along with the product, of course, written in Spanish.

Fortabol - Is also available as another oil-based injectable, which can be found within a dark-brown glass, 10 ml or 50 ml bottle. Each bottle contains 20 mgs of Nandrolone Laurate, with the addition of Vitamin A, or 20 mgs/10 ml, Lot # EG 0696, or 20 mgs/50 ml bottle. The bottle has a white sticker which displays the product's entities in blue, black, red, and white ink. There is a medium blue box on the front with a red stripe located over top. Fortabol has a silver aluminum tear-off lid which conceals a multiple-injection type lid underneath. The accompanying package is identical to the bottle itself. There is no accompanying product insert.

*****Please refer to the photographs of Laurabolin 20, 50, and Fortabol, for full color references.***

Drug Description:

The different variations of Laurabolin are injectable anabolic steriodal compounds, which had been intended for veterinary utilization in animals such as dogs and cats, pigs, lambs and horses. It is available in different strengths, and the Fortabol version also had contained an additional Vitamin A compound. These compounds had produced a long anabolism action, as they had contained the anabolism Estrogen 19-nor-androstenolone, which had acted specifically to have promoted the synthesis of proteins, without the production of undesired secondary effects. Laurabolin and Fortabol also had promoted the building of tissues, and had stimulated the cellular protein synthesis, which had allowed for the prevention of the loss protein through the excretion of urea.

Veterinarians had often administered Laurabolin or Fortabol to animals in efforts to have corrected metabolic deficiencies, slow maturation, malnutrition, anemias, and the after effects of bacterial, viral, or parasitic infections.

As Laurabolin and Fortabol had similar effects as other androlones such as Deca-Durabolin, Anadur and Durabolin (currently, both latter compounds are not available in Mexico), several athletes had often also had engaged in it's properties. The main difference between these mentioned steriodal compounds had been the duration of their effects in the system. In animals, the administration of Laurabolin and Fortabol had displayed long-term and continuous anabolic effects, as these substances had been able to have remained active in the system for approximately 21 days. This characteristic had enabled the promotion of the production of red blood cells, and the maintenance of proper levels of calcium and phosphorous.

Another benefit of Laurabolin or Fortabol, was that it had been relatively lower in price compared to Deca-Durabolin. Consequently, several athletes had claimed that one of the great disadvantages of this veterinarian compound, had been that it had been available in only small mg entities such as 20 to 50 mgs in each milliliter. Another somewhat of a disadvantage of the Fortabol version had also been that it had been poorly soluble in oil, therefore, many athletes had required many cc's of oil in order to have reached usual required injectable quantities. This of course, had often resulted in a more frequent and voluminous dosage administration, which most athletes had discovered to have been inconvenient, and painful. Despite these slight differences, most athletes had chosen the administration of Deca-Durabolin over Laurabolin, if the option had been presented.

The administration of Laurabolin or Fortabol had also been frequently utilized amongst female athletes, as these compounds had been the only steroidal items which had not produced virilizing effects. Also, if these items had been used in conservative, therapeutic dosages, it also had not promoted water or sodium retention. Consequently, if athletes had experienced an improvement of their physical condition and weight gain, it had not been due as a result of water retention. As Laurabolin and Fortabol had been able to have stored more water in the connective tissues, it had also temporarily eased, or even had cured existing pain in joints; which often had allowed sore elbows, shoulders, knees etc., to have been alleviated. If Laurabolin or Fortabol had been utilized in reasonable dosages, it had dramatically improved the nitrogen cortisone to have reached the muscle cells and the connective tissue cells. These compounds not only had improved the nitrogen retention, but also had appeared to have lessened the recuperation time that had generally been required between training periods. Therefore, most athletes had been able to have achieved desirable results which had been similar to those which had been experienced with the use of Deca-Durabolin. *(Please refer to Deca-Durabolin for further information).*

Usual Veterinary Recommendation:

Most veterinarians had administrated Laurabolin or Fortabol intramuscularly in dogs, cats, pigs, lambs or horses at 1 ml x every 20 kg. The maximum dosage had been 20 ml (400 mg). This was not to have been repeated sooner than 21 days, nor administered in gestational, or lactating animals.

Adventitious Dosage and Administration:

These versions which had contained the Nandrolone Laurate ingredient, had been intended for deep intramuscular injection. The best site for this type of injection had been in the gluteus medius muscle area, which had been the upper outer portion of the buttock approximately 2 to 3 inches below the hip bone (iliac crest). Most athletes had wisely alternated the injections from one side to the other, (first injection on the left side, the second time injection administered on the right, or vice versa) not only because it had been somewhat less painful, but had also permitted the area to have slightly "healed", in further attempts to have prevented a thick scar tissue from having potentially formed. The more injections that had been administered, the greater possibility of scar tissue had generally resulted. A common dosage regime of some athletes, has been discussed in the following:

Although one single injection would have been hypothetically sufficient due to Laurabolin's and Fortabol's long duration effect in the system, it unfortunately, had not often been adequate enough to have produced desired athletic or bodybuilding enhancement qualities. Therefore, most athletes had often administered these compounds on a weekly bases, and usually had acquired satisfactory results when sufficient dosages had been injected.

Females:

Female athletes usually had administered approximately 100 to 200 mgs (which if the Laurabolin 20, or Fortabol version had been administered, would have been equivalent to 5 to 10 ml, or 5 to 10 cc's) a week, to ten days. If the Laurabolin 50 version had been administered, this would have been the equivalent to 2 to 4 ml, or 2 to 4 cc's weekly, to every ten days.

Males:

Male athletes generally had administered between 200 to 400 mgs on a weekly basis. Many athletes had claimed that a considerable disadvantage of the Laurabolin 20 or Fortabol version had been administered, that this would have been the equivalent to 10 to 20 mls, or 10 to 20 cc's once a week!!

However, if Laurabolin 50 had been administered instead, it would still have totaled an amount of 4 to 8 ml, or 4 to 8 cc's which would have been required to be injected on a weekly basis. Consequently, an adequate dosage of 2 ml or 2 cc's, twice a week, had warranted desirable results for most administering male athletes.

Side Effects:

As previously mentioned, potential side effects which may have been experienced from these veterinarian steriodal compounds, had been very similar to those associated with the same ill effects from having utilized the Nandrolone Decanoate (Deca-Durabolin). However, there may have also been a numerous amount of other side effects related to the use of a product that had been intended for the use of animals, within human beings. Unfortunately, they may not have been precisely documented, or for that matter, even considered or discovered as ill effects when applied in human utilization.

Some of the known side effects which had been experienced by both female and male athletes had frequently included nausea, leukopenia, symptoms resembling those of a peptic ulcer, acne, edema, excitation, sleeplessness, chills, vomiting, diarrhea, hypertension, prolonged blood clotting time, and an increased libido.

Some of the side effects which had been peculiar to especially females if they had administered Laurabolin or Fortabol in high, excessive amounts included those of virilization such as menstrual irregularities, post-menopausal bleeding, swelling of the breasts, hoarseness or deepening of the voice, enlargement of the clitoris, and water retention.

Some of the side effects which had sometimes been experienced by a few male athletes had included those of impotence, chronic priapism, epididymitis, inhibition of testicular function, oligospermia, and bladder irritability. Potential problems of gynecomastia had usually been rare, as well as the incidence of hair loss. These compounds also had minimal liver toxicity, and only had aromatized in excessive dosages. Laurabolin and Fortabol had an effect on the body's natural hormone level, however, it had not been nearly as pronounced as it had been with other drugs such as Testosterone.

WARNING:

The intent of these products had been indicated for use in veterinarian medicine, therefore, these pharmaceuticals had not been required to have met the same health and safety standards in which human pharmaceuticals had to have surpassed. Consequently, severe side effects may have occurred when applied in human self-administration. However, some other possible side effects may have been experienced which have not been recognized by the athlete, and therefore, had not been documented.

Rating:

Based on a 1 to 5 star scale, with 1 considered low, and 5 considered high, a -- symbol is indicative of no value. This compound of Nandrolone Laurate had rated as the following:

	MALES	FEMALES
Strength Increase	**	****
Mass & Weight Increase	***	***
Side Effects	**	**
Cost Efficiency	***	***

NORANDREN 50 *VETERINARY*

Chemical Name: Nandrolone Decanoate.

Common Generic Name: Norandren 50.

Other Trade Names Found in Mexico: Deca-Durabolin (human).
Norandren 50.

Manufacturer: Norandren 50 - Brovel.

Dosage Form: Norandren 50 - 50 mg/ml.
- 10 ml/50 ml.

Storage: Store at controlled room temperature 15 to 30 degrees C (59 to 86 degrees F). Do not permit to freeze. Protect from light. It is advisable to keep in packaging until use.

Price Range: Norandren 50 - not known.

Type of Drug: Anabolic Steriod.

Ingredient: 50 mgs of Nandrolone Decanoate.

Drug Identification:

Norandren 50 - for injectable administration could not be obtained for illustration and identification purposes. However, this product is still available on a limited basis in some veterinarian stores, and may require several attempts at various outlets.

Drug Description:

Norandren 50 is a sterile solution of Nandrolone Decanoate, which is a derivative of 19-Nortestosterone; considered to be a long acting anabolic agent. It is an oil-based (dileunt is sesame oil), intramuscular injectable. Both the human and veterinary versions of Nandrolone Decanoate, Deca-Durabolin and Norandren 50, had been considered to have been the most widely used steroidal compounds of choice amongst most athletes. The drug itself, is a moderate androgen and a highly anabolic preparation.

The administration of Norandren 50 had frequently proven to have been an excellent product for the promotion of size and strength gains, as it had allowed the muscle cells to have stored more nitrogen than it had released. This had permitted a positive nitrogen balance to have been achieved. It had been well known that a positive nitrogen balance had often been synonymous with muscle growth, as when the muscle cell had been in this phase, it had been able to have accumulated a greater amount of protein than usual. However, a positive nitrogen balance and the protein building effect which had generally accompanied it, had only occurred if enough calories and protein had been additionally supplied. Therefore, athletes had to have ensured that proper protein and caloric intake had also been obtained in efforts to have received the full benefits of the Nandrolone Decanoate compound.

Consequently, at the same time, some athletes had occasionally experienced considerable water retention if they had administered high doses of this drug, which had generally resulted in a smooth and watery-type appearance of the muscles. However, most athletes had claimed that if Norandren 50 had been utilized in conservative dosages, it had dramatically improved the nitrogen cortisone to have reached the muscle cells and the connective tissue cells. As the compound of Norandren 50 had also been able to have stored more water in the connective tissues, it had been also able to have temporarily eased, or even had cured existing pain in joints; which had allowed sore elbows, shoulders, knees etc., to have been alleviated. The administration of Norandren 50 had not only improved the nitrogen retention, but many athletes had claimed that it had also improved the recuperation time between training periods.

Although Norandren 50 had an effect on the body's natural hormone levels, it's effects had not been as great as those which had been frequently experienced from the exogenous administration of Testosterones. Unfortunately, the substance of Nandrolone Decanoate had possessed very stubborn metabolites, which had often appeared in steroidal compound testing, even as long as 18 months after it had last been administrated. This, along with the Norandren 50's vast gaining popularity, had generally contributed to it's presence on steroid testing, to have been greater than any other compound. Obviously, most athletes had not engaged in the administration of Norandren 50 in competitions where drug testing had been prevalent. Even though Norandren 50 had been increasingly difficult to obtain, it had still remained to have been the number one choice as a steroidal compound; amongst athletes who had not required substance testing prior to a competition.

Usual Veterinary Recommendation:

The usual veterinary application had been for cattle, 20 mgs every 10 kg of weight, every 21 days intramuscularly.

Adventitious Dosage and Administration:

The use of Norandren 50 had been intended for deep intramuscular injection. The best site for this type of injection had primarily been in the gluteus medius muscle area, which had been the upper outer portion of the buttock, approximately 2 to 3 inches below the hip bone (iliac crest). Most athletes had often alternated injections from one side to the other, (first injection on the left side, the second time injection administered on the right, or vice versa) in attempts to have alleviated pain somewhat, and to possibly allow the area to have slightly "healed". This practice had generally prevented a thick scar tissue from potentially having formed. However, the more injections that had been administered, the greater possibility of scar tissue had often resulted. A common dosage regime of some athletes, has been discussed in the following:

This veterinarian steroid had frequently been administered by many bodybuilders for "cutting and bulking". The utilization of Norandren 50 had also proven to have been beneficial in untested contest preparations. Results had generally been evident from the administration of 2 mgs/pound of body weight. If water retention had become problematic, it had often been counteracted with the additional administration of anti-Estrogenic compounds such as Nolvadex, combined with Proviron.

Females:

Several female athletes had frequently administered dosages of approximately 50 to 100 mgs per week, (5 to 10 cc's, or 5 to 10 mls). The combination of Norandren 50 at approximately 50 mgs or more, (5 + cc's or 5 + mls) weekly, with Oxandrolone (currently, not available in Mexico), at approximately 10+ mgs daily, had also been another favorite stack of steroidal compounds. If the dosage had been generally kept at a relatively low range such as these, then the potential masculization ill-effects had been kept to a low minimum, which of course, had always been ultimately desired by females.

Other also possible stacks that had been utilized by female athletes had sometimes included the administration of Norandren 50 stacked with Winstrol tablets (currently, not available in Mexico), or Primobolan tablets. If women however, had experienced ill-effects even at low dosages of Norandren 50, they had usually discontinued this compound, and had often switched to Deca-Durabolin, or another milder steroidal compound.

Males:

The average dosage for male athletes had generally been in the area of 200 to 400 mgs (4 to 8 cc's, or 4 to 8 mls) per week. Norandren 50 had often been compatibly stacked with practically every other known steroidal drug compound for positive results, as it had appeared to have been an excellent base drug for male athletes, who had engaged in any cycle. Norandren 50 at 200 to 400 mgs (4 to 8 cc's, or 4 to 8 mls) a week, stacked with Metandiabol or Reforvit-B, 15 to 40 mgs (approximately 1/2 to 3/4 cc, or mls) daily, or Norandren 50 to 400 mgs (8 cc's or 8 mls) weekly and Sostenon 250 at 500 mgs (2 cc's or 2 mls) weekly, or greater yet, Norandren 400 mgs (8 cc's or 8 mls) weekly, with Sostenon 250 at 500 mgs (2 cc's or 2 mls) with Metandiabol or Reforvit-B 30 mgs (approximately 1 cc and a bit, as 1 cc is equivalent to 25 mgs) daily, had often produced rapid and strong increases in muscle mass. The anabolic and buildup effect of Norandren 50 to a certain degree, had depended on the dosage. If more than 600 mgs a week had been administered, the risk/benefit factor had been greatly increased, which had generally resulted in greater ill effects, than positive results.

Side Effects:

Some of the known side effects which had been occasionally experienced by both female and male athletes had included nausea, leukopenia, symptoms resembling those of a peptic ulcer, acne, edema, excitation, sleeplessness, chills, vomiting, diarrhea, hypertension, prolonged blood clotting time, and an increased libido.

Some of the side effects which had been peculiar to especially women if they had administered Norandren 50 in high, excessive amounts had included virilization effects such as menstrual irregularities, post-menopausal bleeding, swelling of the breasts, hoarseness or deepening of the voice, enlargement of the clitoris, and water retention.

Males who had also administered Norandren 50, had occasionally experienced adverse effects such as impotence, chronic priapism, epididymitis, inhibition of testicular function, oligospermia, and bladder irritability. Norandren 50's conversion to the dihydro form called dihydronandrolone (not Dihydrotestosterone), through the action of 5-alpha reductase, actually had allowed this compound to have been less androgenic after it had been converted. This entity had enabled this compound to have been less likely to have caused any hair loss, as Nandrolone Decanoatc only had been able to have converted to Estrogen at about 20% of the rate which Testosterone did. This had also greatly reduced the potential for possible gynecomastia. This compound also had minimal liver toxicity, and only had aromatized in excessive dosages. Norandren 50 did have an effect on the body's natural hormone level, however, it had not been nearly as pronounced as it had been with steroidal compounds such as Testosterone.

This substance of Norandren 50, had been intended for the use in veterinarian medicine; therefore, these pharmaceuticals had not been required to have met the same health and safety standards in which human pharmaceuticals had to surpass. Consequently, severe side effects may have occurred when applied in human self-administration. However, some other possible side effects may have been experienced which had not been recognized by the athlete, therefore, had not been documented.

WARNING:

Caution should be practiced in those with cardiac, renal or hepatic disease.

Rating:

Based on a 1 to 5 star scale, with 1 considered low, and 5 considered high, a -- symbol is indicative of no value. This compound of Nandrolone Decanoate had rated as the following:

	MALES	FEMALES
Strength Increase	***	***
Mass & Weight Increase	***	***
Side Effects	***	
Cost Efficiency	Not known	Not known

RALGROW VETERINARY

Chemical Name: Zeranol.

Common Generic Name: Ralgrow.

Other Trade Names Found in Mexico: Currently, just Ralgrow.

Manufacturer: Ralgrow - Pitman-Moore.

Dosage: Ralgrow - 24 small pellets in dosing cartridge.

Storage: Ralgrow pellets should be protected from light and moisture, (keep in the carton and plastic wrap until contents are used), and stored at controlled room temperature 15 to 30 degrees C (59 to 86 degrees F). Do not freeze.

Price Range: Ralgrow - approx. $338.00 pesos for 24 pellet cartridge.

Type of Drug: Anabolic agent.

Ingredient: 72 mgs of Zeranol.

Drug Identification:

Ralgrow - is available in 24 small pellets, which are individually placed within a dispenser, similar to that of a "Russian roulette wheel". The wheel itself, is a dark, reddish-brown color, and the pellets themselves are approximately 1/2" in height, and are somewhat of an off-whitish color. The wheel including the pellets, is packaged in plastic. The Ralgrow box is colorful, with a light gray backing, and Ralgrow's product entities and a picture of the wheel and pellets on the front. There is also a small picture of the animals (a horse, cow, pig, sheep, dog, cat and a chicken) beside the Manufacturer's name, Pitman-Moore. This symbol is the Pitman-Moore company's logo.

*****Please refer to the photographs of Ralgrow, for full color references.***

Drug Description:

Veterinarians had often utilized the compound of Ralgrow in efforts to have induced weight in cattle by having administered these small pellets with a type of device which had injected them behind the animal's ear. Zeranol had acted by having stimulated the pituitary gland in the brain to have produced more of it's own natural Growth Hormone, Somatotropin. Maximum results had often occurred in cattle who had been parasite disease free, from good quality stock, and had been on a good plane of nutrition. The pellets had been packaged within a barrel-type of distributor, similar in appearance to that of a roulette cartridge. In cattle, Ralgrow had appeared to have been effective and generally had been more acceptable for perusal for beef products, as opposed to steroidal compounds.

However, as Ralgrow had often provided adequate results for cattle, unfortunately, the same had not applied for humans. The application of Zeranol had tended to have been only effective in animals with gastric structures, such as those found in cattle. There had also been the possibility, that the weight increase experienced in these animals, may not have necessarily been from increased muscle mass, but perhaps from increased visceral mass.

Therefore, reports that Ralgrow had beneficially provided results in human application may have been somewhat disillusioned, as this substance had usually been crushed and reconstituted with other injectable steroidal compounds; therefore, results had generally been obtained from the latter.

Usual Veterinarian Recommendation:

Usually one pellet had been administered subcutaneously behind the cow's ear, once every four months.

Adventitious Dosage and Administration:

Some athletes, had utilized the compound of Ralgrow by having the small pellets ground into a fine powder substance, and then mixed with either sterile water, cottonseed oil, or into another steriodal injectable. Crushing these pellets had been often achieved by having placed one on the back of a hard surface with a piece of paper or foil cover, and then by having applied pressure with the back of a spoon (much like crushing an aspirin tablet). Once a powder substance had been acquired, it had then been reconstituted with approximately 2 cc's of either oil or sterile water, and poured into the back of an open sterile syringe. This had then been shaken together vigorously. After the solution had appeared to have been liquefied, it had then been pulled back into the syringe and had been considered ready to have been injected intramuscularly, usually in the gluteal area.

However, these Ralgrow particles could usually have been only crushed to a certain degree, consequently, the injectable syringe size had to have been rather large; approximately an 18 gauge needle or lower, to have accommodated the solution. For virtually all administering athletes, this had often presented a painful, annoying injection, as not only had the needle been large, but often had become clogged, so that added pressure had been necessary to have injected all of this mixture into the injection site.

Females
& Males:

Both genders of athletes usually had not incorporated the compound of Ralgrow into their athletic enhancement regimes. There had been much more effective and safer veterinary compounds available, which had been compatible for human use. However, some athletes had altered the structure of this pellet into an injectable solution by having followed the above methods, usually 3 pellets x 3 times a week.

Side Effects:

As this compound of Zeranol had been frequently utilized and definitely highly unrecommended by many athletes, there had probably been sufficient potential side effects which may had ensued from having utilized a product which had been intended strictly for the use in cattle only.

Some of these side effects may have included gastrointestinal discomfort, and possibly even damage. Other harmful effects could have also become apparent, since Ralgrow had also been an unsterile compound. There had probably been many other associated risks with the administration of Ralgrow within humans, most of which have presumably, been not identified. Cautious athletes often had not engaged in the utilization of this veterinarian product, in efforts to have prevented all conceivable health hazards.

WARNING:

This compound should have been left for the utilization of veterinarians for having increased mass in cattle. Ralgrow had not been considered to have been a sterile product. Consequently, most athletes wisely had not injected unsterile compounds into their systems.

In veterinarian application, it had been advised not to have been used in cattle that had been intended for breeding. Ralgrow pellets had also been cautioned to have been implanted in the ear only. Any other location on an animal, may have resulted in a violation of the law.

Rating:

Based on a 1 to 5 star scale, with 1 considered low, and 5 considered high, a -- symbol is indicative of no value. This compound of Zeranol had rated as the following:

	MALES	FEMALES
Side Effects	*****	*****
Cost Efficiency	***	**

SYNOVEX*-H *VETERINARY*

Chemical Name: Testosterone Propionate, Estradiol Benzoate.

Common Generic Name: Synovex*-H.

Other Trade Names Found in Mexico: Currently, just Synovex*-H.

Manufacturer: Synovex*-H - Syntex.

Dosage Form: Synovex*-H - 50 pellets.

Storage: Synovex*-H pellets should be protected from light and moisture, (keep in the carton until

	contents are used), and stored at controlled room temperature 15 to 30 degrees C (59 to 86 degrees F).
Price Range:	Synovex*-H - approx. $724.00 pesos for 50 pellets.
Type of Drug:	Hormone Implant.
Ingredient:	200 mgs Testosterone Propionate, 20 mgs Estradiol benzoate.

Drug Identification:

Synovex*-H - pellets are available in 5 disks of 10 pellets each, for a total of 50 pellets in each box. The pellets are approximately 3" in height, and are of a whitish-colored nature. They are embedded separately into a light blue dispenser, similar to the nature of a "Russian roulette cartridge". Plastic then conceals all five dispensers. Lot # 040513. The accompanying package is black and white, with a yellow line through the upper third portion. Synovex*-H's entities are displayed on the front, including the manufacturer's name of Syntex, along with Syntex's symbol. A package insert is included in the package, along with the pellets.

*****Please refer to the photograph of Synovex-H* for full color references.***

Drug Description:

Synovex*-H had been intended for the veterinarian application for administration in efforts to have increased weight gain, and feed efficiency in heifers. Evidently, the correct ratio for maximal growth had been 10:1:1, which, for every ten parts Testosterone, there had been ideally an additional one part Estrogen, and one part Progesterone. Cattle had frequently grown larger with the addition of Estrogen.

Recently, there have been studies which had indicated that the steroids which had been more easily converted into Estrogen (aromatization), had in turn, caused more IGF-1 to have been produced in the body. Similarly, as when males had became older, there had been more aromatization in the body, as the levels of Testosterone had easily readily converted to Estrogen. Increased Estrogen levels had then lead to an increase of over 50% in the number of androgen receptors. Consequently, female athletes who had engaged in the administration of steroidal compounds, had generally displayed greater comparative androgenic and anabolic effects, then the male athletes. Evidently, female athletes had experienced these benefits due to the increased levels of Estrogen within their bodies; which had increased the amount of androgen receptors throughout the body.

Therefore, many athletes had engaged in the preparation of a topical solution of Synovex*-H, through the application aided by the DMSO compound or through an intramuscular injection. These practices had often enhanced mass increases, then just the sole utilization of the Testosterone compound. Unfortunately, a few male athletes had encountered problems with gynecomastia along with their period of great growth due to the additional amount of administered Estrogen. The additional amount of Estrogen had often also caused the brain to have shut down the stimulating hormones, which had been responsible for the Testosterone secretion, therefore, the testicles had frequently shrunk down in size.

To many athletes, this 10:1:1 ratio had appeared to have been tempting, however, the additional administration of Estrogen had been able to have caused alot of harm, especially to the immune system in both athletic genders.

Consequently, a few athletes had intelligently discovered a way to have removed the Estrogen from the 10:1:1 ratio, in attempts to have lessened the problematic Estrogenic adverse effects. Some athletes had been successfully able to have extracted the Estrogen from the Synovex*-H compound by the addition of approximately 50 ml of diethyl ether to the ground up mixture of approximately 2 to 3 implants. After this combination had been mixed together well, the filtrate had then been allowed to have slowly evaporated, until crystals had started to form. These crystal had usually been the Estradiol Benzoate extract.

When athletes had observed the formation of these crystals in the ether solution, it had then been placed in the freezer overnight, as the cold had aided the Estrogen to have crystallized and precipitate out of the solution. The ether on the other hand, did not freeze. The next morning, the Estriol had crystallized, and had risen to the top. These crystals had then been filtered out and had been either scraped away, or had been left to have evaporated completely, having left behind highly pure concentrated Testosterone Propionate crystals. These remaining crystals had then been placed in a 200 degree F oven for a few hours, in further efforts to have removed any residual ether. Athletes had been cautious to have only had placed completely dry Testosterone Propionate crystals which had ideally been dried at room temperature, due to the easy flammability characteristics of ether.

Although this practice had not removed all of the Estradiol Benzoate from the Synovex*-H compound, it had sufficed most athletes who primarily had only desired the Testosterone substance within this combination. If male athletes had utilized Synovex*-H without having extracted the Estrogen, it had often resulted in severe gynecomastia.

Usual Veterinarian Recommendation:

Usually one pellet had been administered subcutaneously behind the cow's ear. Synovex*-H had generally been administered once in a lifetime, one pellet per animal, 10 mg per 185-400 kg. The maximal growth potential had been accomplished by the dosage of 10:1:1, which had meant that every ten parts of Testosterone, there had ideally been one part Estrogen and one part Progesterone.

Adventitious Dosage and Administration:

Some athletes had utilized the veterinarian Synovex*-H compound by having ground up the small pellets into a fine powder substance, and having this mixed with either sterile water, cottonseed oil, or into another steriodal injectable. Crushing these pellets had been achieved by having placed one on the back of a hard surface with a piece of paper or foil cover, and then having had applied pressure with the back of a spoon (much like crushing an aspirin tablet). Once a powder substance had been achieved, it had then been reconstituted with approximately 2 cc's of either oil or sterile water, and poured into the back of an open sterile syringe. Then this combination had been shaken together vigorously. After the solution had appeared to have been liquefied, it was then pulled back into the syringe, ready to have been injected intramuscularly, usually in the gluteal area.

However, since the Synovex*-H particles could only have been crushed to a certain degree, the injectable syringe size usually had to have been rather large; approximately an 18 gauge needle or lower, to have accommodated the solution. This often had provided a painful, annoying injection as not only had the needle been large, but often it had become clogged, so that added pressure had been additionally required to have injected all this mixture into the injection site.

The compound of Synovex*-H had originally been intended for veterinarian utilization, however, several athletes had altered the pellet form into a solution for deep intramuscular injection. However, since the administration of Testosterone Propionate slightly had swelled the site of injection, several lagging bodyparts such as the arms, shoulders, and the calf areas had been often substituted for this injection. Despite this temporary benefit, these areas had become usually much too painful and inconvenient for repeated injection use, especially since a large needle of an 18 gauge or lower had to have been used for administration. Consequently, the best site for the injection of Synovex-H, had been primarily in the gluteus medius muscle area, which had been the upper outer portion of the buttock, approximately 2 to 3 inches below the hip bone (iliac crest). Most athletes had alternated the injections from one side to the other, (first injection on the left side, the second time injection administered on the right, or vice versa) to slightly have alleviated pain, which had also often allowed the area to have slightly "healed". This practice had also often prevented a thick scar tissue from potentially having formed. However, the more injections that had been administered, the greater possibility of scar tissue had frequently resulted.

Another method which some athletes had engaged in efforts to have avoided painful intramuscular injections, had been conceivable by the assistance of the DMSO compound. Dimethyl sulfoxide (DMSO) had been one of few substances which had been fully absorbed through the skin, which had allowed the skin to have become permeable to other substances which could have been distributed through the body.

One possible way in which many athletes had applied this compound topically, had been by finely having ground up 2 to 3 pellets by having placed them on the back of a hard surface with a piece of paper or foil cover, and then pressure had been applied with the back of a spoon (much like crushing an aspirin tablet). Then, it had been mixed with a half a teaspoon of DMSO gel, a thin layer had then been applied to the skin, and finally, the selected area had been covered with a piece of "Saran" plastic wrap. This had allowed for a "warming" of this mixture, which had further enabled for quicker absorption into the system. It had been important that it had been applied, and NOT rubbed into the skin. One or two applications had usually sufficed. Athletes had generally claimed that it had been best to apply for approximately 20 to 40 minutes in efforts to have achieved the full effect. A common dosage regime of some athletes has been discussed in the following:

Females:

Female athletes had occasionally utilized the adjusted version of Synovex*-H, in the range of 25 to 50 mgs (1 to 2 cc's, or 1 to 2 mls), every 5 to 7 days. If dosages or frequency intervals had exceeded these amounts, better results had usually been obtained. However, this had often resulted in the dramatic increase of potential virilization side effects.

Therefore, many female athletes had been careful to have limited the duration of intake; which had not exceeded 8 to 10 weeks. Instead, this dosage had been supplemented by mild and mostly anabolic steriodal compounds such as Primobolan, Durabolan, and Anadur (the latter two compounds, are currently not available in Mexico). This stack had been administered in order to have promoted the synthesis of protein.

Males:

Some male athletes had entertained the adjusted version of Synovex*-H in initiating dosages in the range of 50 to 100 mgs (2 to 4 cc's, or 2 to 4 mls), on alternate days. Many male athletes had claimed that this had been advantageous due to the rapid initial effect of the Propionate-ester, as a several week duration could have been started with this compound. Most male athletes had been careful in only having administered conservative dosages of this compound, as there had still been a small degree of Estradiol Benzoate left having remained within this altered compound.

Anxious users who had been impatient for the depot steroids to have taken effect, had sometimes injected Primoteston Depot 250 mgs (1 cc, or 1 ml), and 50 mgs of Synovex*-H, at 50 mgs, at the beginning of the cycle. Then, when the effect of the Testosterone Propionate had decreased, another 50 mgs had been injected, usually within a two to three day duration. Two days after that, elevated Testosterone levels which had been caused by the Synovex*-H had often begun to have decreased, which had represented the effect of Enanthate in the system. This characteristic therefore, had frequently eliminated the need of further injections. This had also been indicative of a high Testosterone level, which had been reached and maintained for a long time, due to the depot Testosterone.

Another possible option which had frequently been used for the entire period of intake, had been 50 to 100 mgs every day, or every second day. This dosage had seemed to have lowered the problematic side effect of water retention, which had often been experienced with the Depot Testosterones. Several male athletes had remarked that muscle mass had often been achieved by having administered the altered compound of Synovex*-H at 100 mgs (1/2 cc or 1/2 ml) x 2 days, Winstrol Depot (currently, not available in Mexico) at 50 mgs x 2 days, and Metandiabol or Reforvit-B at 30 mgs x daily. A combination of 100 mg of altered Synovex*-H 100 mgs every 2 to 3 days, either Winstrol Depot 50 mgs (currently, not available in Mexico), per day, or Parabolon 76 mgs every 2 days, and of Oxandrolone 25 mgs daily (these latter two compounds are not currently available in Mexico), had allegedly helped many athletes to have achieved this goal, while also having increased qualitative muscle mass.

Side Effects:

Side effects which had been occasionally reported in implanted heifers had included bulling, vaginal and rectal prolapsed, udder development, ventral edema and elevated tailheads.

The side effects which had been occasionally experienced by some athletes from the administration of the altered compound of Synovex*-H had been similar to those which had been sometimes experienced from other Testosteronal compounds such as Testosterona* 200 and Testosterone Cypionate (currently, not available in Mexico, as a sole entity). The main difference which had separated the altered compound of Synovex*-H from this group, had been the fact that these ill effects had occurred less frequently when they had been administered in lower dosages. Both female and male athletes had similarly experienced an increase in sex drives.

However, if high dosages had been entertained, and there had been a pre-existing predisposition for certain problems such as acne, male pattern baldness, increased facial and body hair, increased libido, and deepening of the voice had often resulted. The possibility of gynecomastia had been been very likely to have resulted from the original form of Synovex*-H, and even slightly with the altered compound. Also, potential water retention had also been low, since the retention of electrolytes and water had been less pronounced.

Several athletes had also administered Testosterone-stimulating compounds such as HCG and Clomid along with Synovex*-H. This had a strong influence on the hypothalamohypophysial testicular axis, which had been able to have suppressed the endogenous hormone production. To combat the problematic and annoying effects of water retention, many athletes had utilized the combination of Nolvadex and Proviron. Liver damage had also been rarely experienced due to the minimal toxic influence that Synovex*-H had displayed on the liver.

Consequently, there may also have been a numerous amount of other side effects which had been related to the use of a product such as Synovex*-H, which had been intended for the use of animals, but instead, had been utilized by human beings. Unfortunately, these adverse effects may not have been precisely documented, or for that matter, even discovered as ill effects when administered for human utilization.

WARNING:

For veterinarian administration, it had been cautioned that Synovex*-H only be implanted in the ear only; as any other location may have resulted in condemnation of the carcass. It also had been advised not to have been used in cattle that had been breeding.

The intent of these products had been indicated for use in veterinarian medicine, therefore, these products had not been required to have met the same health and safety standards in which human pharmaceuticals had to have surpassed. Consequently, severe side effects may have occurred when applied in human self-administration.

Rating:

Based on a 1 to 5 star scale, with 1 considered low, and 5 considered high, this compound of has rated as the following:

	MALES	FEMALES
Strength Increase	***	**
Mass & Weight Increase	***	*
Side Effects	***	****
Cost Efficiency	***	***

TESTOSTERONA 200 *VETERINARY*

Chemical Name: Testosterone Enanthate.

Common Generic Name: Testosterone Enanthate.

Other Trade Names Found in Mexico: Currently, just Testosterona 200.

Manufacturers: Testosterona 200 - Brovel.

Dosage Form: Testosterona 200 - 200 mg/cc x 10 ml bottle.

Storage: Testosterona 200 injectables should be protected from light, (keep in the carton until contents are used), and stored at controlled room temperature 15 to 30 degrees C (59 to 86 degrees F). Do not freeze.

Price Range: Testosterona 200 - approx. $120.00 pesos for 200 mg/cc x 10 ml bottle.

Type of Drug: Anabolic Hormone.

Ingredient: 200 mg of Testosterone Enanthate.

Drug Identification:

Testosterona 200 - is available as an oil-based injectable solution which is distributed in a dark brown 10 ml bottle. The top has a silver aluminum tear-off lid, which conceals a multiple injection-type rubber top. The label is a white and yellow sticker stating the product's entities in black ink, along with the manufacturer Brovel, and Brovel's symbol. Lot # 9695. The box which it is packaged within, looks identical to thc label on the bottle. A Spanish product insert also accompanies the 200 mg/cc 10 ml bottles.

Please refer to the photograph of Testosterona 200 for full color references.

Drug Description:

Testosterona 200 is a synthetic veterinarian version of the naturally occurring androgen, Testosterone. In veterinarian use, it often had been administered in efforts to have treated animals who had been suffering from hypogonadism, breast tumors in female dogs, and to gave increased the osteous in male animals who had been primarily affected by maturation and weakness. The utilization of Testosterona 200 had further developed muscle tissue and had accelerated the recuperation time of sustained fractures.

Testosterona 200 is a long acting injectable Testosterone which had been commonly utilized by many athletes due to it's mass building characteristics. However, similar to all Testosterones, it had also been able to have aromatized easily, and had been moderately toxic to the liver. However, a distinct advantage of the administration of Testosterona 200, had been that it had a very strong androgenic effect combined with an intense anabolic component. This had often resulted in an increased amount of strength and mass, generally within a short time interval.

Consequently, the rapid and strong weight and mass increase had been often associated with distinct water retention, due to a withholding of electrolytes and water. Many athletes had been able to have achieved mass and an increase of strength with the administration of Testosterona 200, however, only a very few had been able to have retained their size after they had discontinued the compound. This had been a common reason why some athletes unfortunately, had often refused to take a break from a Testosterona 200 cycle. This negative practice had undoubtedly, often had increased the athlete's potential of having acquired risks which had generally been associated with steriodal compound use.

Several athletes had claimed that some advantages of the water retention had included temporary relief from problems with knee, elbow and shoulder joint pain, and intervertibral disk erosion. Unfortunately, however, many athletes had additionally experienced after a few weeks of having administered Testosterona 200, a flat, puffy appearance had generally been displayed by the muscles. Another problem had been that the conversion rate to Estrogen had been very high, which had permitted the body to have stored more fat, or had suffered from other feminization symptoms such as gynecomastia. Consequently, the athlete's predisposition had often determined whether or not these had been problematic. Generally, if they had posed to have been a problem, most athletes additionally had administered the combination of Nolvadex and Proviron at a dosage level of approximately 500 mgs or greater per week. This had allegedly kept the side effects at a minimum.

The administration of Testosterona 200 had also demonstrated a strong influence on the hypothalamohypophysial testicular axis, as the hypophysis had been inhibited by a positive feedback, which had generally lead to a negative influence on the endogenic Testosterone production. High dosages of Testosterona 200 which had been taken over a prolonged time interval, had frequently resulted in a reversible interruption or even a reduction of the sperm count in the testes. Inevitably, the testes had also often been reduced to a smaller size. Again, to have avoided these potential occurrences, several males athletes had engaged in the administration of HCG for an interval of every 6 to 8 weeks, at 5000 I.U.'s every fifth day, over a period of 10 days (a total of 3 injections), in efforts to have reduced this problem.

Allegedly, the self-administration of the veterinary compound of Testosterona 200 had produced results for every athlete who had utilized it. Reportedly, it had strongly promoted the regeneration process, which had encouraged an increased feeling of well-being, and an increase in energy levels. Some athletes had claimed that this characteristic had often been the explanation of the additional increase in intense training and exercise allotment, which had been accompanied by the increase of strength and mass without the usual associated lethargy. Usually, it had been common to have experienced an exorbitant, strong pump during training, as an increased blood volume accompanied by a high oxygen supply, and a high quantity of red blood cells had been particularly responsible for this feeling of a "Steroid pump". The administration of extremely large doses of Testosterona 200 had usually resulted in a tremendous pump sensation, which had been mostly experienced in the both the upper thigh and calf regions. Athletes had stated that this feeling could have been provoked from the slightest activity, such as having climbed a flight of stairs or even by having ridden a stationary bike.

Testosterona 200 along with Testosterone Cypionate (currently, not available as a sole entity in Mexico), and Sostenon 250, had appeared to have been the primary steroids of choice amongst several athletes. The compound of Testosterona 200 had been long-acting and therefore, had been able to have remained in the system for one to two weeks, which had depended upon the body's metabolism and initial hormone level. This characteristic had enabled for a longer interval between injections, and consequently, could have been injected anywhere from once a week, to once every two weeks, and still had been able to have remained very effective. This of course, had provided much more convenience, less expense, and a much more comfortable injection cycle for several self-administering steroidal compound athletes.

Usual Veterinarian Recommendation & Application:

Veterinarians had often administered the compound of Testosterona 200 intramuscularly in cattle, lambs and pigs, in dosages of 0.5 to 1.5 ml. This dosage had been repeated if required after 3 to 4 weeks.

Adventitious Dose and Administration:

The compound of Testosterona 200 had been intended for deep intramuscular injection. The best site for this type of injection had been in the gluteus medius muscle area, which had been the upper outer portion of the buttock, approximately 2 to 3 inches below the hip bone (iliac crest). Many self-administering athletes had alternated injections from one side to the other, (first injection on the left side, the second time injection administered on the right, or vice versa) in attempts to have alleviated pain, and also to have permitted the injection area to have slightly "healed". This practice often had prevented a thick scar tissue from potentially having formed. However, the more injections that had been administered, the greater possibility of scar tissue had also frequently resulted. A common dosage regime of some athletes, has been discussed in the following:

If the compound of Testosterona 200 had been accidentally frozen, the crystallization of the substance could have been normalized once the product had been reheated. If this had occurred, athletes had been careful to slightly have heated and shaken the contents.

Steriod novices had wisely avoided all Testosterone compounds, and had utilized milder steriodal substances to have initiate their enhancement ventures. Consequently, once these compounds had become somewhat ineffective, then the entertainment of a stronger anabolic such as Testosterona 200 had then possibly been considered.

Females:

Similarly, female athletes usually had not administered Testosterone steriodal compounds, as it generally had not been well tolerated, as severe side effects of virilization had frequently occurred. However, a few female athletes who had been willing to have neglected the risk/benefit ratio, and had indulged in this compound anyway, a maximum of 250 mgs, (which is 1 ampule of Testosterona 200) every 7 to 10 days had been used. If higher and more frequent injections had been entertained, then the greater potential of having acquired male characteristics had greatly prevailed.

Males:

Male athletes had been able to have tolerated this compound rather easily, and often had encouraged it's effects of increased strength, mass, aggressiveness and stamina. Often, the more advanced male athlete had administered either Testosterona 200 alone, or in combination with other steriodal compounds.

Singularly, there had been a wide range of dose administration having ranged from 500 mgs (2 ampules of Testosterona 200), all the way up to 3000 mgs (6 ampules of Testosterona 200) per day! However, the latter range had been somewhat extreme and unnecessary, as Testosterona 200 had a plasma half-life time in the blood of a week, and had been able to have remained in the system for approximately 7 to 10 days.

Consequently, the range for the most sensible dosages had generally varied between 250 to 1000 mgs (1 to 4 x 250 ampules, or 1 to 4 cc's) a week. Dosages which had exceeded these amounts had usually been unnecessary. If the dosage had been at a minimum of 250 to 500 mgs (1 to 2 x 250 ampules, or 1 to 2 cc's), it had generally been administered all at once, usually once a week or once every ten days. Dosages that had been higher than this range, had often been equally divided into two injection intervals per week, or every ten days, by most male athletes.

Most often athletes had determined the proper amount of required dose, by the following variables; age, goals, steriodal stack, temperament, and of course, financial situation. The latter had generally been considered by most athletes, due to the quantity of Testosterona 200 which usually had to have been required to have been administered, had often caused this steriodal compound to have become very expensive

Testosterona 200 had been primarily combined with many other steriodal compounds, in order to have gained size and mass. As Testosterona 200 is an androgen, it had somewhat of a synergetic effect with the anabolic steriodal compounds, which had resulted in the bonding with several receptors.

Several athletes had remarked that Testosterona 200 had stacked exceptionally well with Anapolon, Metandiabol or Reforvit B, (veterinary products), Deca-Durabolin or Norandren 50 (also a veterinary product) and Parabolan (currently, not found in Mexico).

Another common utilized stack amongst some male athletes had been Anapolon 100 mgs (2 x 50 mg tablets) a day, Deca-Durabolin or Norandren 50 (veterinary product) at 200 mgs (2 x 1 ml redi-jects) a week, along with Testosterona 200 to 500 mgs (Testosterona 200 at 2 x 250 mg ampules) a week. Also, Metandiabol or Reforvit B (veterinary products) at 40 mgs (approximately 1 1/2 to 3/4 cc's) daily, had also sometimes replaced the Anapolon dosage after about six weeks.

Another feasible combination had occasionally included Testosterona 200 at 500 mgs (Testosterona 200 at 2 x 250 mgs ampules, or 2 cc's) weekly, with Metandiabol or Reforvit B (veterinary products), at approximately 1 1/2 to 3/4 cc's per week, or Anapolon 2 tablets daily, in efforts to have kept water retention at a minimum. Testosterona 200 combined with Oxandrolone or Winstrol (both are currently not found in Mexico), had permitted the increase of strength and mass, without the associated bodyweight increase.

At the conclusion of a Testosterona 200 cycle, the administration of Testosterone-stimulating compounds such as Gonadotropyl, Gonakor, or Profasi (HCG), Omifin or Serofene (Clomid), Nolvadex and anti-catabolic substances such as Spiropent or Ephedrine (currently, not available in Mexico), or even Human Growth Hormone (Biotropin, Genotropin, Humatrope, Nanorm, Norditropin, Saizen or Protropin) had also been frequently necessarily entertained. The administration of these compounds had additionally aided in having absorbed the catabolic phase; which had helped in the elevation of the endogenic Testosterone level. Consequently, these compounds had also reduced the potential strength and mass loss, which had been usually inevitable.

Several athletes had claimed that having slowly tapered down the dosages of Testosterona 200 had not, unfortunately, helped to have maintained the acquired strength and mass increases. Another preventative measure had been the possibility of having had switched to milder steriodal compounds such as Deca-Durabolin, Primobolan Depot, or Winstrol (currently, not available in Mexico). Consequently, the discontinuation of these compounds had usually permitted most athletes to have retained the acquired gains.

Side Effects:

Some of the side effects which some animals had occasionally experienced from the administration of Testosterona 200 had included excessive sexual stimulation, and the long administration of exaggerated dosages had sometimes caused inhibition of the testicular function with a decrease in oligospermia ejaculation. If this product had been administered in animals that had been too young, it had often prevented the normal sexual development and maturation of the animal.

Some of the side effects which had been associated with the veterinarian compound of Testosterona 200 when it had been utilized by humans had included the side effects which had been primarily the distinct androgenic effects, and the probability of increased water retention.

Other side effects experienced by some athletes had also included acne, which had been predominantly harsher on the chest, back, arms, and shoulder areas, than on the face. This had often been a recognizable indication of the administration of Testosterones, including Testosterona 200. However, sometimes a type of rebound effect had occurred, and these side effects had not generally appeared until after the discontinuation of the Testosterone. Testosterona 200 had been only slightly toxic when it had been administered in reasonable quantities. Although had been broken down through the liver, the liver values changes had not occurred as often as experienced with the oral 17-alpha alkylated steriodal compounds.

A few male athletes sometimes especially had experienced feminization effects such as gynecomastia, testicular atrophy, reduced spermatogenesis and increased aggressiveness. Some athletes had also encountered the experience of hair loss and further deepening of the voice.

Most female athletes had generally avoided Testosterone steriodal compounds such as Testosterona 200 due to potential masculizational traits. These androgen-linked side effects of virilization had included acne vulgaris, increased facial and body hair growth, male pattern baldness, a hoarseness or deepening of the voice, menstrual irregularities, increased clitorial size, and a great increase in sex drive. Some of these side effects had been somewhat irreversible such as the increased facial and body hair growth, increased libido, male pattern baldness, however, often once damage had occurred to the voice and clitoris, it had often been of a permanent nature. Depending on the quantity of Testosterone administered by a female athlete, and if the cycle had been completely terminated before these had become evident, had sometimes resulted in a lessening effect of these associated problems.

However, there may also have been a numerous amount of other side effects related to the utilization of a product that had been intended for the use in animals, but instead, had been utilized by human beings. Unfortunately, they may not have all been precisely documented, or for that matter, even recognized as ill effects in human application.

WARNING:

In veterinarian medicine, the compound of Testosterona 200 had not been administered in animals within 60 days of having been slaughtered.

If hypertension had become elevated at the initiation of Testosterona 200, or if an athlete had a predisposition for high blood pressure, they routinely had it monitored by a competent physician, or had learned to have taken blood pressure readings themselves. Usually, any pharmacy or Clinic had offered to have taught these instructions. An antihypertensive compound such as Catapresan (available in Mexico) had also been sometimes prescribed to have helped kept the blood pressure within normal limits.

Rating:

Based on a 1 to 5 star scale, with 1 considered low, and 5 considered high, a -- symbol is indicative of no value. This compound of Testosterone Enanthate had rated as the following:

	MALES	FEMALES
Strength Increase	****	**
Mass & Weight Increase	****	**
Side Effects	***	*****
Cost Efficiency	**	**

TESTOSTERONA 25 & 50 *VETERINARY*

Chemical Name: Testosterone Propionate.

Common Generic Name: Testosterone Propionate.

Other Trade Names Found in Mexico: Testosterona 25.
Testosterona 50.

Manufacturers: Testosterona 25 - Brovel.
Testosterona 50 - Brovel.
Ara-Test - Aranda Laboratories (N.L.M.)

Dosage Form: Testosterona 25 - 25 mg/cc x 10 ml bottle.
Testosterona 50 - 50 mg/cc x 10 ml bottle.
Ara-Test - 25 mg/cc x 10 ml bottle (N.L.M.)

Storage: Testosterona 25 & 50 injectables should be protected from light, (keep in the carton until contents are used), and stored at controlled room temperature 15 to 30 degrees C (59 to 86 degrees F). Do not freeze.

Price Range: Testosterona 25 - approx. $30.00 pesos for 25 mg/cc x 10 ml bottle.
Testosterona 50 - approx. $35.00 pesos for 50 mg/cc x 10 ml bottle.

Type of Drug: Anabolic Hormone.

Ingredient: 25 or 50 mg of Testosterone Propionate.

Drug Identification:

Testosterona 25 & 50 - are oil-based injectable solutions which are distributed in dark brown 10 ml bottles. The top has a silver aluminum tear-off lid, and a multiple injection-type top. The label is a white, yellow and black sticker stating the product's entities, along with the manufacturer Brovel, and Brovel's symbol. Lot # 1195. The boxes which they are packaged within, look identical to the bottles with the exception of Testosterona 50, as a new colorful package has been recently displayed along with the Testosterona 50 bottle. This box had been primarily shades of ascending colors of blue, with "50" displayed within a yellow slanted rectangle, and the product's entities written in both white and black ink. A package insert accompanies both the 25 mg/cc and 50 mg/cc 10 ml bottles.

Ara-Test - as an injectable administration solution, could not be obtained for illustration and identification purposes. The manufacturers of the compound Ara-Test had recently stopped producing the injectable solution product. However, some farmacias may still have a few of these products still located upon their shelves. The compound of Ara-Test may be difficult to find, and will be obsolete in the near future.

*****Please refer to the photographs of Testosterona* 25 & 50 for full color references.***

Drug Description:

Veterinarians had used Testosterona 25 & 50 as an aid in the treatment of androgenic hormone deficiency, which had usually been experienced by castrated horses. It had also been utilized to have treated geldings that had showed signs of muscle weakness, poor appetite, and a lack of competitive spirit. Veterinarians had also commonly used Testosterona 25 & 50 to successfully have treated mares, who had shown excessive estrus.

Testosterona 25 & 50, along with Testosterone Cypionate (currently, not available in Mexico as a sole entity), and Enanthate, had also been frequently used by many athletes in attempts to have increased both strength and muscle mass. This compound of Testosterone Propionate, had been highly androgenic and also had been able to have acted very quickly once it had been administered intramuscularly into the system. Unfortunately, Testosterona 25 & 50 only had a duration effect of 1 to 2 days, which had usually been dependent upon the type of esters, and on the amount administered. Therefore, many athletes had to have administered this veterinarian steriodal compound to have achieved and maintained positive effects. Athletes had claimed that these inconvenient frequent injections, usually within a short time period, had frequently resulted in painful, swollen injection sites. Some other distinct advantages of this oil-based compound had been however, that water retention had occurred at a much lower rate, and an increase in energy levels had also been apparent; which often had transpired in a better pump, associated with a slight increase in strength.

Another positive aspect of Testosterona 25 & 50 had been that it's androgenic side effects could have been curbed much easier, which had permitted this type of Testosterone to have been compatible for several females athletes. Consequently, many of the ill effects which some female athletes had experienced, had easily been kept at a minimum, by only having administered proper low doses of Testosterona 25 & 50. This had usually been accomplished by having increased the time intervals between the injections so that the Testosterone level could have fallen; which had generally resulted in an accumulation of androgens. Therefore, the androgenic effects included in Testosterona 25 & 50, had allowed for improved regeneration, without the virilization symptoms, for female athletes who had wished to have ventured with a Testosterone compound.

Male athletes who similarly had not been afraid of the intake of Testosterone due to it's potential side effects; which had been often much less pronounced, also had administered Testosterona 25 & 50. This had often been due to the fact that the weekly dose of Testosterona 25 & 50, had generally been much lower than that with depot Testosterones. Also, when compared with Testosterona 200 and Testosterone Cypionate, (currently, not available as a sole entity in Mexico), Testostcrona 25 & 50 had been considered to have been a much "milder" Testosterone substance which had generally been better tolerated in the body.

Male athletes who had wished to have ignored having obtained possible side effects, and had chosen to have administered Testosterones on a daily basis, had often decided to have injected Testosterona 25 & 50. Many of these athletes had claimed that a successful method in having acquired positive effects from Testosterona 25 & 50 had been achieved by regularly having administered this compound in relative small quantities.

Bodybuilders had utilized the compound of Testosterona 25 & 50 mostly in preparation for competition, due to the fact that a restriction in calories had frequently been combined with Testosterone to help maintain maximum muscle mass and density. Several athletes had claimed that this Testosterone compound had always proven to have been effective for these entities, as it not only had accomplished these requirements, but at the same time, also had lowered potential water retention problems.

Testosterona 25 & 50 had also been combined with Epitestosterone, to have rendered negative test results, when doping tests for competitions had been mandatory. Six had been the threshold value for a positive doping test. The administration of Testosterona 25 & 50 had prevented a positive test result, as Testosterone Propionate's value in the urine had been able to have decreased faster than the Testosterone concentration in the blood.

Usual Veterinarian Recommendation & Application:

The usual veterinarian recommendation for horses had been 3 to 5 ml per 454 kg of bodyweight administered every week for 3 to 5 weeks.

Adventitious Dose and Administration:

Testosterona 25 & 50 had been intended for deep intramuscular injection. However, since Testosterone Propionate slightly had swelled the site of injection, several lagging bodyparts such as the arms, shoulders, and the calf areas had been substituted for this injection. Despite this temporary benefit, these areas had become usually much too painful and inconvenient for repeated injection use. Consequently, the best site for the injection of Testosterona 25 & 50, had been in the gluteus medius muscle area, which again, had been the upper outer portion of the buttock, which is approximately 2 to 3 inches below the hip bone (iliac crest). Most athletes had alternated the injections from one side to the other, (first injection on the left side, the second time injection administered on the right, or vice versa) to slightly have alleviated pain, which had also often allowed the area to have slightly "healed". This practice had also often prevented a thick scar tissue from potentially having formed. However, the more injections that had been administered, the greater possibility of scar tissue had frequently resulted. A common dosage regime of some athletes had been discussed in the following:

Females:

Female athletes had usually used Testosterona 25 & 50, in the range of 25 to 50 mgs (1 to 2 cc's, or 1 to 2 mls), every 5 to 7 days. If dosages or frequency intervals had exceeded these amounts, better results had usually been obtained. However, this had often resulted in the dramatic increase of potential virilization side effects.

Therefore, many female athletes had been careful to have limited the duration of intake; which had not exceeded 8 to 10 weeks. Instead, this dosage had been supplemented by mild and mostly anabolic steriodal compounds such as Primobolan, Durabolan, and Anadur (the latter two compounds, are currently not available in Mexico). This stack had been administered in efforts to have promoted the synthesis of protein.

Males:

An initiating dosage had usually been kept in the range of 50 to 100 mgs (2 to 4 cc's, or 2 to 4 mls), on alternate days. Many male athletes had claimed that this had been advantageous due to the rapid initial effect of the Propionate-ester, as a several week duration could have been started with this compound.

Anxious users who had been impatient for the depot steroids to have taken effect, had sometimes injected Primoteston Depot 250 mgs (1 cc, or 1 ml), and 50 mgs of Testosterona 25 or 50, at 50 mgs (if 25 had been used, then 2 cc's, if the 50 had been used, then 1 cc), at the beginning of the cycle. Then, when the effect of the Testosterona had decreased, another 50 mgs had been injected, usually within a two day duration. Two days after that, elevated Testosterone levels which had been caused by the

Testosterona, had begun to have decreased, which had represented the effect of Enanthate in the system; therefore, this had frequently eliminated the need of further injections. This had also been indicative of a high Testosterone level, which had been reached and maintained for a long time, due to the depot Testosterone.

If Anapolon had been prcviously utilized for a six week duration, and the favored weight increase had been obtained, then several male athletes often had chosen to have switched to Testosterona. This had mostly been preferred due to the Anapolon collapse of its effects once it had been discontinued; that had required a quick elevated Testosterone level; which had been able to have been accomplished by having had used Testosterona.

Another possible option which had frequently been utilized for the entire period of intake, had been 50 to 100 mgs every day, or every second day. This dosage had seemed to have lowered the problematic side effect of water retention, which had often been experienced with the Depot Testosterones. Several male athletes had remarked that muscle mass had often been achieved by having had administered Testosterona 200 at 100 mgs (1/2 cc or 1/2 ml) x 2 days, Winstrol Depot (currently, not available in Mexico) at 50 mgs x 2 days, and Metandiabol or Reforvit B (veterinary products) at 30 mgs x daily.

A combination of 100 mg Testosterona 100 mgs every 2 days, either Winstrol Depot 50 mgs (currently, not available in Mexico), per day, or Parabolon 76 mgs every 2 days, and of Oxandrolone 25 mgs daily (these latter two compounds are not currently available in Mexico), had allegedly helped to have achieved this goal, while also having increased qualitative muscle mass.

Side Effects:

The side effects which had been experienced by the administration of Testosterona 25 & 50, had been similar to those which had been experienced from other Testosteronal compounds such as Testosterona 200 and Testosterone Cypionate (currently, not available in Mexico, as a sole entity). The main difference which had separated Testosterona 25 & 50 from this group, had been the fact that these ill effects had occurred less frequently when they had been administered in lower dosages. Both female and male athletes had similarly experienced an increase in sex drives.

However, if high dosages had been entertained, and there had been a pre-existing predisposition for certain problems such as acne, male pattern baldness; increased facial and body hair, increased libido, and deepening of the voice had often resulted. Despite the high conversion rate of Propionate into Estrogen, the possibility of gynecomastia had been less likely to have resulted from the use of Testosterona 25 & 50, than with the administration of other Testosterones. Also, potential water retention had also been low, since the retention of electrolytes and water had been less pronounced.

Several athletes had also administered Testosterone-stimulating compounds such as HCG and Clomid along with Testosterona 25 & 50. This had a strong influence on the hypothalamohypophysial testicular axis, which had been able to have suppressed the endogenous hormone production. To combat the problematic and annoying effects of water retention, many athletes had utilized the combination of Nolvadex and Proviron. Liver damage had also been rarely experienced due to the minimal toxic influence that Testosterona 25 & 50 had displayed on the liver.

Consequently, there may also have been a numerous amount of other side effects that had been related to the use of a product such as Testosterona 25 & 50, which had been intended for the use of animals, but instead, had been utilized by human beings. Unfortunately, these adverse effects may not have been precisely documented, or for that matter, even discovered as ill effects when utilized for human use.

WARNING:

This product had not been administered 60 days prior to the slaughter of the animal for human consumption. The intent of these products had been indicated for use in veterinarian medicine, therefore, these pharmaceuticals had not been required to have met the same health and safety standards in which human pharmaceuticals had to surpass.

Consequently, severe side effects may have occurred when applied in human self-administration.

Rating:

Based on a 1 to 5 star scale, with 1 considered low, and 5 considered high, a -- symbol is indicative of no value. This compound of Testosterone Propionate has rated as the following:

	MALES	FEMALES
Strength Increase	****	**
Mass & Weight Increase	***	**
Side Effects	**	*****
Cost Efficiency	**	**

VITAMIN B12 VETERINARY

Chemical Name: Cyanocobalamin.

Common Generic Name: Vitamin B12.

Other Trade Names Found in Mexico: Neurofor (human).
Super Vitamina B12 5500.
Hdroxo & Cyano.

Manufacturers: Super Vitamina B12 5500 - Laboratorios Tomei S.A.

	Hdroxo & Cyano	- United Vitamin Labs.
Dosage Form:	Super Vitamina B12 5500	- 5500 mcg/ml x 5 ml bottle. - 5500 mcg/ml x 30 ml bottle.
	Hdroxo & Cyano	- 20 mcg/ml x 10 ml bottle.

Storage: Cyanocobalamin injectables should be protected from light, (keep in the carton until contents are used), and stored at controlled room temperature 15 to 30 degrees C (59 to 86 degrees F). Do not freeze.

Price Range:	Super Vitamina B12 5500	- approx. $30.00 pesos for 5500 mcg/ml 5 ml bottle. - approx. $85.00 pesos for 5500 mcg/ml 30 mls.
	Hdroxo & Cyano	- approx. $25.00 pesos for 20 mcg/ml 10 ml bottle.

Type of Drug: Vitamin.

Ingredient: 100 or 5500 mcg/ml Cyanocobalamin.

Drug Identification:

Super Vitamina B12 5500 - is available in both the 5 and 30 ml bottle size, and both contain 5500 mcg/ml of cyancobalamin. Consequently, both bottles are clear glass, with the sticker of red, white and blue with the product's entities written in black. There is also a picture of a rooster and a chicken on the front, along with the Laboratorios Tomei S.A. name, and symbol. The box is identical to the bottle's sticker. The injectable itself is red-colored. There is a Spanish product insert accompanying the product.

Hdroxo & Cyano - is available in a 10 ml bottle, and contains 20 mcg/ml of Cobalamin. It is administered from a dark brown bottle with a white, red and black sticker label, containing the product's entities, and manufacturer on it. Lot # 36770. It also has a silver aluminum tear-off lid, which reveals a rubber multiple injection entry lid underneath. The container in which it comes in is very different. It is a hard clear plastic container, with a red top. The front contains the product's name and a picture of a chicken, both of which are displayed in gold print, which is also edged into the plastic, and is easily felt with the fingertips. The injectable itself is also red-colored.

*****Please refer to both the Super Vitamina B12 5500, and the Hdroxo & Cyano photographs for full color references.***

Drug Description:

Veterinarians had utilized the Vitamin B12 compound in animals in efforts to have also treat anemia. However, it had been more commonly used as a "supportive" vitamin, in larger animals such as cattle, who had acquired their vitamin absorption from bacteria which had been found within their stomach; or in horses who had been "colicky". It had also been administered to treat Vitamin B12 deficiencies, maintain correct functions of the nervous system when there had been changes in the animals surrounding environment, and to have increased appetites. Veterinarian Vitamin B12 had also been administered via subcutaneously, intramuscularly, or intravenously.

Accordingly, Vitamin B12 for utilization in humans, had been essential to growth, in regenerating red blood cells, and in having maintained a healthy nervous system. It had also been known to have provided a general well feeling, as it had been able to have increased energy levels. Vitamin B12 also had been able to have utilized fats, carbohydrates and proteins properly. Some other known values of Vitamin B12 had included the improvement of concentration, memory and balance, relief from irritability, and the ability to have increased appetite levels. Vitamin B12 is quantitatively, and had been absorbed into the system very quickly from either intramuscular, or deep subcutaneous injections. It had not been well assimilated through the stomach, therefore, Vitamin B12 had provided the best results when it had been administered by injection measures.

The average human diet had been able to have supplied approximately 5 to 15 mcgs a day of Vitamin B12, which had been available for absorption after normal digestion. Vitamin B12 had been found only in foods of animal origin, therefore, it had been not present in plants. Consequently, strict vegetarians had often suffered from deficiencies of this vitamin, which inevitably had frequently lead to pernicious anemia.

Athletes often had utilized Vitamin B12 for it's ability to have increased the appetite, and for having increased energy levels. This characteristic had especially been important when athletes had been required to have ingested numerous amounts of calories, in efforts to have achieved gains in strength and weight. Steriod cycles also had depended on the proper and abundant caloric intakes of protein, carbohydrates and fats. Increased energy levels also had aided many athletes in daily functioning, and training regiments.

However, since the human pharmaceutical of Vitamin B12 had been easily obtainable, and just as inexpensive, most athletes had chosen to have acquired this compound through a farmacia.

Usual Veterinarian Recommendation:

The usual dosage for large animals had been approximately 1 to 3 ml (or 1000 mcg), per 100 lbs, once to twice weekly. This had also been administered by subcutaneous, intramuscular, or intravenous injections.

Horses	5 ml.
Pigs	2 - 5 ml.
Dogs & Cats	0.5 to 1 ml.
Roosters	0.5 ml.

Adventitious Dosage and Administration:

The use of Super Vitamina B12 5500 had been intended for intramuscular or deep subcutaneous injection. The best site for this type of intramuscular injection, had been in the gluteus medius muscle area, which had been the upper outer portion of the buttock, approximately 2 to 3 inches below the hip bone (iliac crest). Most athletes had also alternated the injections from one side to the other, (first injection on the left side, the second time injection administered on the right, or vice versa) in attempts to have alleviated pain somewhat, and to let the area slightly "heal". This practice had sometimes allotted for the prevention of a thick scar tissue from potentially having formed. However, the more injections that athletes had administered, the greater possibility of scar tissue had often resulted. Subcutaneous injections, which had been just underneath the layer of skin, had usually been best administered in the outer surface of the arms and forearms. Some athletes had often easily accomplished this by having gathered the skin in a pinch-like fashion, then having injected the substance within this grasped area. A common dosage regime of some athletes, has been discussed in the following:

Females
& Males:
Usually one injection of 11,000 mcgs (2 cc's of Super Vitamina B12 5500, or 550 cc's of Hdroxo & Cyano, which is the equivalent of 55 x 10 mls bottles!!) every second day, x one week on, one week off, for three dosing sessions had sufficed many athletes who for some reason or other could not have obtained the human version of this compound. Obviously, the Hdroxo & Cyano veterinary version of Vitamin B12, had not been intended for "larger" users such as "humans", (intended for small animals such as chickens, hamsters etc.), due to the quantity that would have required to have been administered to have received any effect.

Side Effects:

Although there had been no known side effects that had posed to have been a threat to an animal's health, there may have been the possibility due to the incidence of having utilized a veterinarian Vitamin B12 compound for human application. Consequently, the following had been cited from the applicable "human" version of Vitamin B12:

Some of the more common side effects which had been associated with the parenteral administration of Vitamin B12 had included those of pulmonary edema, congestive heart failure early in treatment, peripheral vascular thrombosis, diarrhea, itching, and a swelling sensation of the entire body.

WARNING:

No overdosage had been reported with Vitamin B12. However, Anaphylactic shock and death had been reported after parenteral vitamin B12 administration (in clinical human Vitamin B12 application). No warning indications had been acknowledged for veterinarian utilization.

Athletes had generally investigated clinically if they had a sensitivity to this compound, before they had indulged in self-administration. Clinically, this had often been obtained through a competent physician by an intradermal testing dose. However, these results still had applied and had been warranted efficacious to the veterinarian version of Vitamin B12.

Rating:

Based on a 1 to 5 star scale, with 1 considered low, and 5 considered high, a -- symbol is indicative of no value. This compound of Cyanocobalamin has rated as the following:

	MALES	FEMALES
Strength Increase	*	*
Mass & Weight Increase	*	*
Fat Burner	*	*
Contest Preparation	*	*
Appetite Stimulant	*****	*****
Side Effects	*	*
Cost Efficiency	*	*

SUMMARY OF HUMAN ANABOLICS CURRENTLY AVAILABLE IN MEXICO:

CHEMICAL NAME: *Spironolactone.*
COMMON TRADE NAME: *Aldactone.*
TRADE NAMES FOUND IN MEXICO, CENTRAL AMERICA:
Aldactone
MANUFACTURER:
Searle.

CHEMICAL NAME: *Oxymetholone.*
COMMON TRADE NAME: *Anadrol 50.*
TRADE NAMES FOUND IN MEXICO, CENTRAL AMERICA:
Anapolon 50 (available for institutional use only)
MANUFACTURER:
Syntex.

CHEMICAL NAME: *Clenbuterol Hydrocloride.*
COMMON TRADE NAME: *Clenbuterol.*
TRADE NAMES FOUND IN MEXICO, CENTRAL AMERICA:
Spiropent
MANUFACTURER:
Prome.

CHEMICAL NAME: *Clomiphene Citrate.*
COMMON TRADE NAME: *Clomid.*
TRADE NAMES FOUND IN MEXICO, CENTRAL AMERICA:

	MANUFACTURER:
Omifin	*Hoechs.*
Serofene	*Serono.*

CHEMICAL NAME: *Co-Enzyme B12.*
COMMON TRADE NAME: *Co-Enzyme B12.*
TRADE NAMES FOUND IN MEXICO, CENTRAL AMERICA:
Maxibol
MANUFACTURER:
Roussel Hoechs.

CHEMICAL NAME: *Cyclofenil.*
COMMON TRADE NAME: *Cyclofenil.*
TRADE NAMES FOUND IN MEXICO, CENTRAL AMERICA:
Fertodur

MANUFACTURER:
Schering.

CHEMICAL NAME: *Liothyronine Sodium.*
COMMON TRADE NAME: *Cytomel.*
TRADE NAMES FOUND IN MEXICO, CENTRAL AMERICA:
Cynomel

MANUFACTURER:
SmithKline Beecham.

CHEMICAL NAME: *Phenformin.*
COMMON TRADE NAME: *Debeone.*
TRADE NAMES FOUND IN MEXICO, CENTRAL AMERICA:
Debeone

MANUFACTURER:
Armstrong.

CHEMICAL NAME: *Nandrolone Decanoate.*
COMMON TRADE NAME: *Deca-Durabolin.*
TRADE NAMES FOUND IN MEXICO, CENTRAL AMERICA:
Deca-Durabolin

MANUFACTURER:
Organon.

CHEMICAL NAME: *Triamterene Hydrochlorothiazide.*
COMMON TRADE NAME: *Dyazide.*
TRADE NAMES FOUND IN MEXICO, CENTRAL AMERICA:
Dyazide

MANUFACTURER:
Armstrong.

CHEMICAL NAME: *Fluoxymesterone.*
COMMON TRADE NAME: *Halotestin.*
TRADE NAMES FOUND IN MEXICO, CENTRAL AMERICA:
Stenox

MANUFACTURER:
Atlantis Laboratories.

CHEMICAL NAME: *Chorionic Gonadotropin.*
COMMON TRADE NAME: *HCG (Human Chorionic Gonadotropin).*

TRADE NAMES FOUND IN MEXICO, CENTRAL AMERICA:	MANUFACTURER:
Gonadotropyl	*Roussel*
Gonakor	*Sanfer*
Profasi	*Serono.*

CHEMICAL NAME: *Somatropin.*
COMMON TRADE NAME: *Human Growth Hormone.*

TRADE NAMES FOUND IN MEXICO, CENTRAL AMERICA:	MANUFACTURER:
Genotropin	*Pharma*
Humatrope	*Eli Lilly Labs*
Nordtropin	*PISA*
Saizen	*Serono*
Biotropin (made for institional use)	*Biotec Labs.*

CHEMICAL NAME: *Somatrem.*
COMMON TRADE NAME: *Human Growth Hormone.*

TRADE NAMES FOUND IN MEXICO, CENTRAL AMERICA:	MANUFACTURER:
Protropin	*Genentech.*

CHEMICAL NAME: *Furosemide.*
COMMON TRADE NAME: *Lasix.*

TRADE NAMES FOUND IN MEXICO, CENTRAL AMERICA:	MANUFACTURER:
Lasix	*Hoechs.*

CHEMICAL NAME: *Levothyroxine Sodium.*
COMMON TRADE NAME: *L-Thyroxine.*

TRADE NAMES FOUND IN MEXICO, CENTRAL AMERICA:	MANUFACTURER:
Eutirox	*Merck.*
Tiroidine	*Rudefsa.*

CHEMICAL NAME: *Naproxen.*
COMMON TRADE NAME: *Naprosyn.*
TRADE NAMES FOUND IN MEXICO, CENTRAL AMERICA:
Naxen

MANUFACTURER:
Syntex.

CHEMICAL NAME: *Cyanocobalamin.*
COMMON TRADE NAME: *Neurofor.*
TRADE NAMES FOUND IN MEXICO, CENTRAL AMERICA:
Neurofor

MANUFACTURER:
Roussel Hoechs.

CHEMICAL NAME: *Tamoxifen Citrate.*
COMMON TRADE NAME: *Nolvadex.*
TRADE NAMES FOUND IN MEXICO, CENTRAL AMERICA:
Nolvadex

MANUFACTURER:
Zeneca.

CHEMICAL NAME: *Nalbuphine HCI.*
COMMON TRADE NAME: *Nubain.*
TRADE NAMES FOUND IN MEXICO, CENTRAL AMERICA:
Nubain

MANUFACTURER:
Rhone.

CHEMICAL NAME: *Methenolone Enanthate.*
COMMON TRADE NAME: *Primobolan Depot.*
TRADE NAMES FOUND IN MEXICO, CENTRAL AMERICA:
Primobolan Depot

MANUFACTURER:
Schering.

CHEMICAL NAME: *Methenolone Acetate.*
COMMON TRADE NAME: *Primobolan Tablets.*
TRADE NAMES FOUND IN MEXICO, CENTRAL AMERICA:
Primobolan

MANUFACTURER:
Schering.

CHEMICAL NAME: *Mesterolone.*
COMMON TRADE NAME: *Proviron.*
TRADE NAMES FOUND IN MEXICO, CENTRAL AMERICA: *Proviron*
MANUFACTURER: *Schering.*

CHEMICAL NAME: *Testosterone Propionate, Testosterone Cypionate, Dihydrotesterone.*
COMMON TRADE NAME: *Sten.*
TRADE NAMES FOUND IN MEXICO, CENTRAL AMERICA: *Sten*
MANUFACTURER: *Atlantis.*

CHEMICAL NAME: *Testosterone Propionate, Testosterone Phenylpropionate, Testosterone Isocaproate, Testosterone Decanoate.*
COMMON TRADE NAME: *Sustanon.*
TRADE NAMES FOUND IN MEXICO, CENTRAL AMERICA: *Sostenon 250*
MANUFACTURER: *Organon.*

CHEMICAL NAME: *Testosterone Enanthate.*
COMMON TRADE NAME: *Testosterone Enanthate.*
TRADE NAMES FOUND IN MEXICO, CENTRAL AMERICA: *Primoteston Depot*
MANUFACTURER: *Schering.*

HUMAN ANABOLIC STEROIDS NO LONGER MANUFACTURED IN MEXICO:

CHEMICAL NAME: *Spironolactone/Hydrochlorthiazide.*
COMMON TRADE NAME: *Aldactazide.*
TRADE NAMES NO LONGER FOUND IN MEXICO, CENTRAL AMERICA: *Aldactazide*
MANUFACTURER: *Searle.*

CHEMICAL NAME: *Testosterone Acetate, Testosterone Valerate, Testosterone Undecanoate.*
COMMON TRADE NAME: *Andriol.*
TRADE NAMES NO LONGER FOUND IN MEXICO, CENTRAL AMERICA:

	MANUFACTURER:
Depotestostarona	*Syntex.*

CHEMICAL NAME: *Clenbuterol Hydrocloride.*
COMMON TRADE NAME: *Clenbuterol.*
TRADE NAMES NO LONGER FOUND IN MEXICO, CENTRAL AMERICA:

	MANUFACTURER:
Novegam	*Chinoin.*

CHEMICAL NAME: *Clomiphene Citrate.*
COMMON TRADE NAME: *Clomid.*
TRADE NAMES NO LONGER FOUND IN MEXICO, CENTRAL AMERICA:

	MANUFACTURER:
Omifin	*Merrell.*

CHEMICAL NAME: *Cyclofenil.*
COMMON TRADE NAME: *Cyclofenil.*
TRADE NAMES NO LONGER FOUND IN MEXICO, CENTRAL AMERICA:

	MANUFACTURER:
Fertodur	*Global Medical.*

CHEMICAL NAME: *Nandrolone Decanoate.*
COMMON TRADE NAME: *Deca-Durabolin.*
TRADE NAMES NO LONGER FOUND IN MEXICO, CENTRAL AMERICA:

	MANUFACTURER:
Deca-Ject	*Unknown.*

CHEMICAL NAME: *Triamterene Hydrochlorothiazide.*
COMMON TRADE NAME: *Dyazide.*
TRADE NAMES NO LONGER FOUND IN MEXICO, CENTRAL AMERICA:

	MANUFACTURER:
Dyazide	*SmithKline Beecham.*

CHEMICAL NAME: *Chorionic Gonadotropin.*
COMMON TRADE NAME: *HCG (Human Chorionic Gonadotropin).*
TRADE NAMES NO LONGER FOUND IN MEXICO, CENTRAL AMERICA:

TRADE NAME	MANUFACTURER:
Pregnyl	*Organon.*

CHEMICAL NAME: *Tamoxifen Citrate.*
COMMON TRADE NAME: *Nolvadex.*
TRADE NAMES NO LONGER FOUND IN MEXICO, CENTRAL AMERICA:

TRADE NAME	MANUFACTURER:
Crioxifeno	*Cryo Pharma*
Tamoxan	*Tecnimede PL: Kener*
Taxus	*Andromaco*
Tenofen	*Tecnofarma.*

CHEMICAL NAME: *Somatropin.*
COMMON TRADE NAME: *Human Growth Hormone.*
TRADE NAMES NO LONGER FOUND IN MEXICO, CENTRAL AMERICA:

TRADE NAME	MANUFACTURER:
Nanorm (made for institional use)	*Unknown.*

CHEMICAL NAME: *Methandrostenolone.*
COMMON TRADE NAME: *Restauvit.*
TRADE NAMES NO LONGER FOUND IN MEXICO, CENTRAL AMERICA:

TRADE NAME	MANUFACTURER:
Restauvit	*Ciba*
Restauvit	*Rugby Labs.*

CHEMICAL NAME: *Testosterone Enanthate.*
COMMON TRADE NAME: *Testosterone Enanthate.*
TRADE NAMES NO LONGER FOUND IN MEXICO, CENTRAL AMERICA:

TRADE NAME	MANUFACTURER:
Delatestril	*Brovel.*

CHEMICAL NAME: *Testosterone Propionate.*
COMMON TRADE NAME: *Testosterone Propionate.*
TRADE NAMES NO LONGER FOUND IN MEXICO, CENTRAL AMERICA:

	MANUFACTURER:
Oreton	*Goldline.*

CHEMICAL NAME: *Stenbolone Acetate.*
COMMON TRADE NAME: *Stenbolone.*
TRADE NAMES NO LONGER FOUND IN MEXICO, CENTRAL AMERICA:

	MANUFACTURER:
Anatrofin	*Syntex.*

SUMMARY OF VETERINARY ANABOLIC STEROIDS CURRENTLY AVAILABLE IN MEXICO:

CHEMICAL NAME: *Nandrolone Decanoate.*
TRADE NAME: *Deca-Durabolin.*
TRADE NAMES FOUND IN MEXICO, CENTRAL AMERICA:

	MANUFACTURER:
Norandren 50	*Brovel.*

CHEMICAL NAME: *Methandrostenolone/methandienone.*
COMMON TRADE NAME: *Dianabol.*
TRADE NAMES FOUND IN MEXICO, CENTRAL AMERICA:

	MANUFACTURER:
Metandiabol	*Quimber.*
Reforvit B	*Oeffler.*

CHEMICAL NAME: *Boldenone Undecylenate.*
COMMON TRADE NAME: *Equipoise.*
TRADE NAMES FOUND IN MEXICO, CENTRAL AMERICA:

	MANUFACTURER:
*Equi-Gan**	*Laboratorios Tornie, S.A.*

Crecibol — *Unipharm (International) S.A.*

Maxi-Gan — *Mital Pharma S.A.*

CHEMICAL NAME: *Nandrolone Laurate.*
COMMON TRADE NAME: *Laurabolin.*

TRADE NAMES FOUND IN MEXICO, CENTRAL AMERICA:	MANUFACTURER:
Laurabolin 20	*Intervet*
Laurabolin 50	*Intervet.*
Fortabol	*Parfarm, S. A.*

CHEMICAL NAME: *Zeranol.*
COMMON TRADE NAME: *Ralgrow.*

TRADE NAMES FOUND IN MEXICO, CENTRAL AMERICA:	MANUFACTURER:
Ralgrow	*Pittman Moore.*

CHEMICAL NAME: *Testosterone Propionate, Testosterone Phenylpropionate, Testosterone Isocaproate, Testosterone Decanoate.*
COMMON TRADE NAME: *Sostenon 250.*

TRADE NAMES FOUND IN MEXICO, CENTRAL AMERICA:	MANUFACTURER:
Deposterona *	*Syntex.*

CHEMICAL NAME: *Progesterone, Estrogen and Testosterone Cypionate.*
COMMON TRADE NAME: *Synovex*-H*

TRADE NAMES FOUND IN MEXICO, CENTRAL AMERICA:	MANUFACTURER:
Synovex-H*	*Syntex.*

CHEMICAL NAME: *Testosterone Enanthate.*
COMMON TRADE NAME: *Testosterone Enanthate.*

TRADE NAMES FOUND IN MEXICO, CENTRAL AMERICA:	MANUFACTURER:
Testosterona 200	*Brovel.*

CHEMICAL NAME: *Testosterone Propionate.*
COMMON TRADE NAME: *Testosterone Propionate.*
TRADE NAMES FOUND IN MEXICO, CENTRAL AMERICA:

TRADE NAME	MANUFACTURER:
Testosterona 25	*Brovel*
Testosterona 50	*Brovel*
Ara-Test	*Aranda Laboratories.*

CHEMICAL NAME: *Cyanobalamin.*
COMMON TRADE NAME: *Vitamin B12..*
TRADE NAMES FOUND IN MEXICO, CENTRAL AMERICA:

TRADE NAME	MANUFACTURER:
Super Vitamina B12 5500	*Laboratorios Tomei SA*
Hdroxo & Cyano	*United Vitamin Labs.*

VETERINARY ANABOLIC STERIODS NO LONGER MANUFACTURED IN MEXICO, CENTRAL AMERICA:

CHEMICAL NAME: *Boldenone Undecylenate.*
COMMON TRADE NAME: *Equipoise.*
TRADE NAMES NO LONGER FOUND IN MEXICO, CENTRAL AMERICA:

TRADE NAME	MANUFACTURER:
Equipoise	*Squibb*
Equipoise	*Solvay Vet.*

CHEMICAL NAME: *Trenbolone Acetate.*
COMMON TRADE NAME: *Finaplix.*
TRADE NAMES NO LONGER FOUND IN MEXICO, CENTRAL AMERICA:

TRADE NAME	MANUFACTURER:
Finaplix	*Roussel.*

CHEMICAL NAME: *Nandrolone Laurate.*
COMMON TRADE NAME: *Nandrolabolin.*
TRADE NAMES NO LONGER FOUND IN MEXICO, CENTRAL AMERICA:

	MANUFACTURER:
Nandrolabolin	*Unknown.*

CHEMICAL NAME: *Testosterone Propionate.*
COMMON TRADE NAME: *Testosterone Propionate.*
TRADE NAMES NO LONGER FOUND IN MEXICO, CENTRAL AMERICA:

	MANUFACTURER:
Ara-Test	*Aranda Laboratories.*

The prices stated within are current as of December 1996. However, during tourist season (mainly November to April), many farmacias and veterinarian stores had been known to have increased their prices on pharmaceutical items. These prices have been stated in "pesos", therefore, if having utilized Canadian currency, this amount had simply been approximately divided by 5 (or what the current exchange rate had been at the time), and if American currency had been used, this amount had been divided by approximately 7 (or again, what the current exchange rate had been at the time). For simplicity measures, (N.L.M.) had implied that a particular item had been either "No Longer Manufactured", or no longer available for sale from a farmacia or veterinarian store.

THE UTILIZATION/STACKING OF ANABOLIC/ANDROGENIC STEROIDS

Contrary to the negative media sensationalism, anabolic/androgenic steroids have been effective; especially when they had been utilized in a sensible and proper manner. Most athletes therefore, generally had cycled steroidal regimes for a 8 to 12 week period, followed by an abstinence duration for approximately the same interval. Several athletes had also reported that having stacked different steroidal products during this regiment course had provided the most productive results.

These desired results had been further amplified when athletes had initiated their regimes by having started with a relatively low dosage of one or more steroidal product, then had slowly increased the dosage and often had added other compatible compounds to the regiment. Since oral steroidal compounds usually had become effective within several days, this characteristic had resulted in a rapid saturation of the receptors; therefore, most athletes had limited oral administration to less than 8 weeks. In the meantime, injectable steroidal compounds had been also administered in efforts to have further supplemented the anabolic/androgenic effects. Many athletes had indicated that a combination of two or three steroidal compounds administered in moderate dosages; had been more effective and had a longer duration of effect, as opposed to one steroid which had been utilized in high dosages.

Most athletes had claimed that the correct combination, had often permitted a synergetic effect if particular attention had been paid in the selection of steroids which had different influences on the factors of strength, tissue buildup, and recovery. Therefore, many athletes had often chosen a compound which had been primarily utilized for each of these requirements. For example, an athlete may have chosen a stack of Deca-Durabolin or Norandren 50 (veterinary), or Primobolan Depot for strength increase, which also had anabolic characteristics, Sostenon 250 for an increase in mass, and the promotion of recovery, and Gonakor, or Gondotrophyl, or Profasi (HCG), or Proviron in efforts to have restarted the body's own production of Testosterone, and possibly Spiropent to slowly have tapered off the cycle. A gradual and even reduction of the doses at the termination of the cycle had also aided in the normalizing of the body functions; and in the preparation for a termination of the intake. The differences in compounds had also allowed for the stimulation of various receptor types over a limited period, which had allegedly lead to the best results. Several athletes had indicated that these acquired effects could have been maintained for a several month duration if the steroidal combination had been completely changed before the end of 8 weeks had arrived.

However, having provided examples of the various stacks which some athletes had sometimes employed, would have been rather pointless. For example, most examples which have been observed in various magazines, and other steroid-related books, have cited products which have been generally unavailable to most athletes. This of course, had not allowed the suggested stack to be as effective with missing items, or if the products had been obtainable, they generally had a very high possibility of having been counterfeited. Therefore, the likelihood of these stacks having produced any type of beneficial effect had been very low, even if all recommended items had been obtainable. Consequently, instead of having illustrated possible steroidal compound stacking tables which probably would have rendered "unapplicable" to most athletes, the suggestion of common sense has instead been recommended. If an athlete had been positively certain that a steroidal product had been legit (usually decided by factors outlined within this book), then depending upon which items had been obtained, he/she had been able to have constituted an efficacious stacking cycle, by merely having identified each product's characteristic (again, stated within each compound's identification within this book), and having decided an appropriate combination cycle from there. This advice had been extremely advantageous to most athletes, as each cycle had then been individualized according to the available steroidal item, the athlete's financial circumstance, and of course, the athlete's health.

HUMAN & VETERINARY PHARMACEUTICAL ILLUSTRATIONS

DIURETICS: Aldactone* 100 & Aldactone*-A

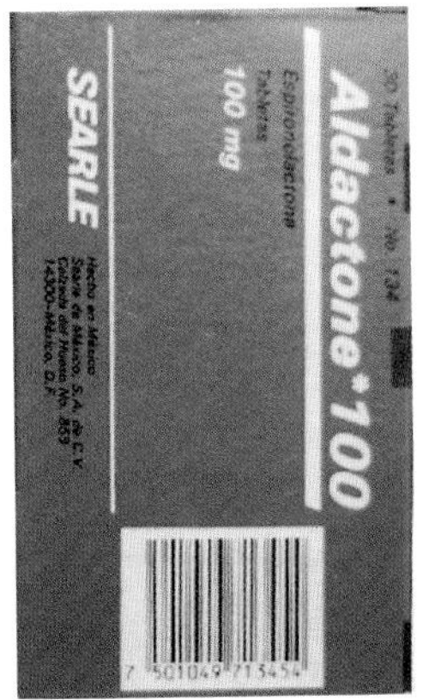

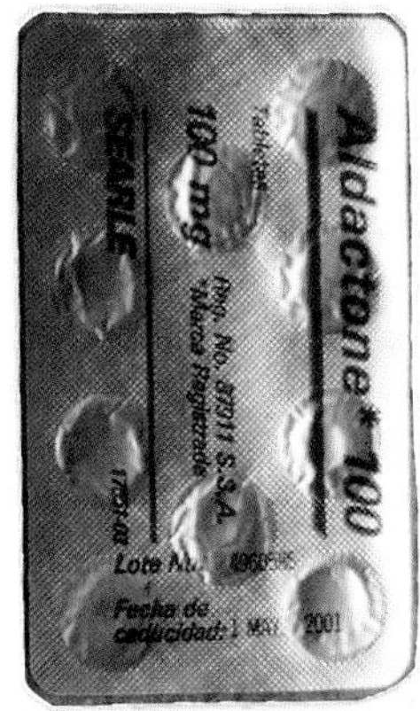

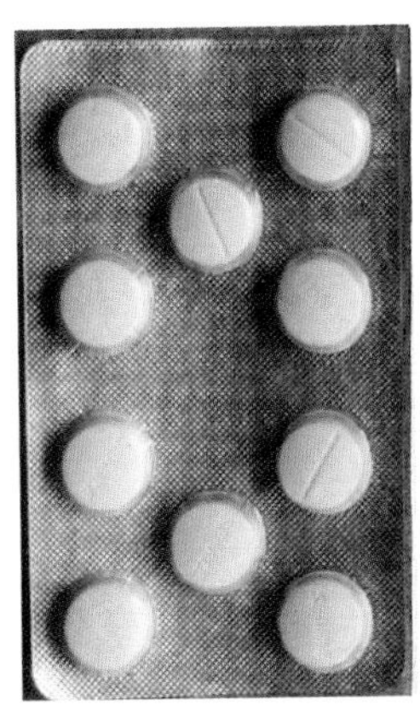

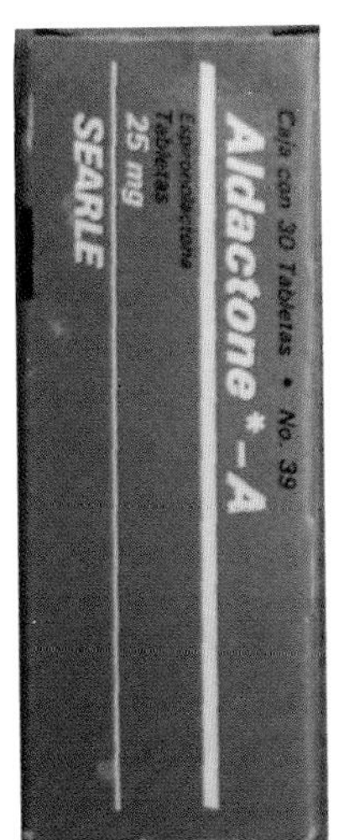

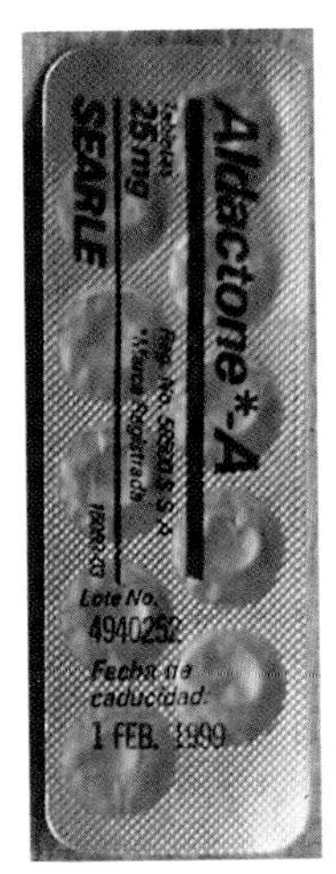

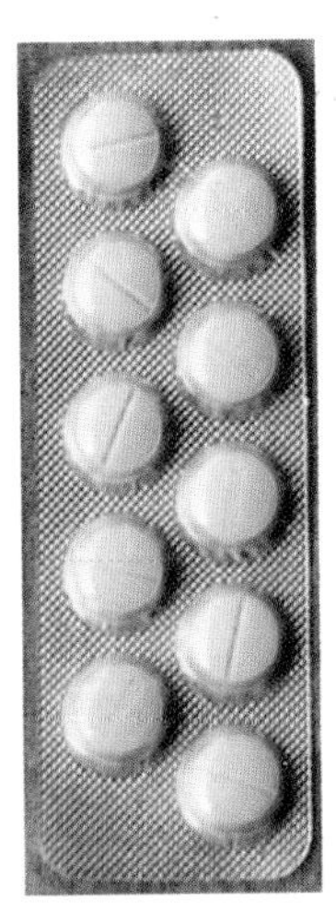

DIURETICS: Lasix & Dyazide

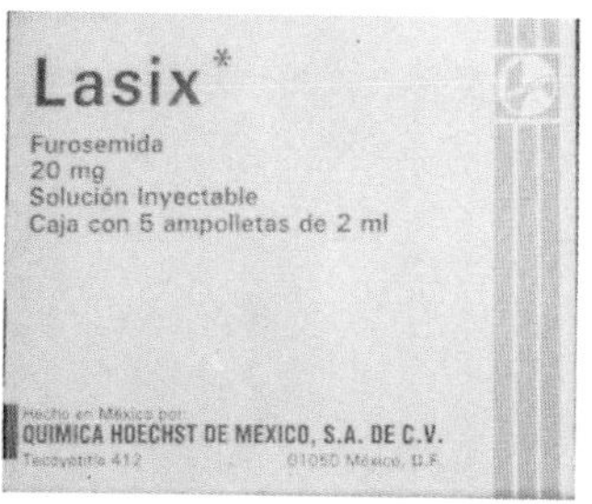

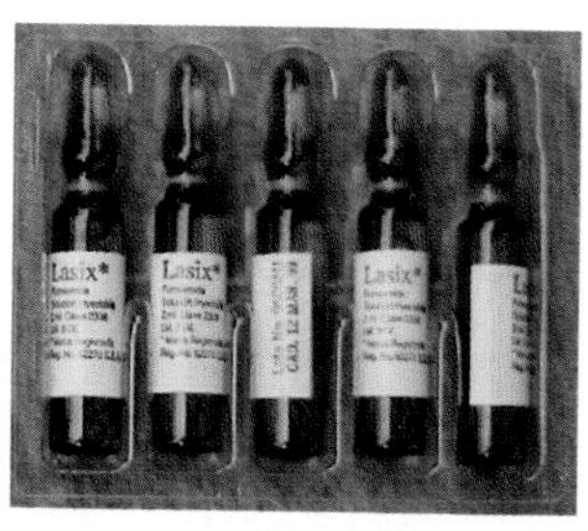

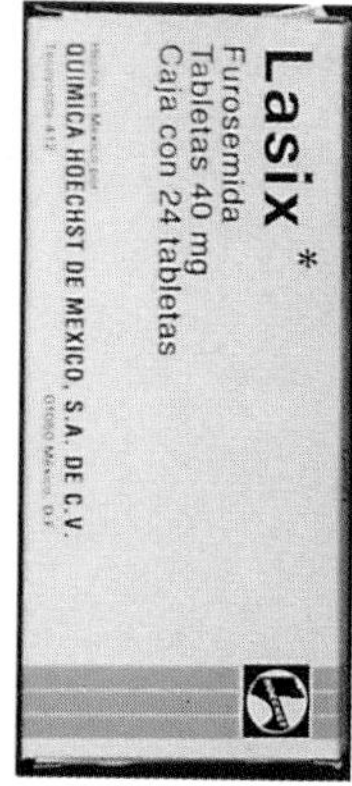

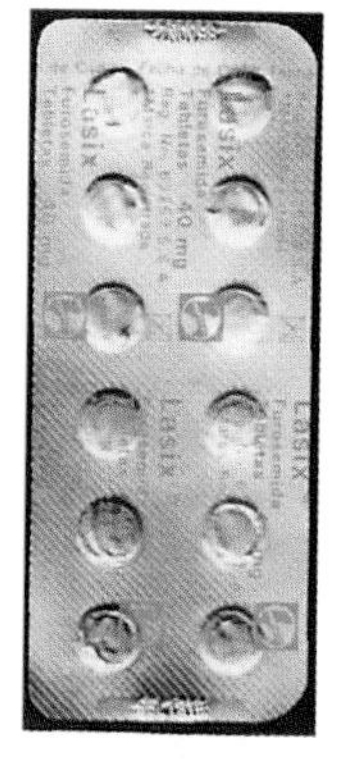

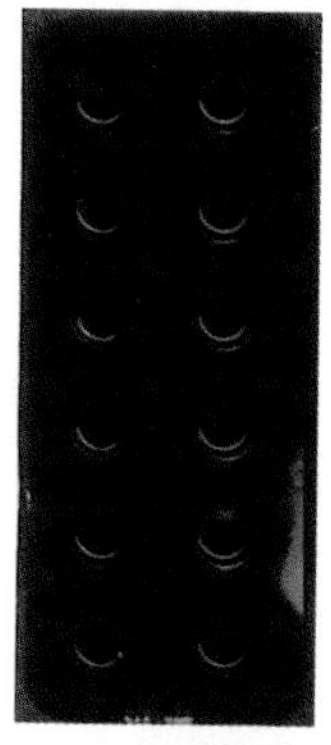

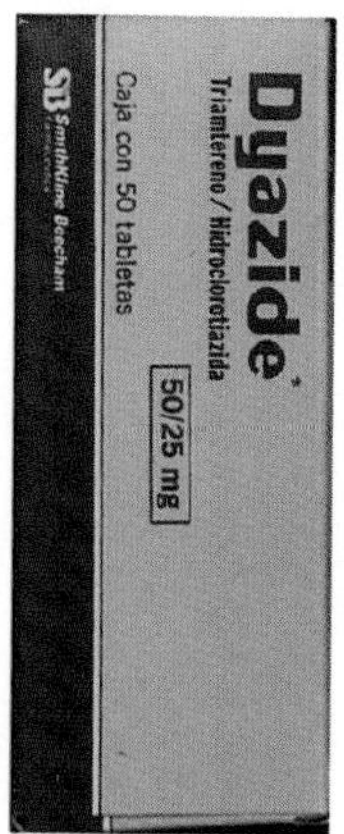

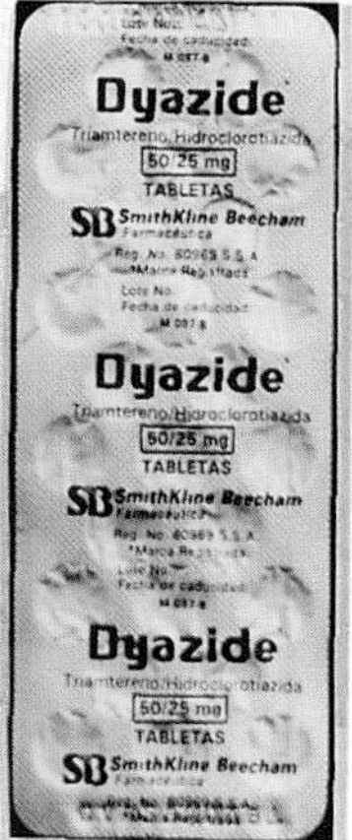

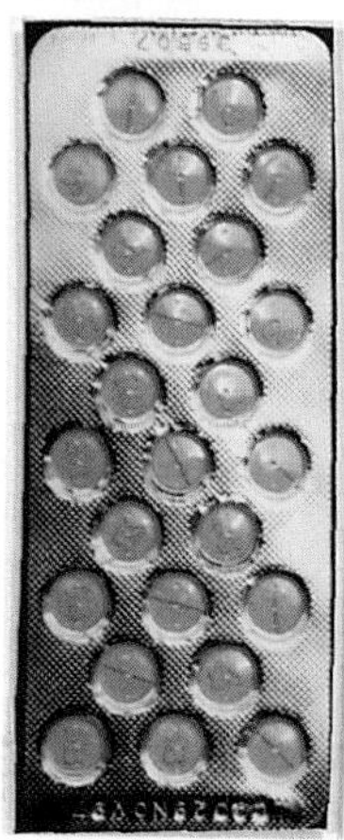

ANTI-INFLAMMATORIES: Naxen

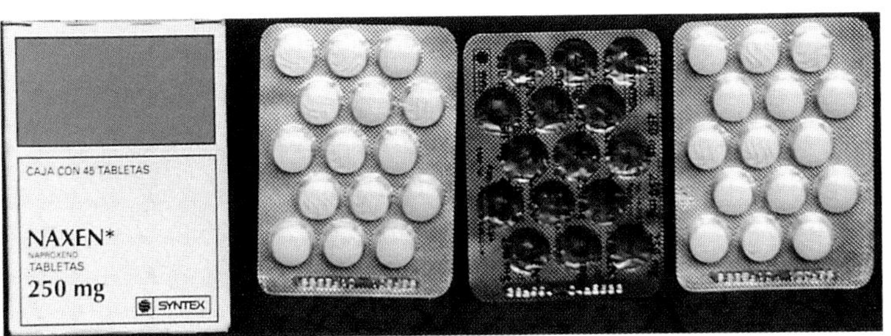

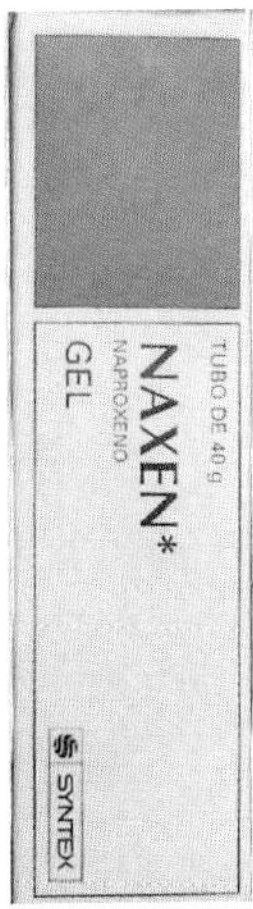

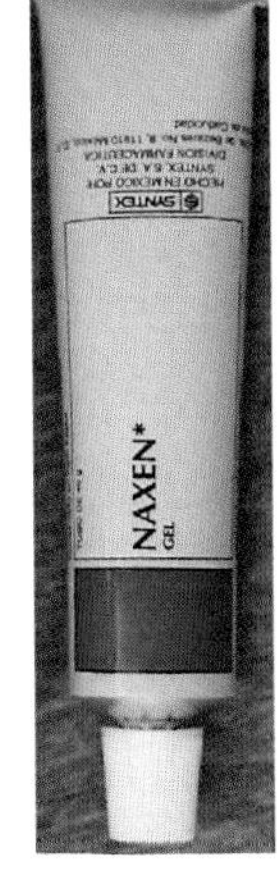

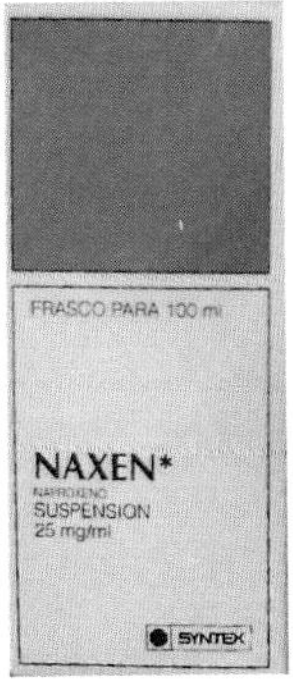

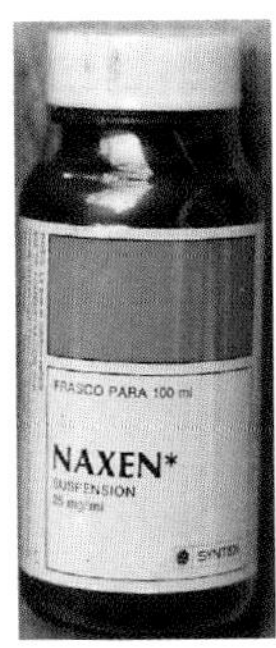

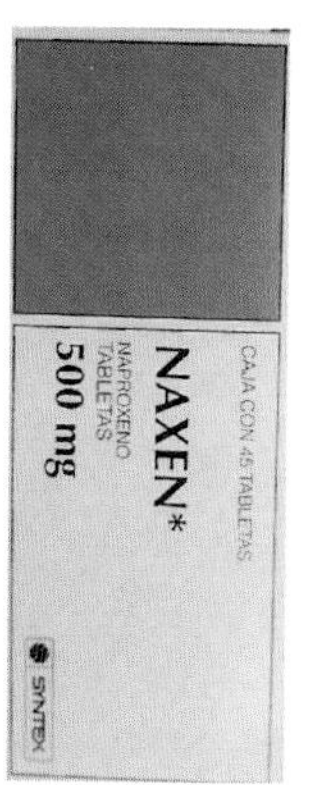

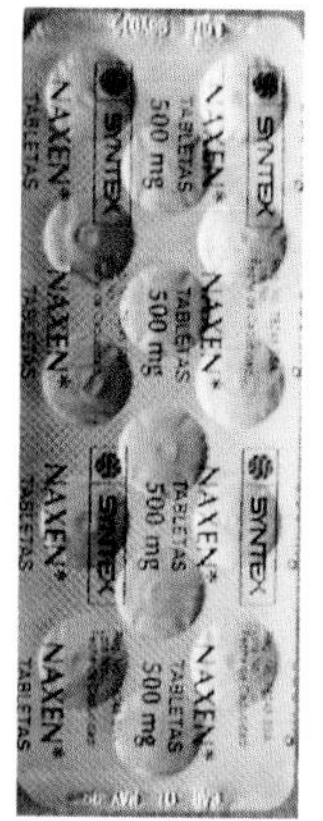

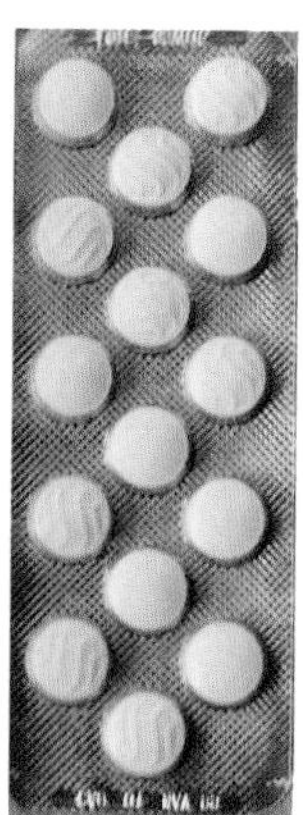

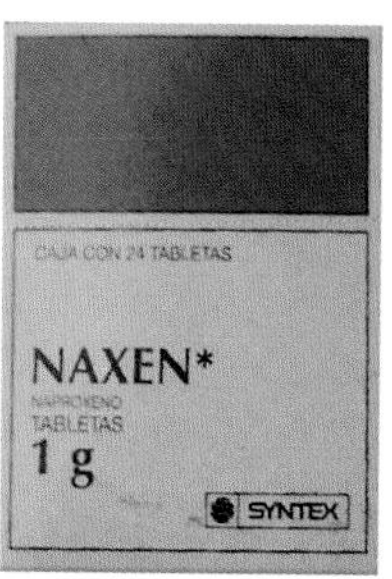

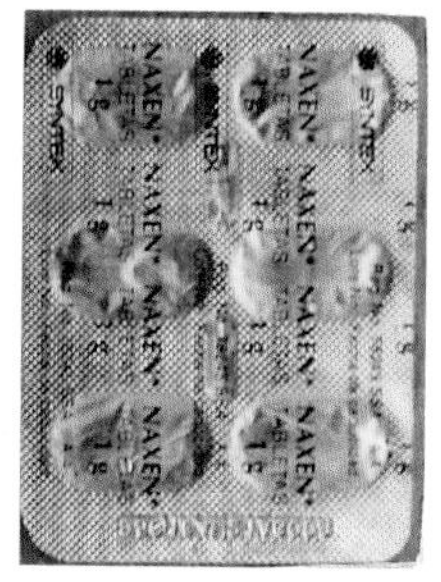

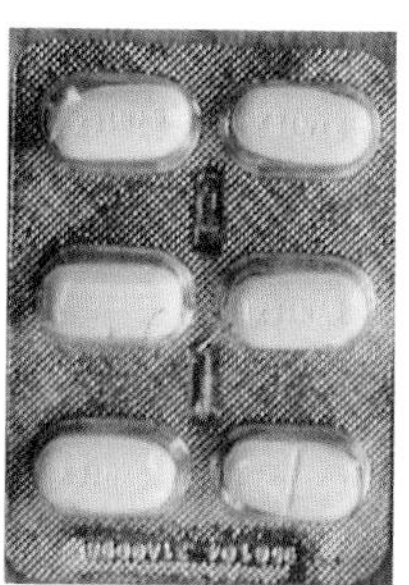

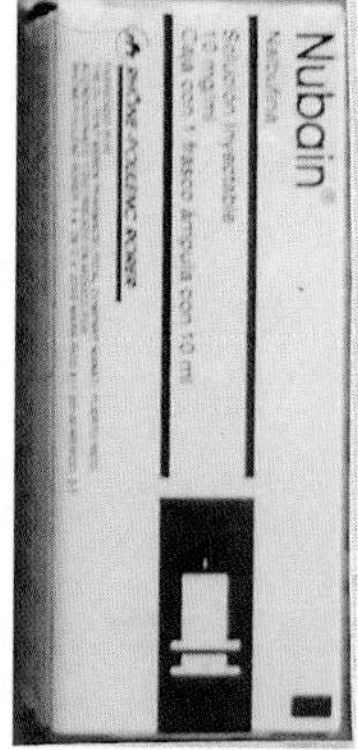

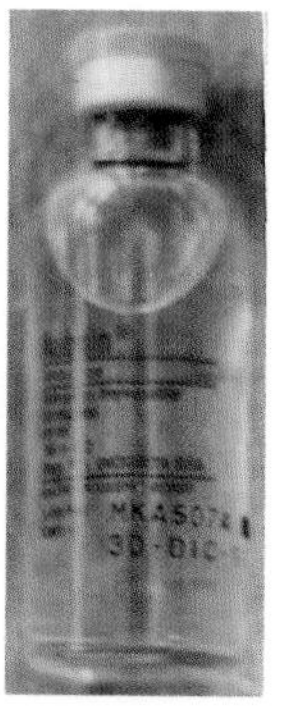

PAIN RELIEVER: Nubain

ANTI-HYPERGLYCEMIC AGENTS:

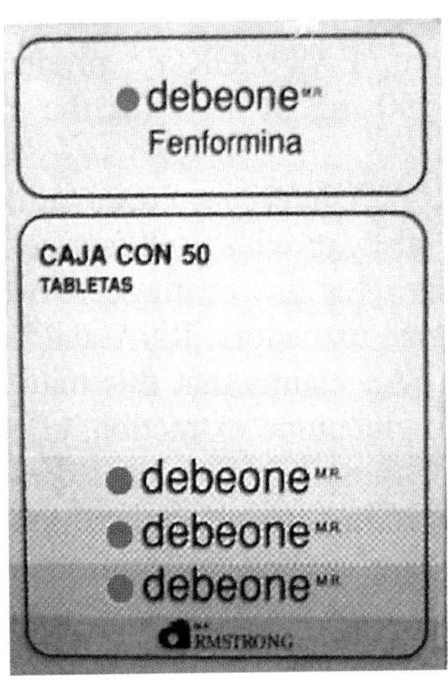

PHENFORMIN: Debeone

METFORMIN: Glucophage

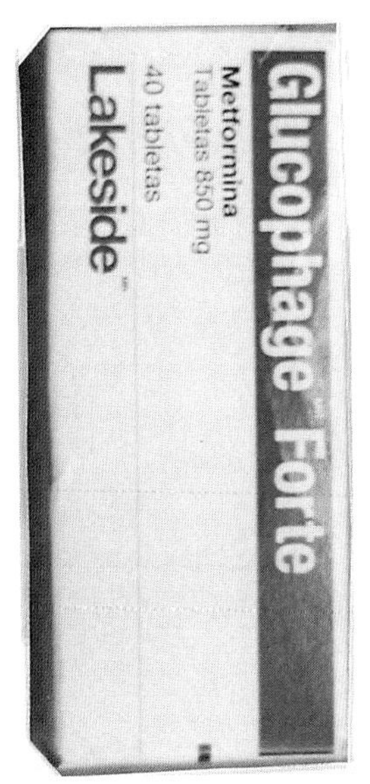

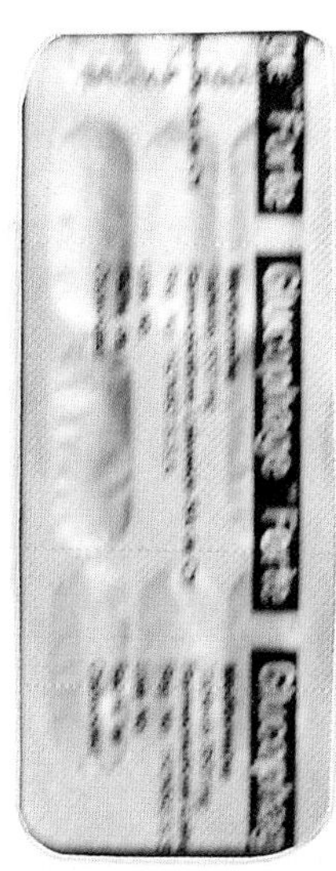

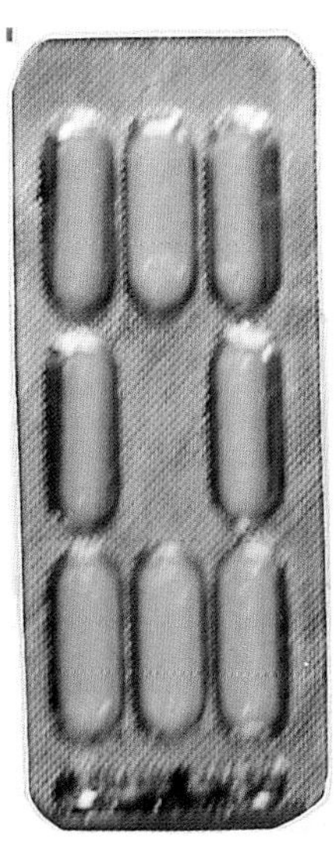

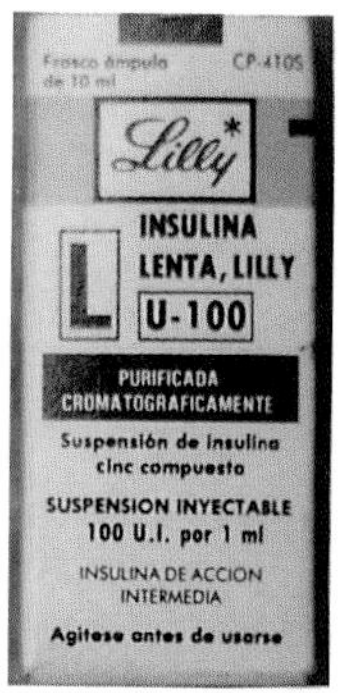

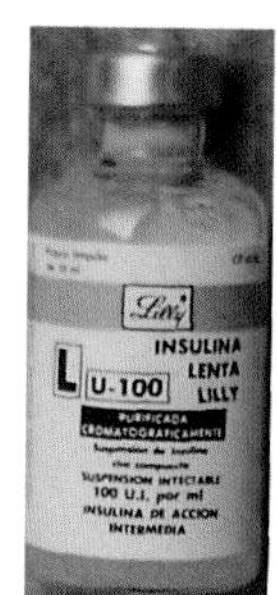

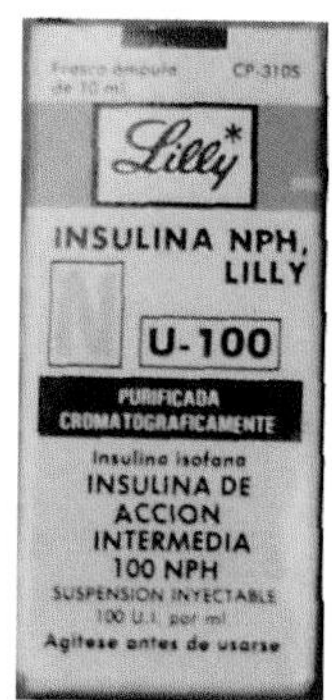

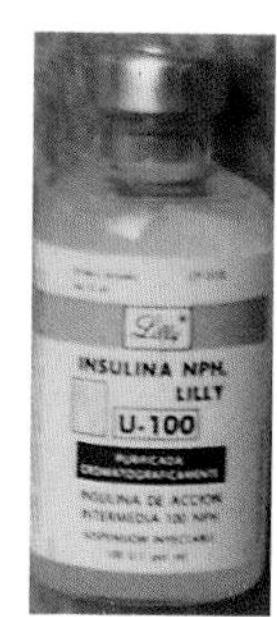

HUMAN INSULINS: Berigiobina*P, Humulin L & N, Seroglubin

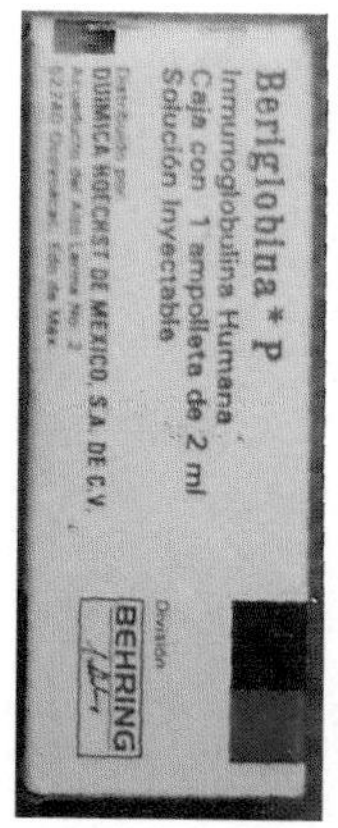

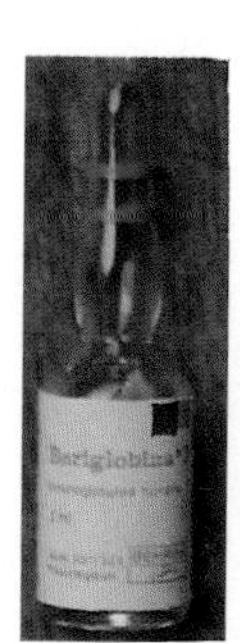

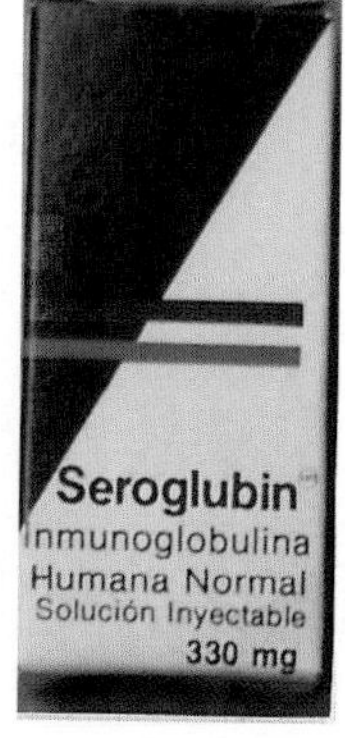

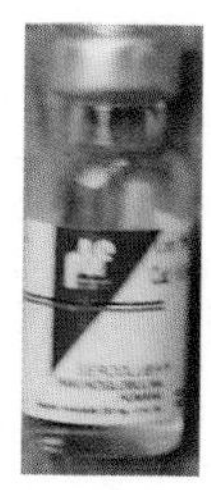

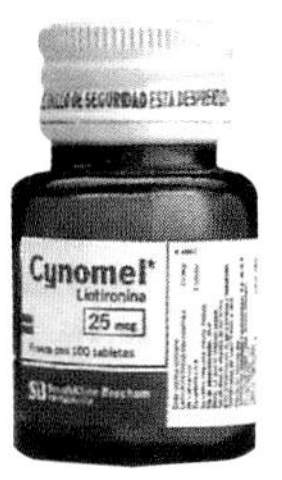

THYROID MEDICATIONS:

T-3: Cynomel

T-4: Eutirox & Tiroidine

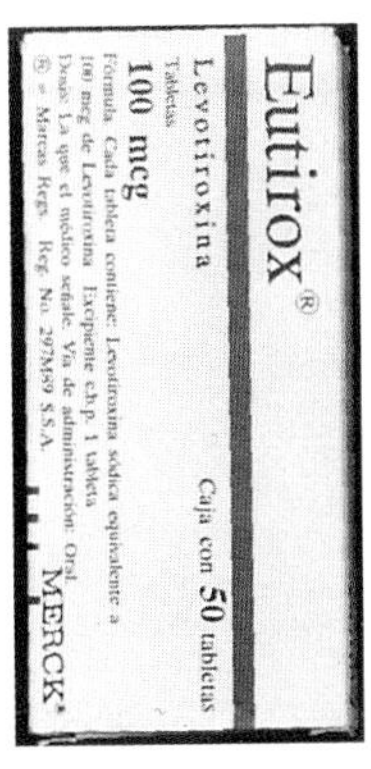

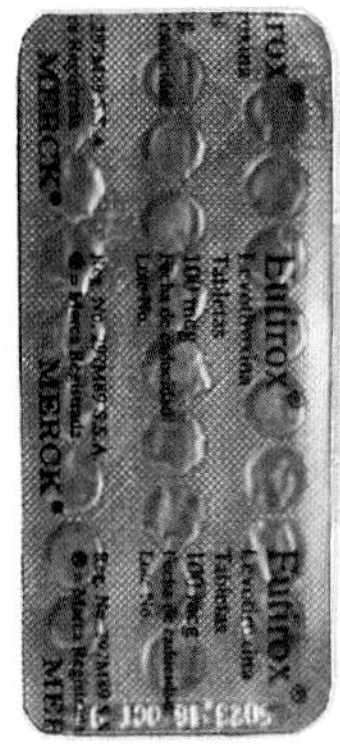

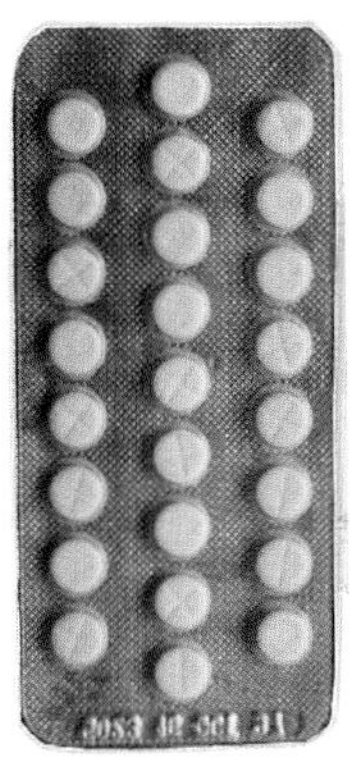

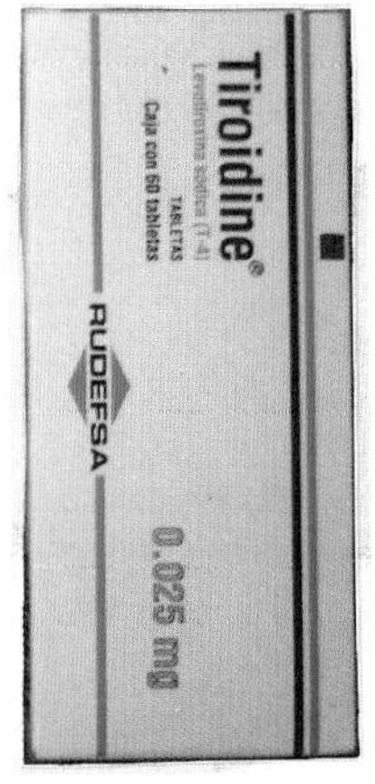

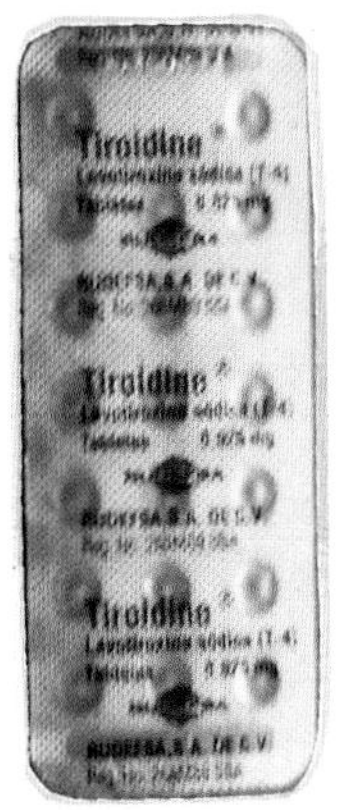

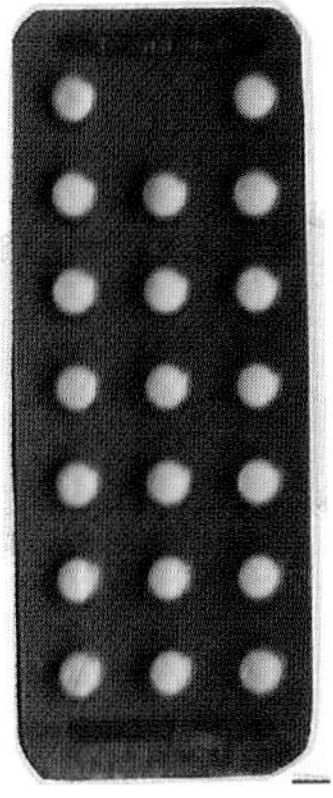

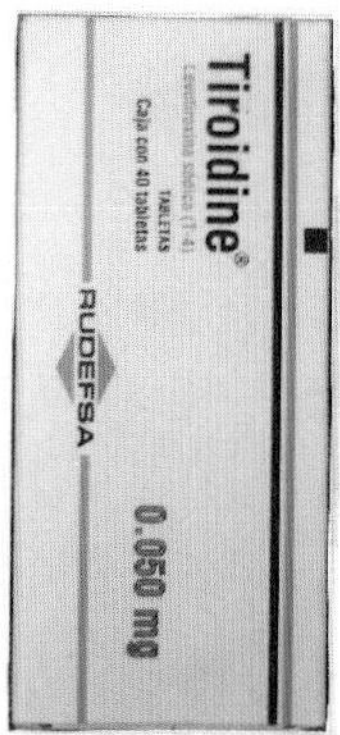
Tiroidine®
Caja con 40 tabletas
RUDEFSA
0.050 mg

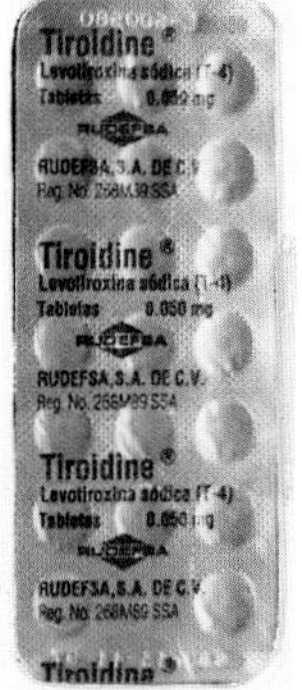
Tiroidine®
Levotiroxina sódica (T-4)
Tabletas 0.050 mg
RUDEFSA
RUDEFSA, S.A. DE C.V.
Reg. No. 266M89 SSA

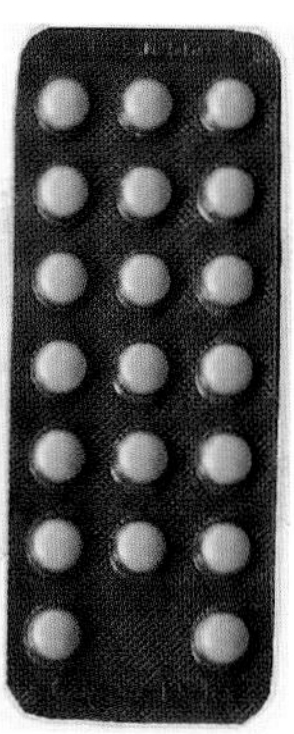

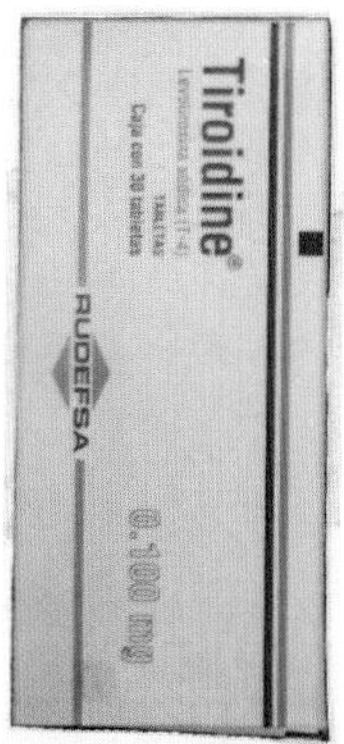
Tiroidine®
Caja con 30 tabletas
RUDEFSA
0.100 mg

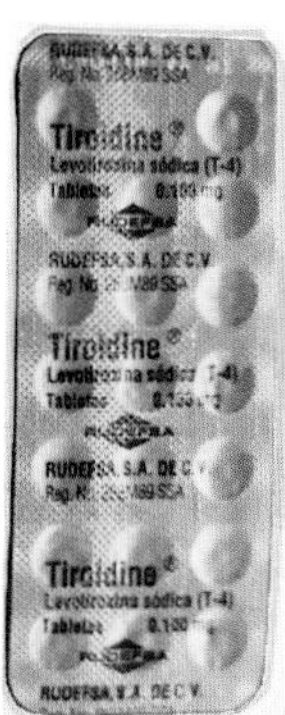
Tiroidine®
Levotiroxina sódica (T-4)
Tabletas
RUDEFSA
RUDEFSA, S.A. DE C.V.

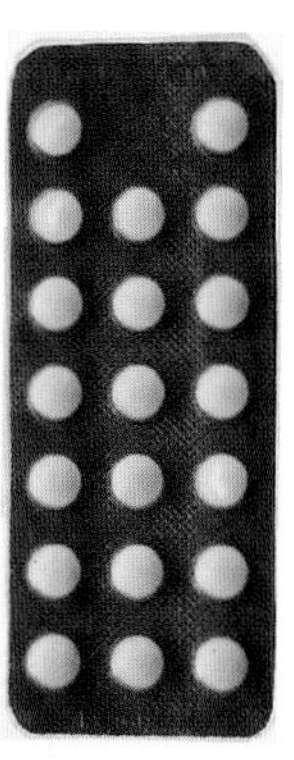

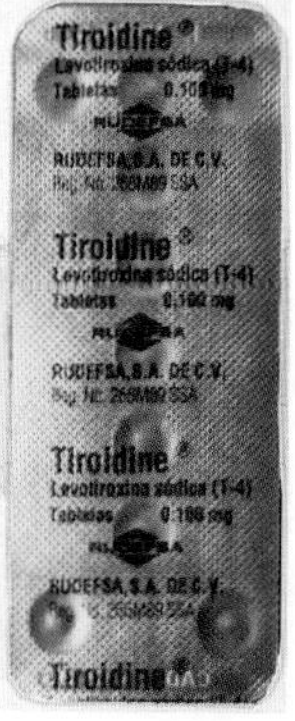
Tiroidine®
Tabletas 0.100 mg
RUDEFSA
RUDEFSA, S.A. DE C.V.
Reg. No. 266M89 SSA

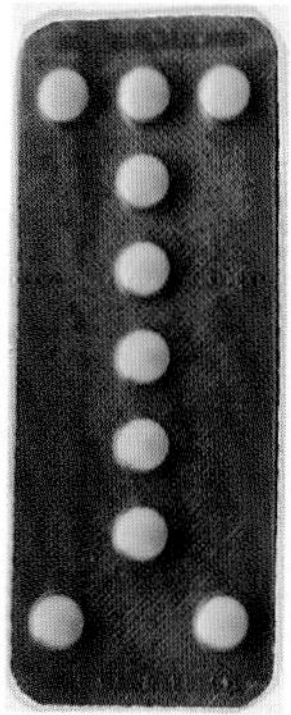

BETA-2-ATAGONIST: Spiropent

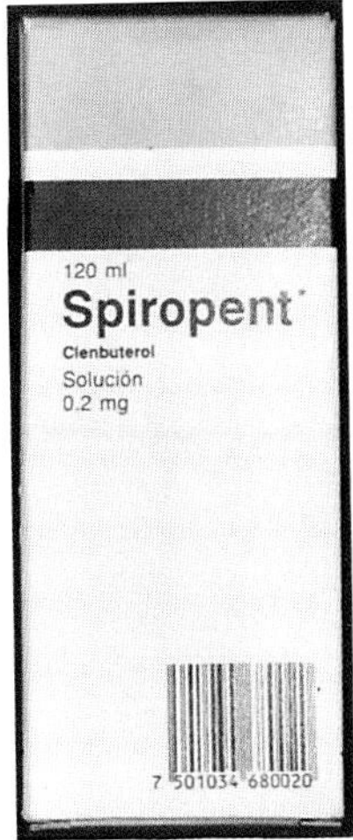

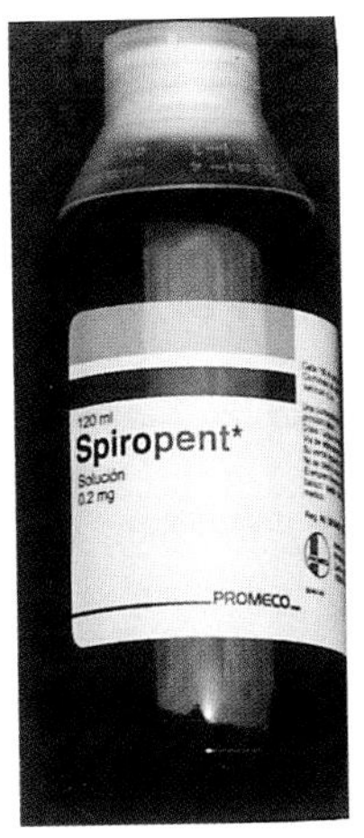

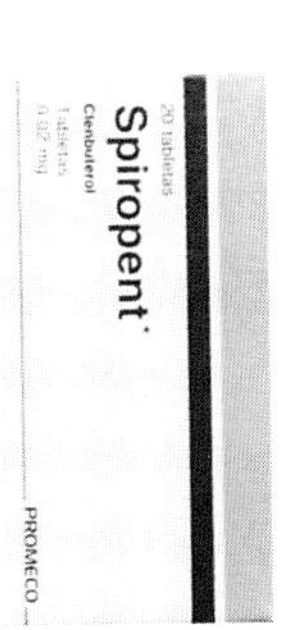

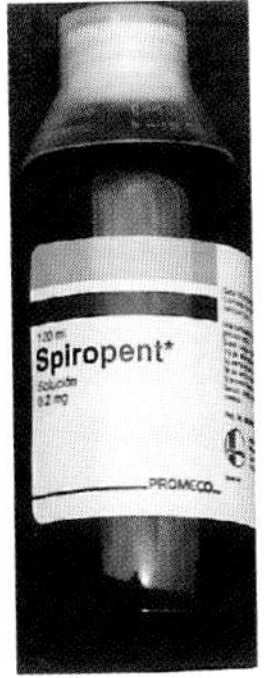

SYNTHETIC HUMAN GROWTH HORMONE: Humatrope Saizen

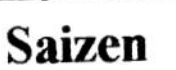

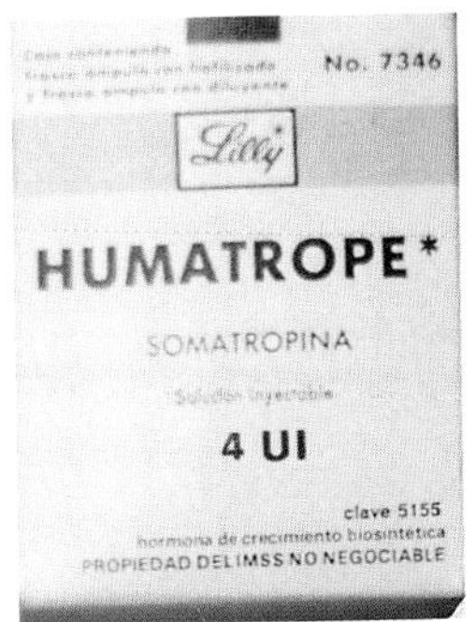

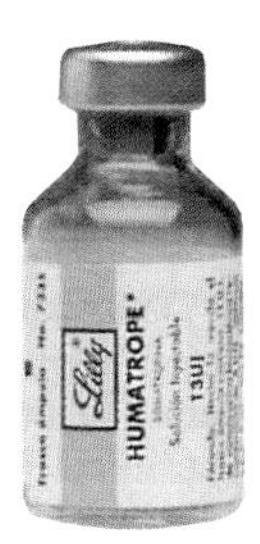

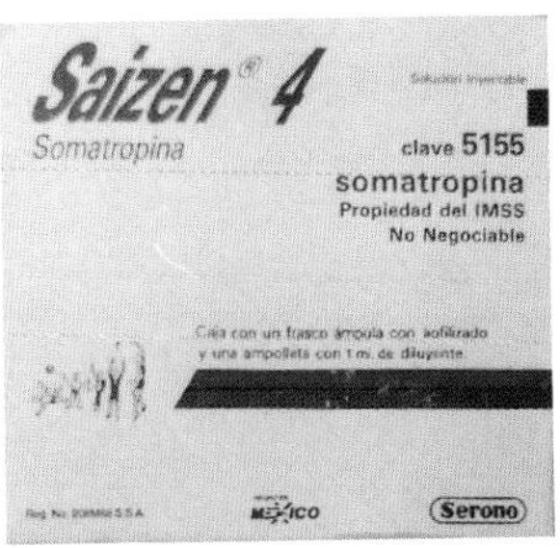

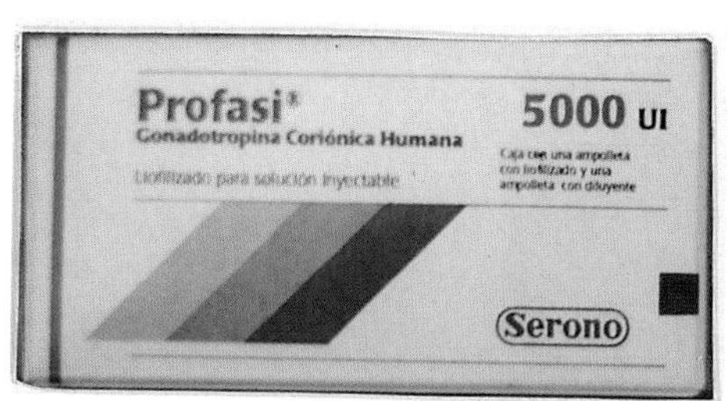

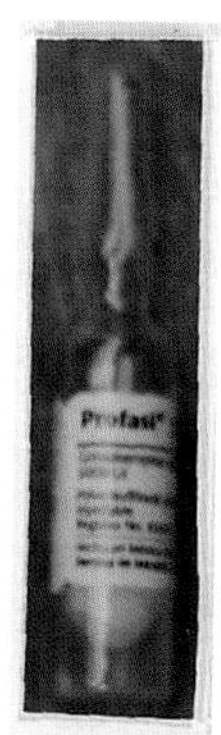

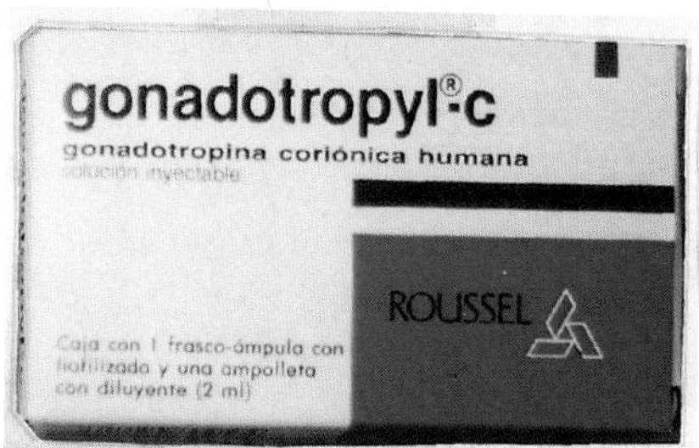

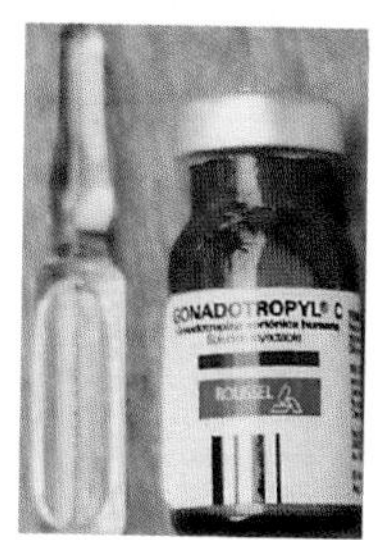

MIMICS THE NATURAL LUTEINIZING HORMONE:
(HCG): Profasi, Gonakor
Gonadotrophyl-C

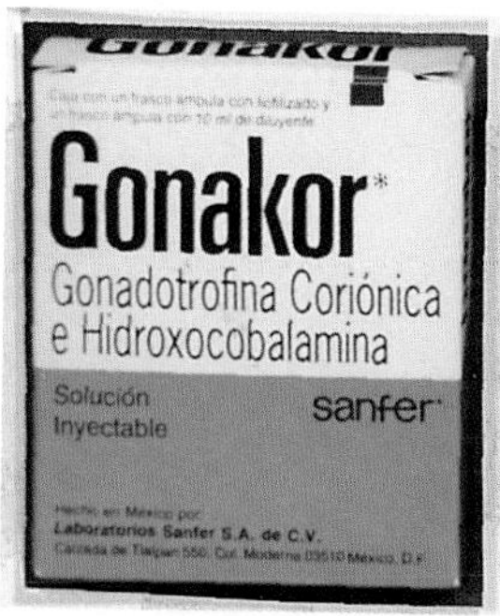

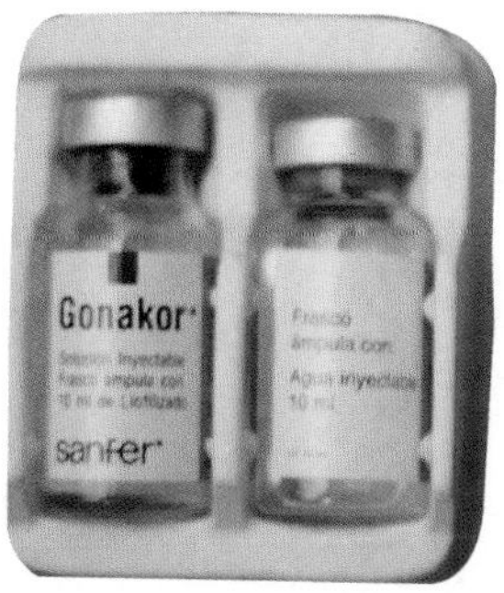

SYNTHETIC ESTROGEN:
(CLOMID): Omifin

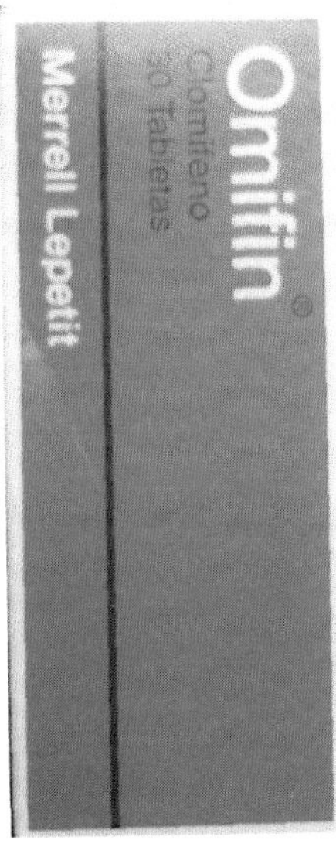

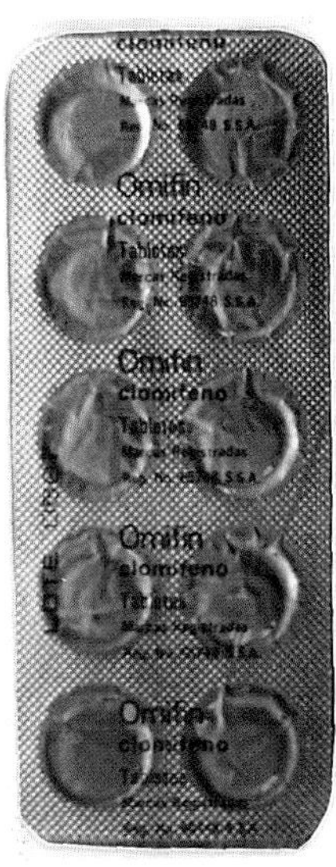

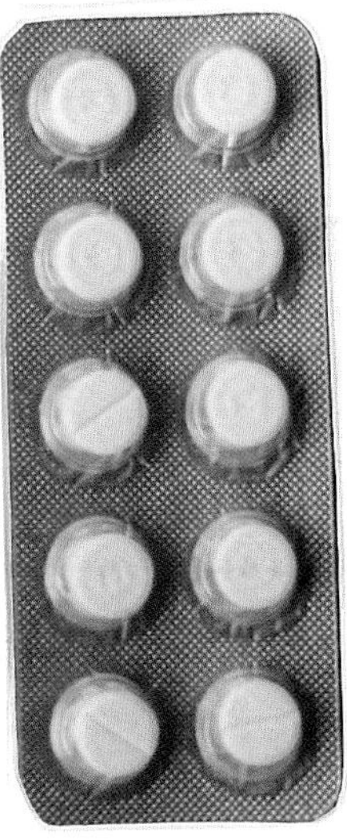

MILD ANTI-ESTROGEN:
(CYCLOFENIL): Fertodur

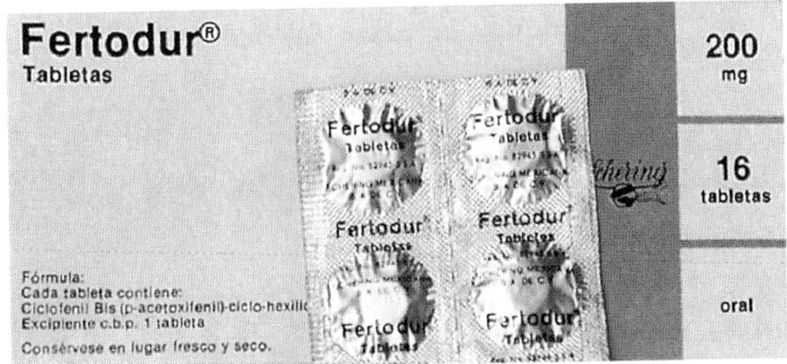

ANTI-ESTROGEN: Nolvadex

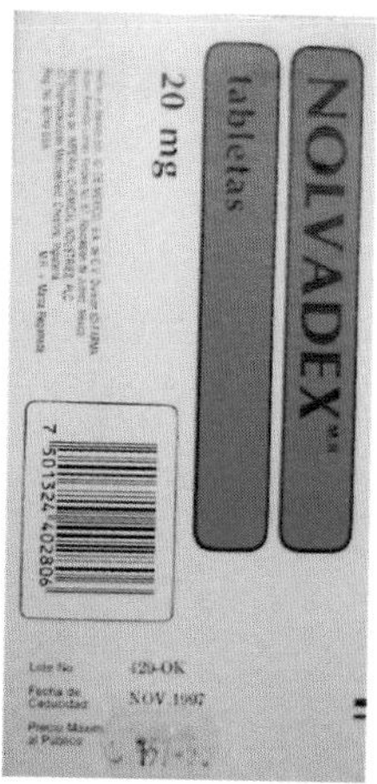

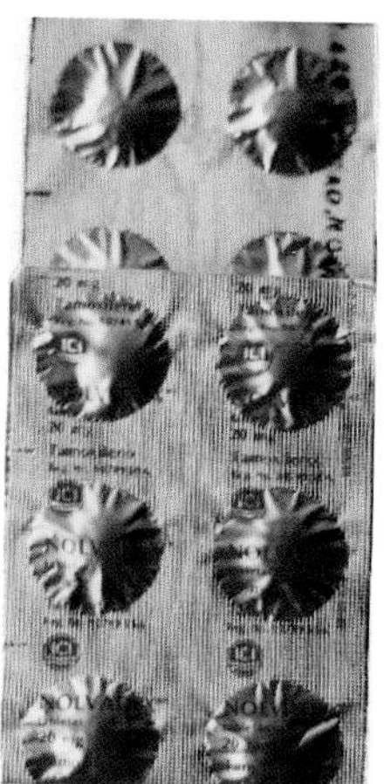

ESTROGEN ANTAGONIST: Proviron

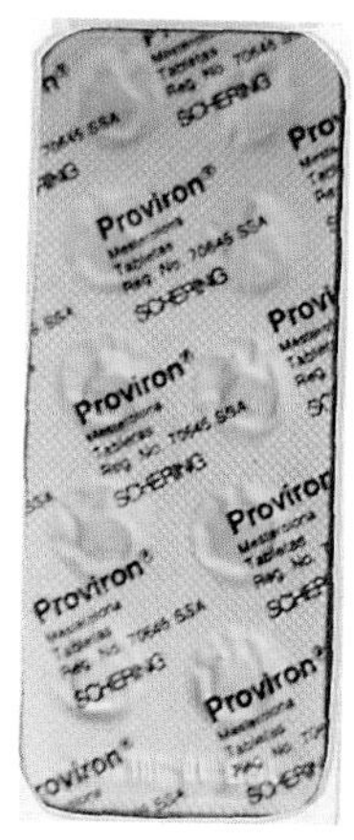

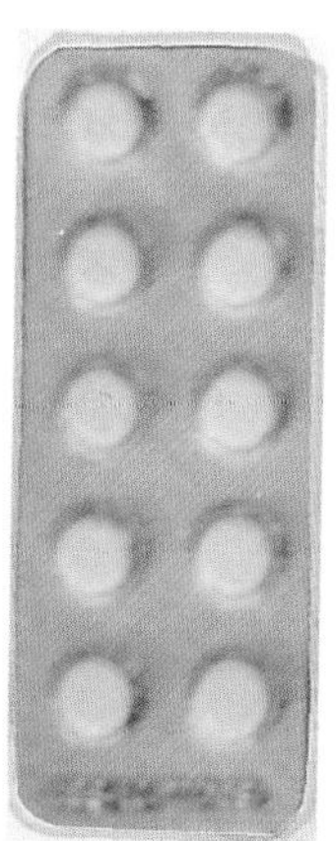

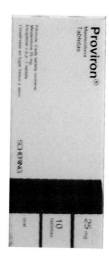

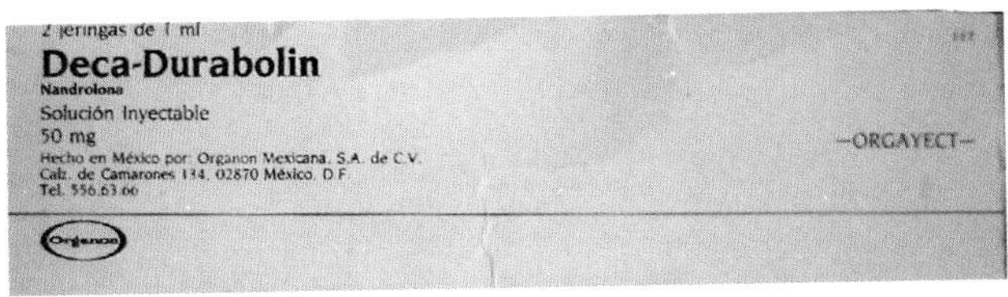

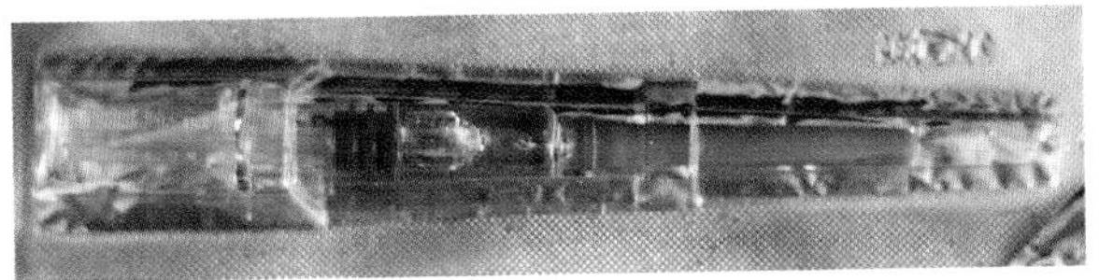

ANABOLIC STEROID: Deca-Durabolin

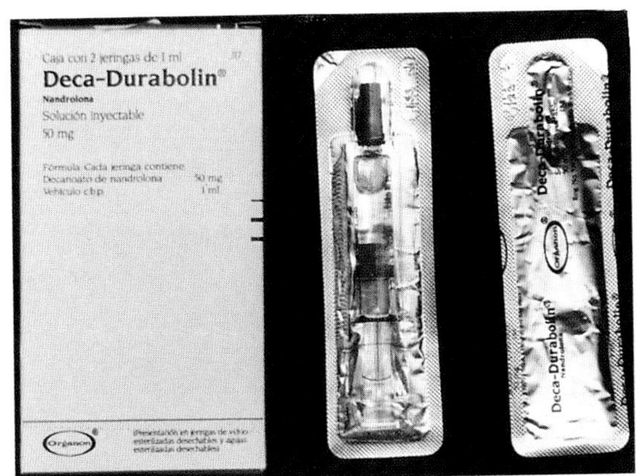

ANABOLIC STEROIDS: Primobolan Depot
Primobolan Tablets

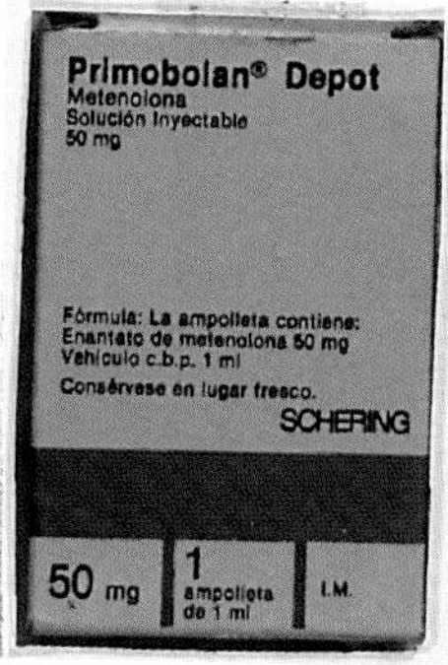

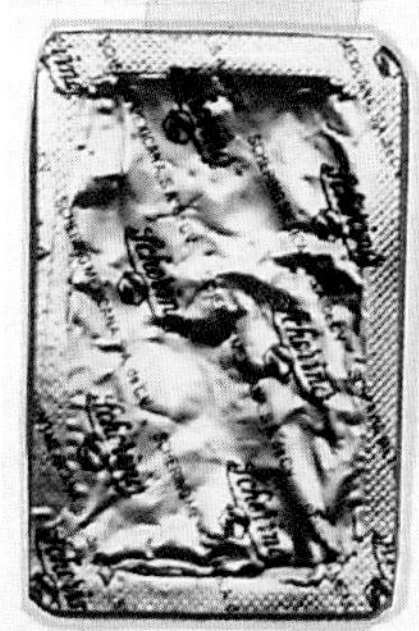

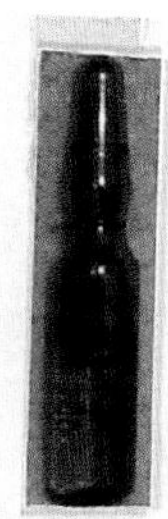

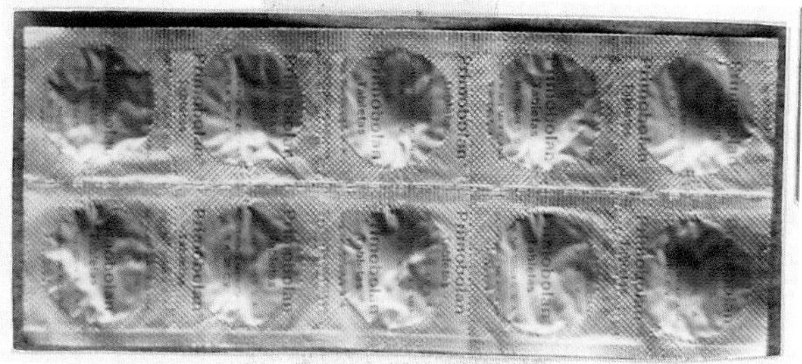

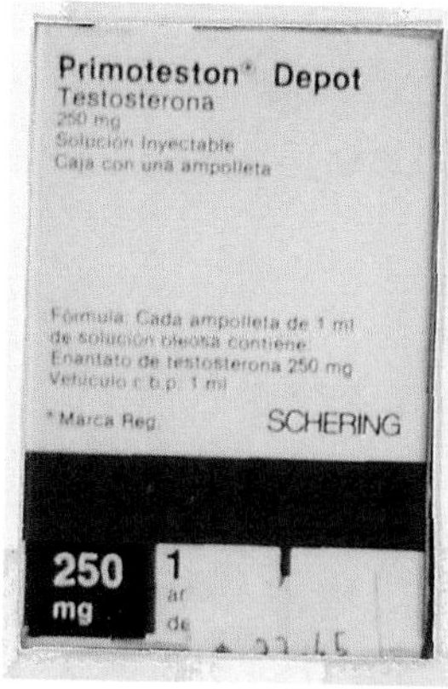

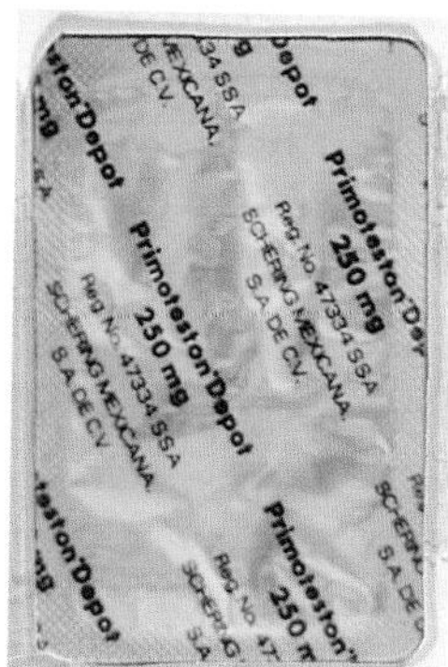

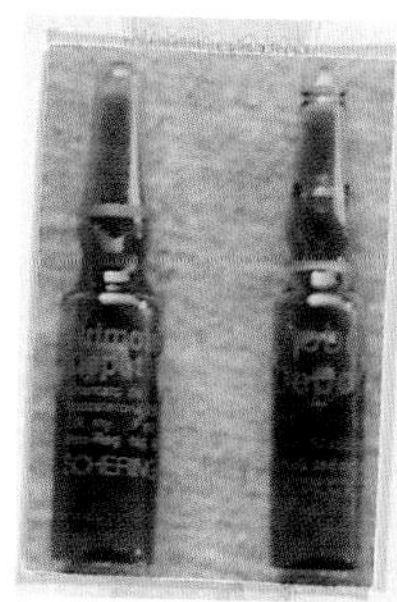

ANDROGENIC STEROID: Sostenon 250

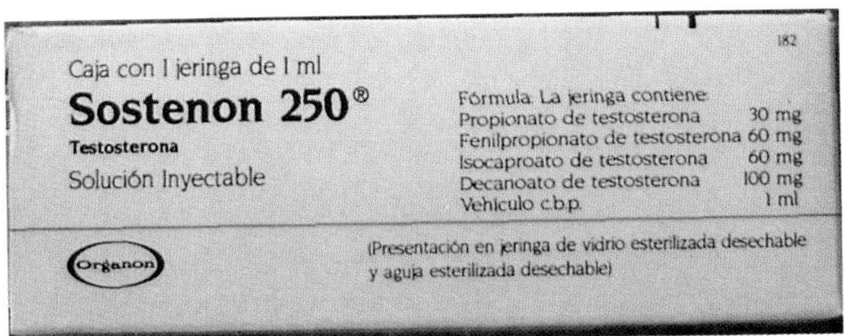

182
Caja con 1 jeringa de 1 ml
Sostenon 250®
Testosterona
Solución Inyectable
Fórmula: La jeringa contiene:
Propionato de testosterona 30 mg
Fenilpropionato de testosterona 60 mg
Isocaproato de testosterona 60 mg
Decanoato de testosterona 100 mg
Vehículo c.b.p. 1 ml
Organon
(Presentación en jeringa de vidrio esterilizada desechable
y aguja esterilizada desechable)

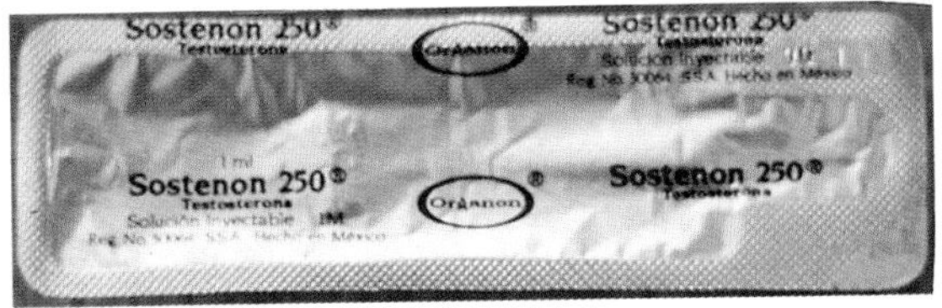

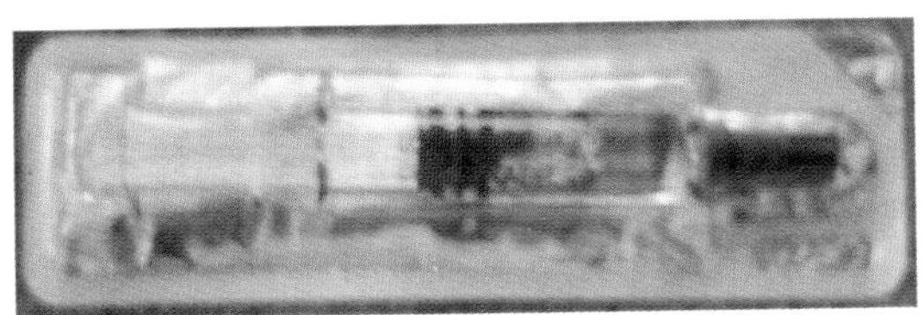

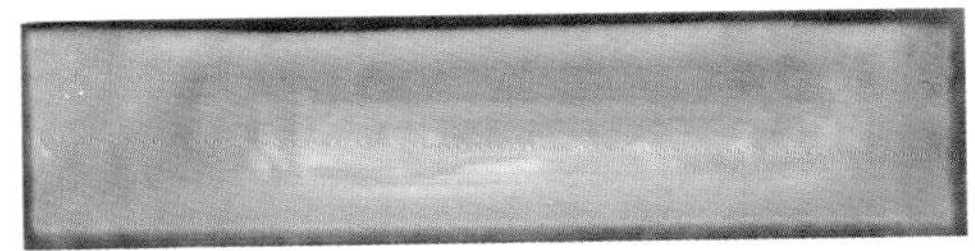

ANABOLIC & ANDROGENIC STEROID: Anapolon

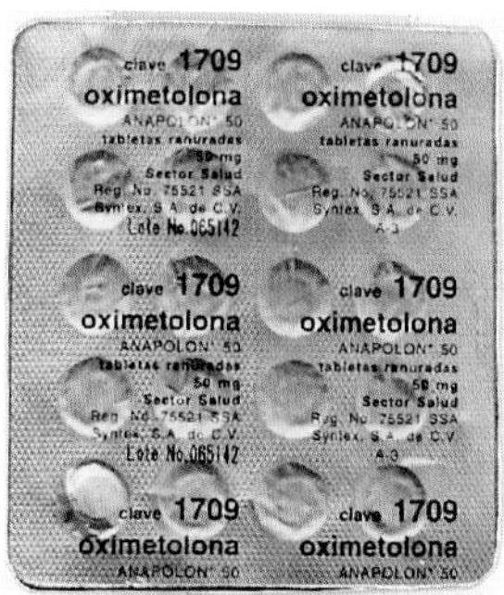

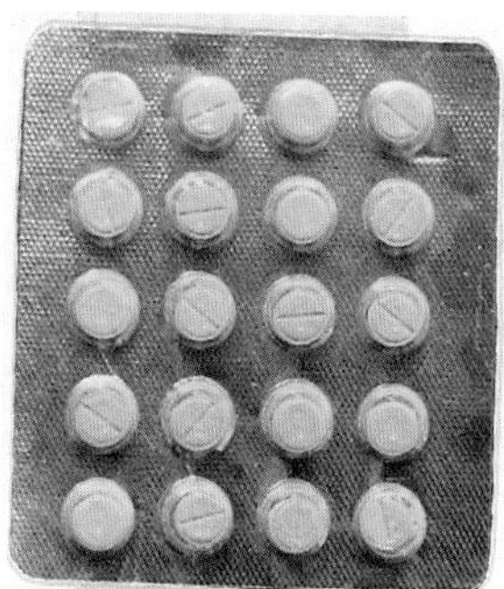

ANDROGENIC STEROID: Stenox

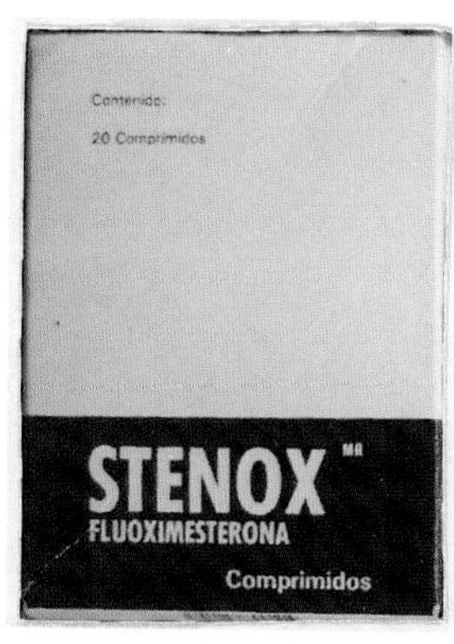

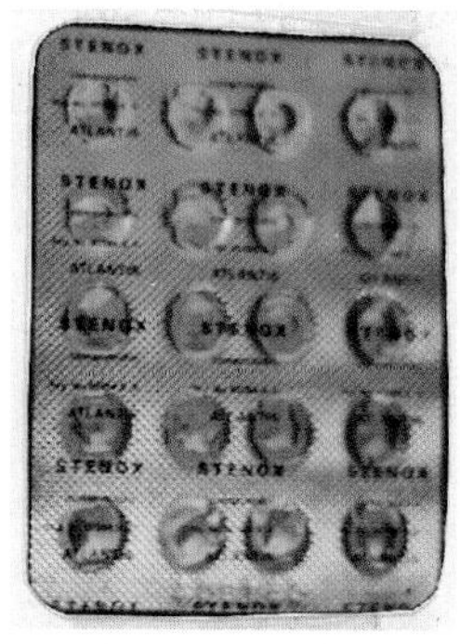

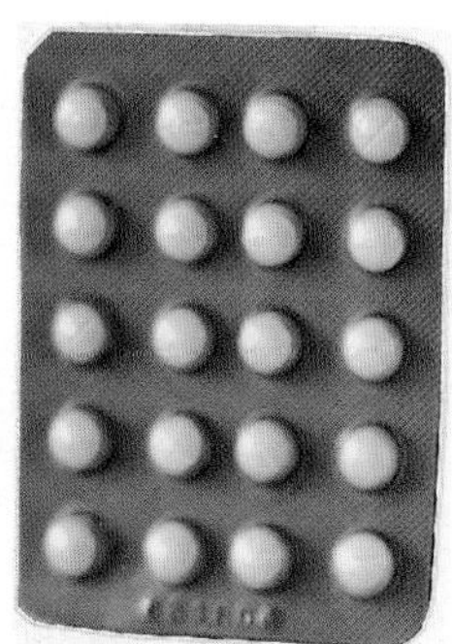

HUMAN CO-ENZYME B12: Maxibol

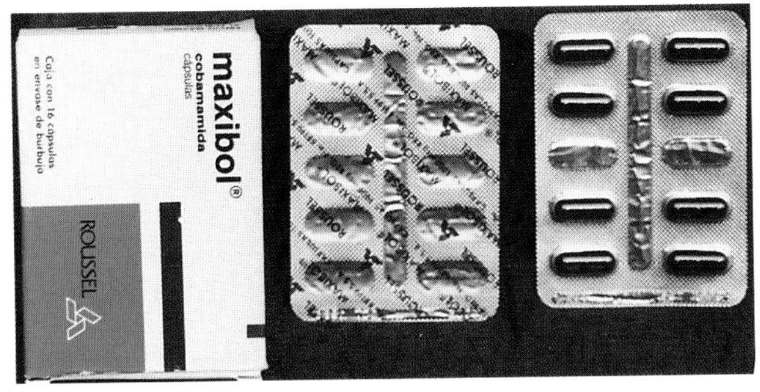

HUMAN VITAMIN B12: Neurofor

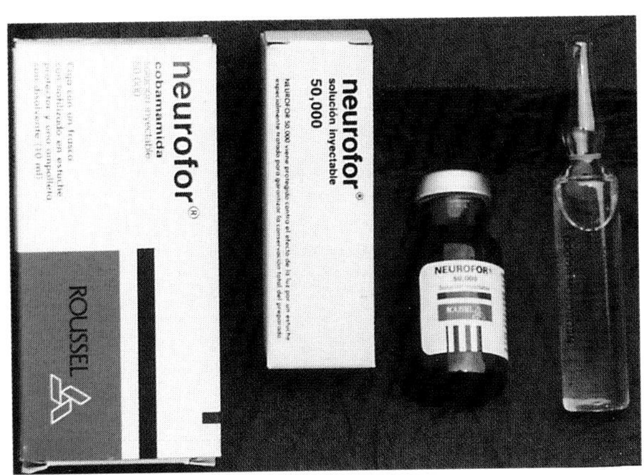

VETERINARY:

ANDROGENIC STEROID: Deposterona*

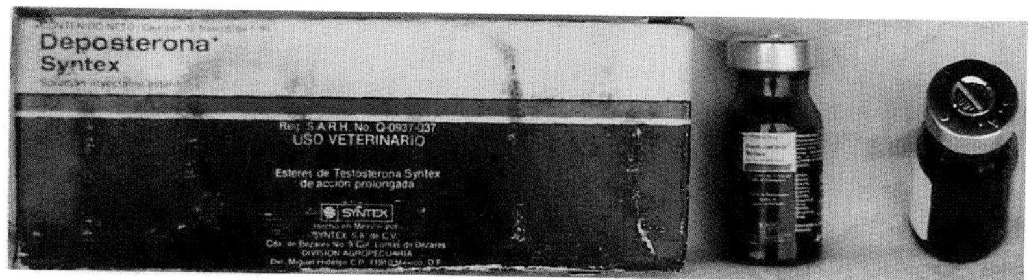

Be careful not to confuse with Progesterona*, which does not contain any Testosterone.

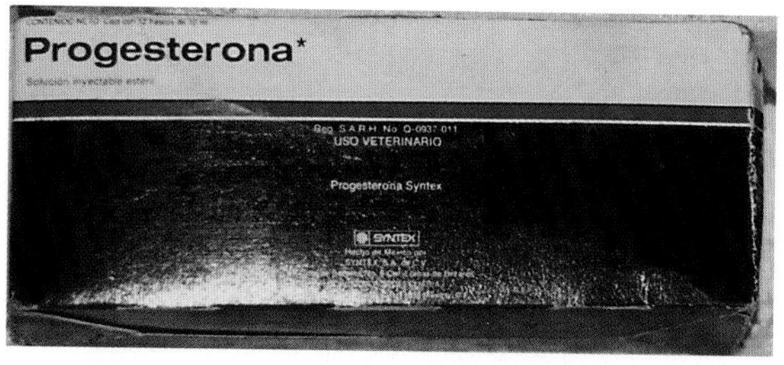

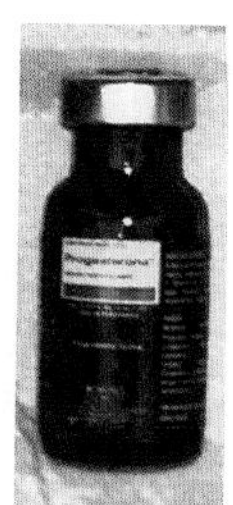

STRONG ANABOLIC, MILD ANDROGENIC STEROID: (Equipoise):

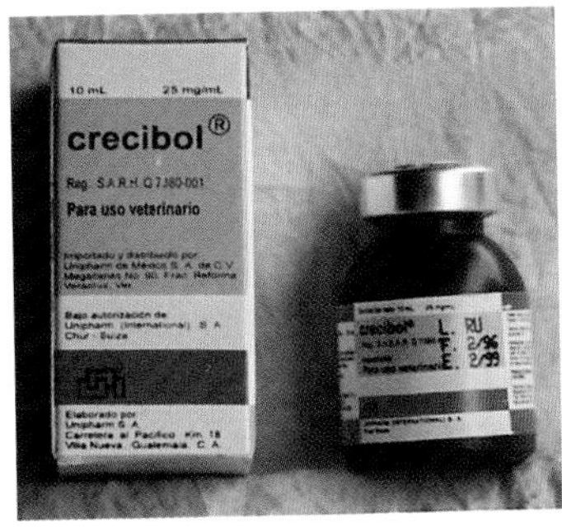

Crecibol

Equi-Gan

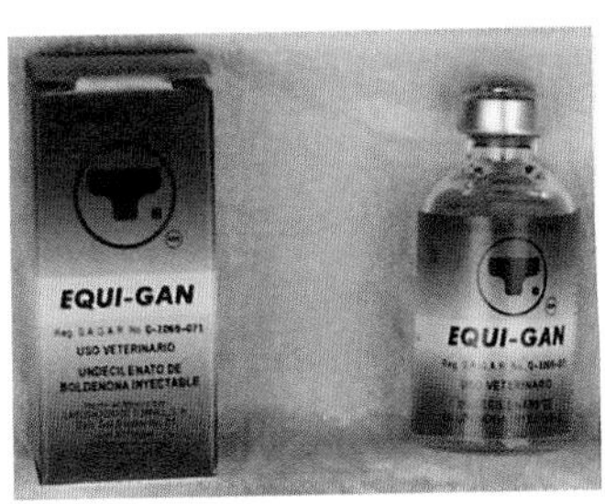

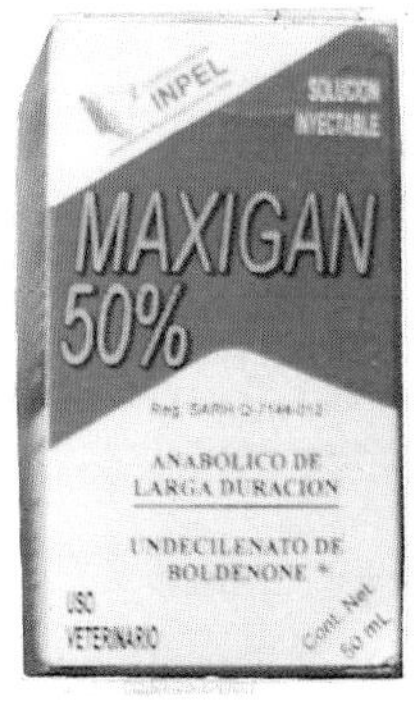

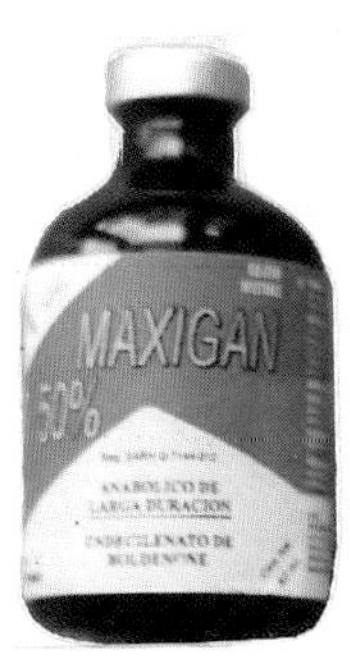

Maxigan

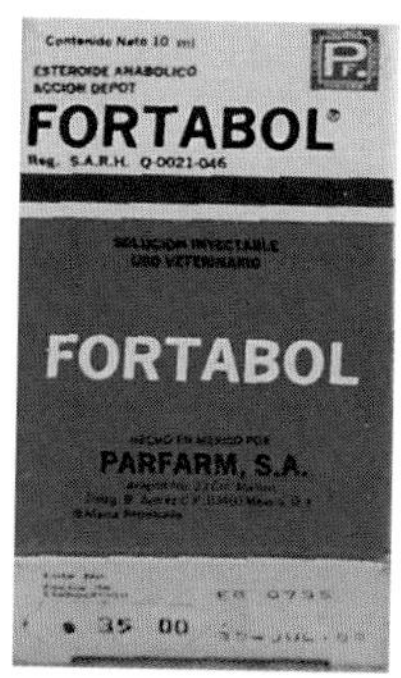

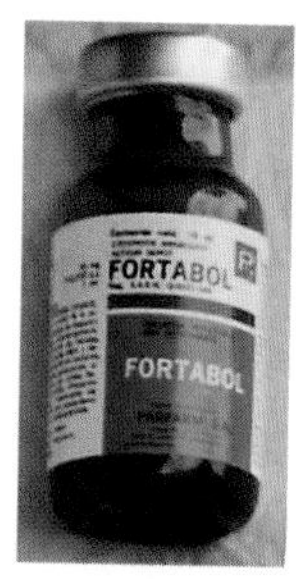

ANABOLIC STEROID:

Fortabol and Laurabolin

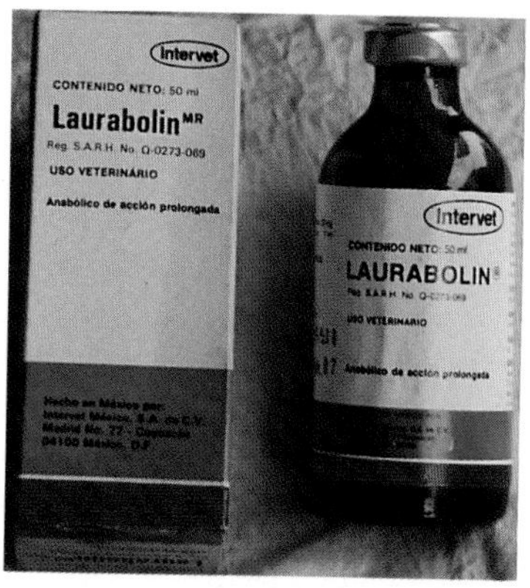

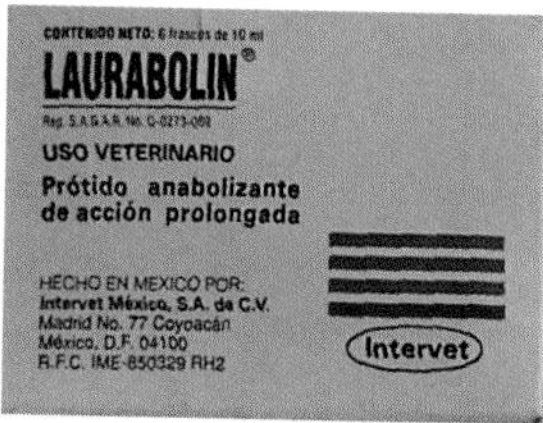

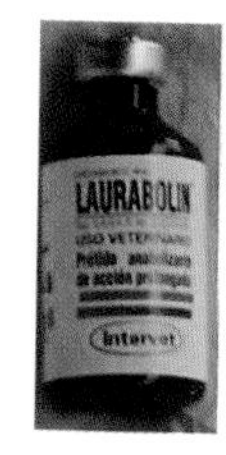

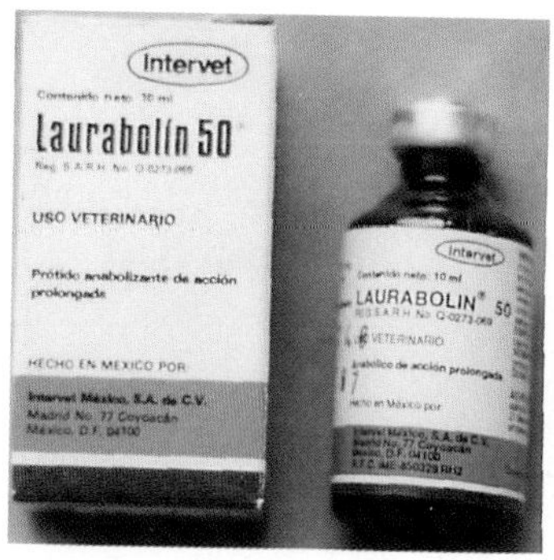

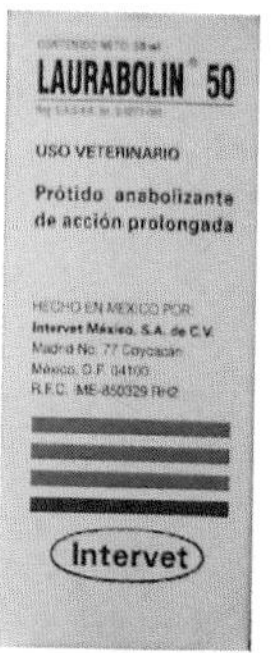

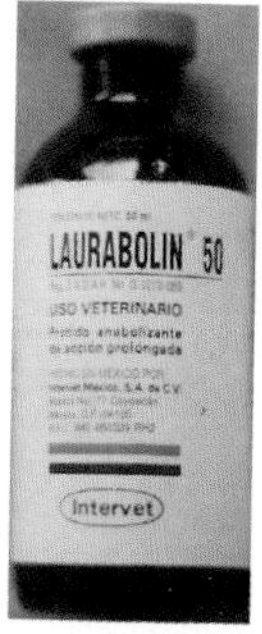

ANABOLIC AGENT: Ralgrow

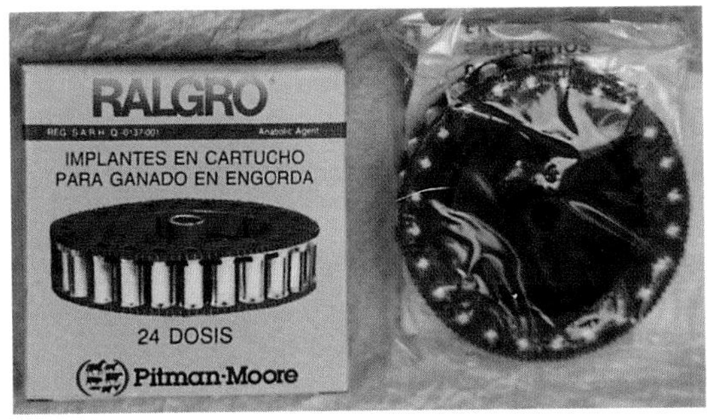

HORMONE IMPLANT: Synovex*-H

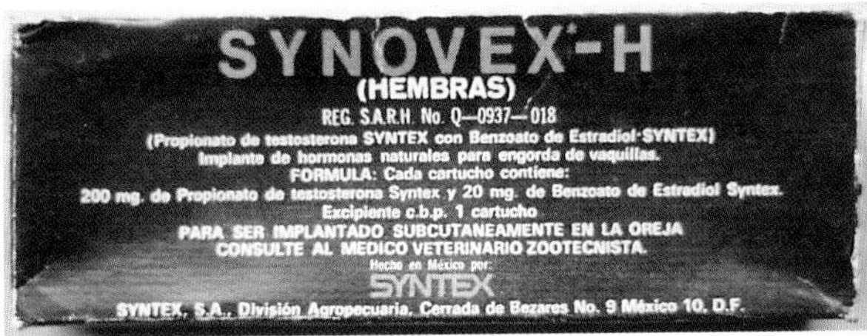

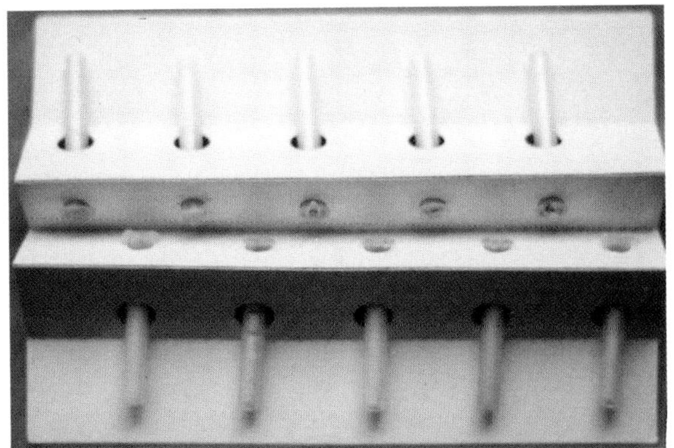

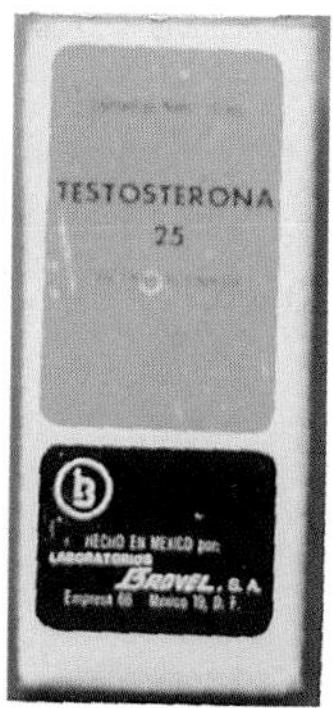

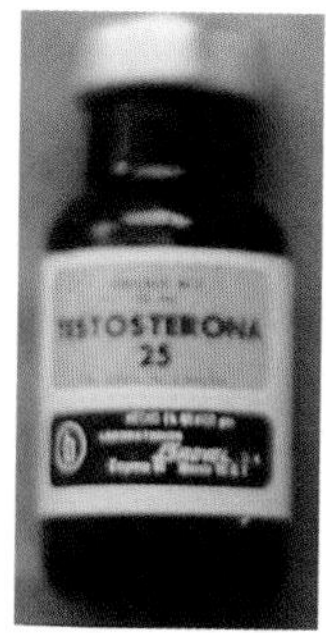

ANABOLIC HORMONE:
Testosterona 25, 50 & 200

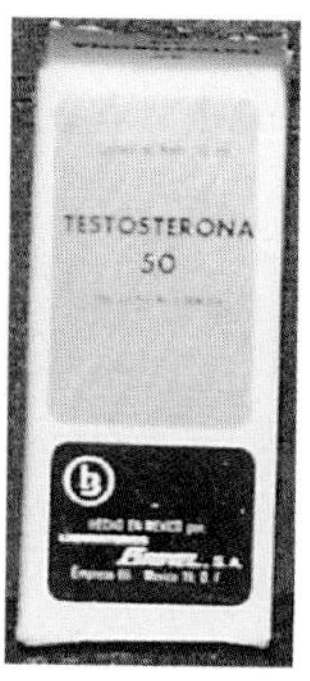

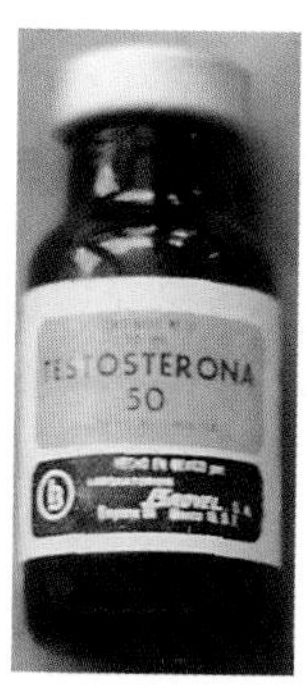

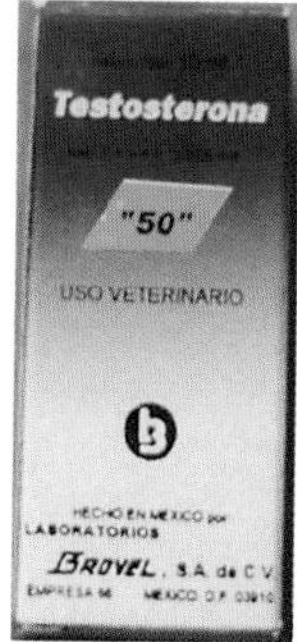

At this juncture, Testosterona 50 is the only product by Brovel with this new packaging.

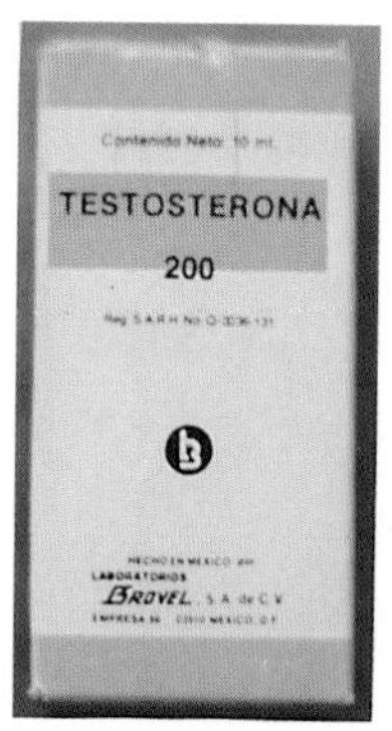

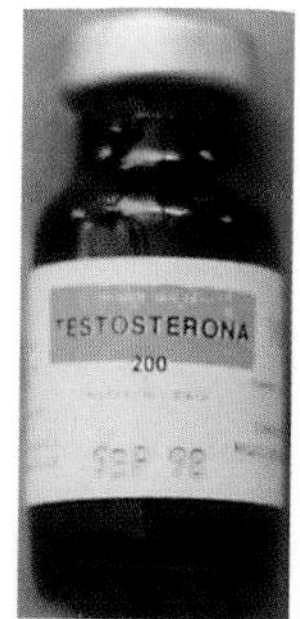

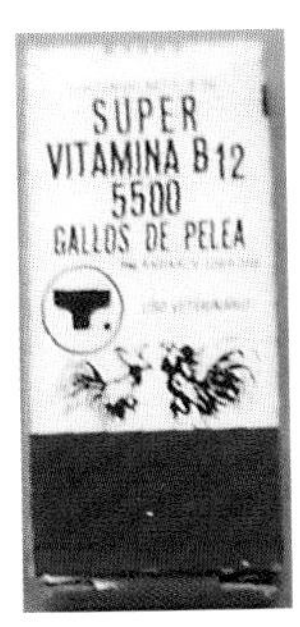

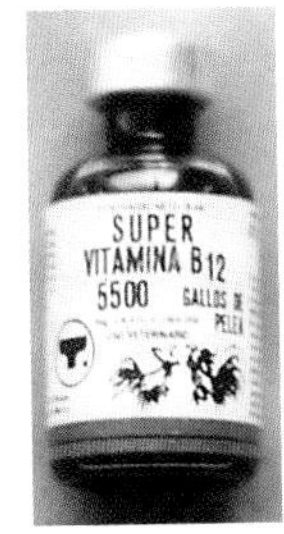

VETERINARY VITAMIN B12:
Super Vitamina B12
Hdroxo & Cyano

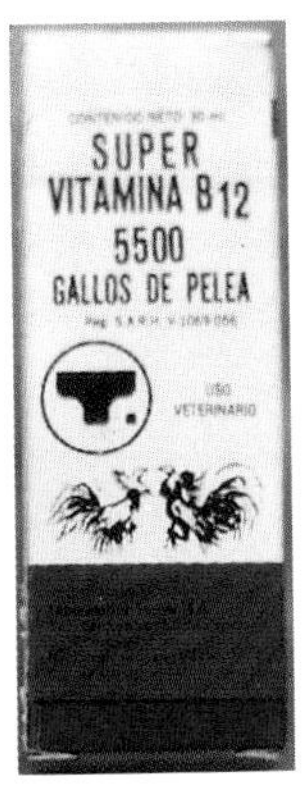

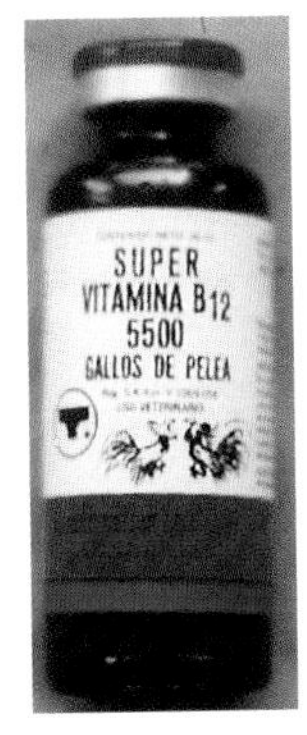

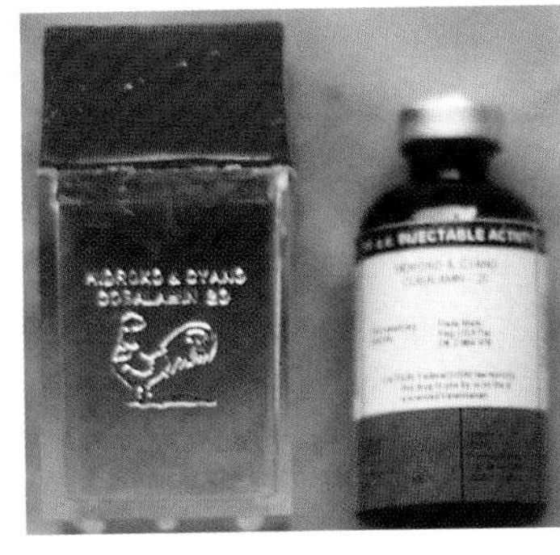

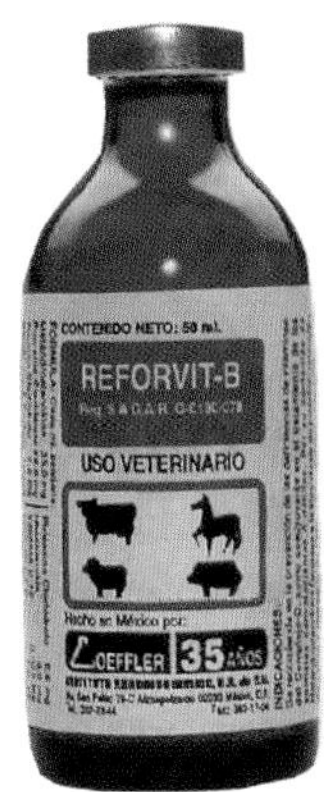

Strong Anabolic and Androgen, with the addition of Vitamin B12: Reforvit-B.

COUNTERFEIT STEROIDS:

The counterfeit market continues to prosper in Canada, the United States, and Mexico, due to continuation of the crackdown on legitimate anabolic steroid preparations. Therefore, most athletes currently have limited options to obtain steroidal compounds. One route, is to travel to another country (such as Mexico) where these substances are able to still be obtained with a written prescription from a licensed physician; or they can be purchased from a veterinarian, usually with no questions asked. Individuals can purchase, own, and use these substances in such countries legally. However, large quantities cannot be brought back into countries which they are not legal, such as Canada and the United States. In Canada and the United States, physicians and veterinarians can face very strict disciplinary actions if they are caught prescribing or distributing steroidal compounds to healthy individuals. Consequently, this is why it is very difficult to obtain these substances from the medical profession. Therefore, unfortunately, approximately 95% of athletes are forced to resort to the "black market", if they wish to self-prescribe, and self-administer steroids. The black market source often includes friends, acquaintances, co-workers, or steroid dealers, who most seldom do not have a great deal of knowledge of the products being exchanged, except for the concept of financial gain. Therefore, not only is the athlete faced with the reality of self medicine, but with also with the risk of administering unknown substances which often take place of what should be, real steroidal compounds.

Due to the fact that the possession and distribution of steroids is illegal in most countries, there is of course, is a great demand for these substances. Many crafty individuals therefore, embark on this dilemma, and quickly make great financial strides, at the expense, and often the health, of trusting athletes. Counterfeits, which are illegal copies of original pharmaceutical steroids, are often clandestinely manufactured. Sometimes, the counterfeit item is identical to the original product in appearance, but usually, there is always some discrepancy. Most pharmaceutical companies employ a sigma, which is very difficult for the average, and most often, even for the professional counterfeiter to copy. Some pharmaceutical companies change the appearance of their products either by label, bottle, ampules, packaging, or by print, to attempt to discourage prospective copiers. However, most athletes are not familiar with what the proper compound should look like, therefore, do not usually question the authenticity of acquired substances. Sometimes, the actual substance itself is not even close to what the compound should be, either in percentage, or the actual ingredients themselves. Usually, the compounds are diluted, or employed by other products which do not contain any androgenic or anabolic properties at all. However, since some of the counterfeit items may contain an actual source of steroid, even though it may not be the drug which is listed on the label, but for many desperate individuals, it is better than nothing at all. Some counterfeits are considered to be good ones and others as bad. Good counterfeits are items which contain some legit ingredient which may produce some results. Bad counterfeits are items which do not contain any active ingredients at all. Sometimes, ingredients may even be very harmful if injected or consumed. Another harmful, realistic factor is the nonsterility of these products, which may also impose possible health dangers, since there is no official authority mandating the sanitary manufacturing in which these steroids are being processed.

Athletes who have experienced an abscess, fever-like symptoms, blood poisoning, strong acne, or a very, very, unusually painful injection after administration of a steroidal compound, which had been obtained through the reliance of others, more than likely, is a victim of a counterfeit product.

Female athletes should practice even greater caution when entertaining steroidal compounds from questionable sources. Severe virilization effects may result from improper dosing, or when "non-userfriendly" products such as Stenox are used instead of what was supposed to be a gentler compound such as Spiropent tablets.

In order to avoid the possibility of purchasing, and administering counterfeit products, most athletes utilize the following recommendations:

I. The most obvious option, is to not administer any androgenic, anabolic, or other steroidal compounds to avoid these risks altogether, and dwell upon other legal forms of supplementation, proper nutrition, and train "naturally".

II. However, most athletes decide to enhance their performance by steroidal compounds, therefore, proper care and technique should also be entertained. To obtain legitimate androgenic/anabolic or other steroidal substances, the only absolute guarantee that an athlete has that the purchased products are legit, is unfortunately, if they obtain a prescription and buy them themselves. This can only be done in countries (such as Mexico), where this practice is still legal. However, again, the buyer must beware, as sometimes, the pharmacies themselves also sell counterfeit versions, to also make extra financial gains. To avoid this mishap, an athlete must be extremely educated about the products being purchased, paying particular attention to the price. If the price seems to be somewhat inexpensive, chances are, the product is not real. This can be somewhat tricky, as these versions are very authentic appearing, and one should be able to trust a pharmacist, right? Wrong!!

III. Unfortunately, most athletes are unable to leave their countries to obtain these products on their own, so many lose their money, and risk their health by turning to the black market. However, **95%** of steroids which are available from this source are fake!! For example, multi-injection vials are easily obtainable by counterfeiters, and difficult to check unless a real product is available for comparison. Therefore, usually none of these products are authentic. The stopper on the top of a vial, should also not be able to be turned by hand. The bottles are often wrapped in a plastic film, with are most often in a box with a single vial inside. Also, legit steroids almost always have safety seals, counterfeits may not. Occasionally, some may have a trace of real steroidal substance, but this is very rare. Simply, do not purchase vial products.

IV. The possibility of having laboratory analytical testing of the steroidal substances is a possibility, however, it is expensive, and most athletes do not have the resources to employ this option. However, testing steroids is the *only* way to tell for certain what is the ingredients actually are.

V. Particular attention should be paid to the label and packaging detail, in particular, the expiration date and the batch number which should be imprinted at a later date than the rest of the product's entities, as many manufacturer's initially have several copies of the labels printed in advance. Usually original steroids have this either stamped on, punched in, or burnt in. If these were printed together with the other writing, or can be easily smeared off, it is counterfeit. In addition to the expiration date and batch number of the package, it is also important to check that the they match the exact form of the preparation.

VI. The corners of the labels on the ampules and glass vials should be rounded. If these do not appear to be smoothly edged, chances are the product is not real. In fact, over 90% of the counterfeits are available with square or rectangled corners. The label ends must also not overlap, and it is especially important that the width is matching, however, the height is not as important.

VII. The attached label should also be in a straight line and not crooked, without air bubbles, well felt, flat on the glass, and not easily removable. Counterfeit labels can usually be removed from a glass surface in one piece while the labels on originals can only be torn off in pieces. However, sometimes, the combination of glue is also added to deceive this telltale sign on good counterfeits.

VIII. If more than one ampule is purchased, check for identical symmetrical form, and that the quantity of the solution has the exact same color. An irregular form of the ampule tip or small bubbles in the glass of the ampule is a clear indication that this product is counterfeited. However, since ampules are expensive and difficult to manufacture, there are only a few counterfeit versions available at this juncture.

IX. If the glass ampules are without a label, the imprint on the ampule must not be able to be removed or smeared with a finger. The imprint on the ampule must not be diagonal, and must be easily felt when touched with fingers, as the imprint of original steroidal substances, is often burnt into the glass.

X. The purchase of loose tablets or capsules should never be practiced, even if accompanied by an plastic bag. Most tablets are packaged in plastic blister-like bubbles, or push-through strips. Tablets which easily crumble must definitely be avoided. Legit tablets and capsules are always accompanied with a carton, and a package insert. Institutional products such as Anapolon 50, is an exception to the rule, due to the fact that it is produced for hospital use only. However, even these tablets are administered in push-through strips. If the seller is indicating that the product was dismantled for smuggling purposes, this may well be true, however, may not.

XI. If the offer of a large quantity of a certain steroidal compound is available, chances are that these products are also counterfeit items, as large amounts of legit products are not usually easily, or readily available.

XII. Also, if the price of a particular steroidal product seems to be peculiarly low, the item is not real. Counterfeiters are able to produce vast quantities of illegit products at inexpensive prices, therefore, are able to also sell them at a lesser cost. Legit products do not go on "sale", no matter what the reason. Very seldom will a dealer sacrifice authentic products, and if so, it may be due to avoid the possible legalities of possession of a narcotic.

XIII. Mail order steroids are usually always counterfeit items, if in fact, any are actually mailed back after receipt of a prepayment. An enclosed price list may appear to be legit, but the products themselves are not. Sometimes, even the trade names of the products are even different from the legit products, which should be a clear distinction of deceit.

Common sense should strongly be followed when buying unknown substances from unknown resources. However, the illustrations of the steroidal compound items should be referred to aid in comparing authentic products with possible counterfeits. Consequently, however, potential counterfeiters may also employ these measures, therefore, possibly allowing even for greater difficulty in distinguishing legit products from the illegit. Buyer Beware, and consider the possible risks involved.

ATHLETES AND BANNED SUBSTANCES

The following is a list of stimulants which the NCAA (National Collegiate Athletic Association, and/or USOC (United States Olympic Committee) have included on their banned substance list. If an athlete had tested positive for any of these substances, which have been considered to be ergogenic aids, then immediate disqualification and possible further actions may have been invoked.

This list is unofficial, and may be incomplete; therefore, it may also be possibly slightly inaccurate. To acquire an updated version which are provided regularly by both the USOC and NCAA, an individual can contact The NCAA Drug-Testing/Education Program at (913)339-1906, or the USOC Drug Education Program at their toll-free hotline number of 1-800-233-0393.

This list is a very board list which has been intended to accommodate all athletic ventures. Consequently, sometimes even prescription medications or herbal preparations may not necessarily be a banned substance; however, sometimes they might contain an ingredient which has been disallowed by some organization.

Other specific athletic areas, specifically bodybuilding, also are mandated by other governing officials much like the NCAA, and USOC. Some of the federations and committees also have different regulations; therefore, a variance in the banned substance lists are also common. It is recommended to obtain current update versions of the banned substances list in respect to competition regularities. When entering within a contest, the sponsors will always be able to provide an athlete with this pertinent information.

BLOOD DOPING

Blood doping is a method which some athletes have utilized in attempts to enhance their performance by administering blood or blood-related products. Blood doping is primarily practiced by endurance athletes, as the additional red blood cells (which carry oxygen) had usually increased levels of endurance. However, this technique often had caused the athlete to be presented with potential side effects, as the manipulation of the blood, especially with the process of adding red blood cells (or "red blood cell packing") had often created serious risks which had been due to the high red blood cell concentration. Other side effects which were sometimes experienced by athletes had also included allergic reactions, bacterial contamination, and hepatitis. Also, endurance athletes (such as marathon runners) concentration of red blood cells had been known to have increased; due to the fluid loss during competition. However, the addition of even more red blood cells through doping had often caused the blood to thicken, which had increased the risk of blood clotting, stroke, and heart failure. The NCAA and USOC had also considered the practice of perusing additional (unrequired) blood similar to that of utilizing any other performance-enhancing aid, therefore, blood doping has also been banned by these and possibly other, governing bodies.

The text which appears in bold print are obtainable from Mexico, and have been discussed in this book.

Androgens and Anabolic Steroids:

1. Dehydroepiandrosterone (DHEA).
2. **Fluoxymesterone** (e.g., Halotestin).
3. Methyltestosterone (e.g., Oreton).
4. **Nandrolone** (e.g., Durabolin).
5. Oxandrolone (e.g., Anavar).
6. **Oxymetholone** (e.g., Anadrol).
7. Stanozolol (e.g., Winstrol).
8. **Zeranol** (e.g., Ralgrow).

Adrenergic Bronchodilators:

1. Bitolterol (e.g., Tornalate).
2. Ephedrine
3. Epinephrine (e.g., Primatine Mist, Bronkaid Mist).
4. Isoetharine (e.g., Bronkometer).
5. Isoproterenol (e.g., Isuprel Medihaler-Iso).
6. Metaproterenol (e.g., Alupent, Metaprel).
7. Pirbuterol (e.g., Maxair).

8. Salmeterol (e.g., Serevent).

Beta-Blockers:

1. Acebutolol (e.g., Sectral)
2. Alprenolol (e.g., Aptin).
3. Atenolol (e.g., Tenormin).
4. Betaxolol (e.g., Kerlone).
5. Atenolol and Chlorthalidone (e.g., Tenoretic)
6. Labetolol and Hydrochlorothiazide (e.g., Normozide).
7. Metoprolol (e.g., Lopressor).
8. Metoprolol and Hydrochlorothiazide (e.g., Lopressor HCT).
9. Nadolol (e.g., Corgard).
10. Nadolol and Bendroflumethiazide (e.g., Corzide).
11. Oxprenolol (e.g., Trasicor).
12. Pindolol (e.g., Visken).
13. Pindolol and Hydrochlorothiazide (e.g., Viskazide).
14. Propranolol (e.g., Inderal).
15. Propranolol and Hydrochlorothiazide (e.g., Inderide).
16. Sotaolol (e.g., Sotacor).
17. Timolol (e.g., Blocadren).
18. Timolol and Hydrochlorothiazide (e.g., Timolide).

Diuretics:

1. Acetazolamide (e.g., Diamox).
2. Amiloride (e.g., Midamor).
3. Bendroflumethiazide (e.g., Naturetin).
4. Benzthiazide (e.g., Exna).
5. Bumetanide (e.g., Bumex).
6. Chlorothiazide (e.g., Diuril).
7. Chlorthalidone (e.g., Hygroton).
8. Cyclothiazide (e.g., Anhydron).
9. Ethacrynic Acid (e.g., Edecrin).
10. **Furosemide** (e.g., Lasix).
11. Hydrochlorothiazide (e.g., HydroDIURIL).
12. Hydroflumethiazide (e.g., Saluron).
13. Indapamide (e.g., Lozol).

14. Methyclothiazide (e.g., Aquatensin).
15. Metolazone (e.g., Zaroxolyn).
16. Polythiazide (e.g., Renese).
17. Quinethazone (e.g., Hydromox).
18. **Spironolactone** (e.g., Aldactone).
19. **Triamterene** (e.g., Dyrenium).
20. Trichlormethiazide (e.g., Metahydrin).

Oral adrenergic Bronchodilators:

1. Albuterol (e.g., Proventil, Ventolin, Volmax).
2. **Clenbuterol** (e.g., Spiropent). *Also a veterinary product.*
3. Fenoterol (e.g., Berotec).
4. Terbutaline (e.g., Bricanyl).

Stimulants:

1. Amphetamine.
2. Amphetamines and Dextroamphetamine Resin Complex (e.g. Biphetamine).
3. Benzphetamine (e.g., Didrex).
4. Caffeine (e.g., NoDoz).
5. Caffeine, Citrated.
6. Cocaine.
7. Dextroamphetamine (e.g., Dexedrine).
8. Ephedrine.
9. Isoproterenol (e.g., Isuprel).
10. Metaproterenol (e.g., Alupent, Metaprel).
11. Methamphetamine (e.g., Desoxyn).
12. Methcathionine ("Cat").
13. Methylphenidate (e.g., Ritalin).
14. Pemoline (e.g., Cylert).
15. Phendimetrazine (e.g., Anorex).
16. Phentermine (e.g., Fastin).
17. Phenylpropanolamine (e.g., Dexatrim).
18. Pseudoephedrine (e.g., Sudafed).

The following is a list of Schedule III, No. 834, Banned Substances, under the Narcotic Control Act (specifically in Canada):

1. Androisoxazole.
2. Androstanolone
3. Androstenediol and it's derivatives.
4. Bolandiol and it's derviatives.
5. Bolasterone.
6. Bolazine.
7. Boldenone and it's derivatives.
8. Bolenol.
9. Calusterone.
10. Clostebol and it's derviatives.
11. Drostanolone and it's derviatives.
12. Enestebol.
13. Epitiostanol.
14. Ethylestrenol.
15. Fluoxymesterone.
16. Formebolone.
17. Furazabol.
18. 4-Hydroxy-19-nortestosterone and it's derivatives.
19. Mebolazine.
20. Mesabolone.
21. Mesterolone.
22. Metandienone.
23. Metenolone and it's derivatives.
24. Methandriol.
25. Methyltestosterone and it's derivatives.
26. Metribolone.
27. Mibolerone.
28. Nandrolone and it's derivatives.
29. Norboletone.
30. Norclostebol and it's derivatives.
31. Norethandrolone.
32. Oxabolone and it's derivatives.
33. Oxandrolone.
34. Oxymesterone.
35. Oxymetholone.
36. Prasterone.

37. Quinbolone.
38. Stanozolol.
39. Stenbolone and it's derivatives.
40. Testosterone and it's derivatives.
41. Tibolone.
42. Tiomesterone.
43. Trenbolone and it's derivatives.
44. Zeranol.

LEGALITIES

If an athlete had chosen to have self-administered human or veterinary pharmaceutical products, not only had the possibility of having scarred what may have been an otherwise clean health record, but a criminal record may have transpired as well. Although the practice of having obtained a prescription from a physician, which in turn, pharmaceutical items may have been purchased from a farmacia had been considered to have been "legal", it had not been legal to bring these items back into a country where they have been considered to have been a controlled substance; narcotic contraband.

On October 27th, 1990, in the United States, Congress had passed the *Comprehensive Crime Control Act* of 1990, which had legislated new laws against anabolic steroids. Effective as of March 1st, 1991, *The 1990 Federal Anabolic Steroid Control Act*, which had been signed by President Bush on November 29th, 1990, had included anabolic steroids on the Schedule III of the Controlled Substance Act. In Canada, on June 18, 1992, Schedule G (834) had been amended to also have included anabolic steroids to the Narcotic Control Act. Mr. Denny Degan is the United States FDA National Steriod Coordinator, and Mr. Dann Michols is the Canadian National Pharmaceutical Strategy, Drugs Directorate.

This Act had enabled the classification of these substances to have been under the jurisdiction of the Drug Enforcement Agency (DEA), FBI, Customs, and the U.S. and Canadian Postal Service; and no longer under the care of the Food and Drug Administration (FDA). The solution presented by Congress had been to change the steroidal compounds from the jurisdiction of the FDA, to that of a controlled substance, which would have been punishable under the same laws that had also criminalized cocaine, heroin, methamphetamine, and other associated substances. The Controlled Substances Act of 1970, had previously regulated the manufacturing, distribution and dispensing of drugs which had the potential of being abused. Consequently, "Schedule III" drugs had been the substances which Congress had stated had a potential for abuse. However, this potential had been considered to have been less than that of Schedule I or II drugs.

Drugs under the jurisdiction of the Controlled Substances Act had been divided into five schedules, which had been based on their potential for abuse, physical and psychological dependence. Therefore, the heaviest drugs had been classified under Schedule I, while lightest-weight drugs had been classified under Schedule V. The basic Federal drug law had made it a felony, to have manufactured, distributed, or possessed with intent to have distributed any controlled substance listed within these categories. Most States and Provinces basically had utilized similar approaches for their own drug laws, although the Schedules which had been adopted, had slightly differed from the Federal Schedules. In many cases, the state laws had been more restrictive than federal laws, and as a result, often had imposed additional requirements having ranged from that of the requirement of triplicate prescription forms, to possibly sterner penalties for the conviction of a steroid-related crime.

Schedule III drugs currently have an accepted clinical use in many countries, including the United States and Canada, which may have lead to high psychological dependence, or moderate to low physical dependence, if abused. Clinically, it had been imperative that the physician or medical facility had kept separate records of the purchases, the dispensing of Controlled Substances, and also an inventory had been required to have been taken every 2 years.

In order for a physician to have been able to have written a prescription for a controlled substance, they first had to obtain a DEA#, which had to be presented every time a prescription had been filled. This individualized number had also been kept track of by the the DEA Department. These prescriptions had to be written in ink, and had to include the name and address of the patient, and the name, address and DEA number of the physician. The oral prescriptions (prescriptions relayed over the telephone) had to be promptly committed to writing, and had often only been accepted by pharmacies on a emergency basis. Controlled substance prescriptions could not have been dispensed or refilled more than 6 months after the date the prescription had been issued, or had been refilled more than five times. A written prescription signed by the physician had been required for schedule II drugs, and these prescriptions could not have been refilled. A triplicate order form had been necessary for the transfer of controlled substances in schedule II, and schedule III, and these prescriptions also could not have been refilled. In the United States and Canada, anabolic steroids had been added to the Control Substance list, therefore, they had also required this type of a prescription, if a physician had agreed to have issued one. However, this had not been the case in the country of Mexico, where these substances had not been classified as a Controlled Substance, therefore, most physicians had been able to have written prescriptions without any governmental concerns.

Schedule III had defined anabolic steroids as any drug or hormonal substance, that chemically and pharmacologically had been related to Testosterone (other than Estrogens, progestins, and corticosteroids), which had promoted muscle growth. However, not all steroidal compounds had been under one particular Schedule of the Controlled Substances Act. There had been different penalties for Human Growth Hormone, Clenbuterol and GHB; although Growth Hormone had been in the same classification as Clenbuterol, it would have been prosecuted as a violation of the Federal Food and Drug Act, and possibly handled as a Customs offense, if it had been smuggled.

Some athletes had been optimistic when the new AIDS Bill had transpired, which had allowed patients to obtain medications in foreign countries that had otherwise not been approved by their own country's FDA. However, these hopes had been rapidly suppressed, as even though a prescription could have been obtained for a personal three month supply and legally brought back into an individual's homeland, this Bill had been selective, specifically in the **exclusion** of steroidal medications. Consequently, essentially all athletes who legally had purchased steroidal compounds in Mexico, had to illegally import or smuggle these items back into their home countries. Under the present law, the mere possession of anabolic steroids is a violation of Federal Controlled Substances Act. An individual had broken the law once these items had crossed over the international borders, and primarily could have been subjected to either state, provincial or federal prosecution. If pharmaceutical items had been discovered which had not been declared, they had been considered to have been smuggled, which had been a violation of the law.

Furthermore, there had been a whole different host of laws if an individual(s) had been selling or manufacturing counterfeit steroids. Under the current statutes, an individual(s) who had been selling steroids had been viewed similarly as an individual(s) who had been selling cocaine.

However, the potential penalties may have been greater when dealing with the latter, even though they had both been under the Controlled Substances Act, as there had been different Schedules, but they had been the exact same law. The resulting penalty had been most often dependent upon the quantity of illegal contraband incurred, sophistication of the situation, if there had been the use of violence or weapons, income and if applicable, previous criminal records of the apprehended athlete, etc., etc. In the Federal system, all sentencing had been done pursuant to sentencing guidelines, which the probability of probation had been very slight. In fact, if an individual(s) criminal activity had risen past a certain guideline level, it had been very likely that they would not have been eligible for probation. Consequently, an individual(s) may have also been convicted for steroid-related charges even with the assistance of "superb", high paid legal counsel, regardless of not having any previous criminal records.

According to the United States and Canadian Customs Officials, an individual(s) who had been apprehended while having attempted to have smuggled a small amount of anabolic steroids; for what had appeared to have been for personal use only, had usually not been arrested. However, usually these individual(s) had been issued a citation and a fine, and the steroids had been confiscated. Their names had also been added to a list which had gone into a computer system referred to as NADDIS (Narcotics and Dangerous Drugs Information System). All the names which had been related to an investigation had been placed into this national computer system; which had been available to Federal law enforcement figures, anywhere in the world. Consequently, if an acquaintance had been arrested for steroids in one particular region, and had supplied another individual(s) name from another state or province, that individual(s) local DEA office had been notified, and allowed to have access to any information within the NADDIS computer system.

THE BEST PLACES TO PURCHASE STEROIDS:

Many individuals, primarily athletes, had claimed that all of the "tourist traps" such as Acapulco, Puerto Vallarta, Cancun, Mazatlan, and Cozumel all have had a great variety of both human and veterinary pharmaceutical items that many individuals have chosen from. In actuality, since these products had been either clinical or veterinary, they had been found practically everywhere in Mexico, however, the smaller areas did not appear to have provided as wide of a selection, and the language of English had been less spoken. However, the more popular the location had been to attract tourists, the higher the price of the steroidal products. Many individuals had claimed that it had also been very common for the pharmacist or veterinarian to actually have negotiated on the price of these items. Most clinical pharmaceutical items had required a written prescription from a pharmacist, which had reportedly usually been fairly easy to have obtained with a payment having ranged from $10.00 to $25.00. Consequently, this had not been the case in several smaller areas such as La Mission, Puerto Nuevo and Ensenada, where the majority of the pharmacies had been willing to have provided practically any requested item. Again, depending on the area, also had made a difference in the amount in which the physician would charge.

Individuals did not require a prescription in order to have acquired veterinarian pharmaceuticals. Tijuana had not often been considered as an ideal location for having purchased steroidal compounds, due to the major confiscation of counterfeit steroids that had originated from there. Also since Tijuana had been closely situated to the border and had been notorious for the production and exporting of steroids, it still had a large percentage of pharmacy workers and other individuals who had provided information to Customs Agents about Americans and Canadians, who had purchased steroids.

Many individuals therefore, had chosen to obtain veterinarian pharmaceuticals, which had quite often eliminated the transaction between pharmacy workers (possible informants), as usually these individuals had dealt with the veterinarian directly. Also, many individuals wisely had purchased less than $300.00 from any one location, in attempts to not have attracted possibly suspicion.

Most often, individuals had traveled to Mexico to acquire steroidal compounds as they had been easily obtainable within this country. However, many of these individuals had also attempted to bring these items illegally back to their own homelands, which had often resulted in the following:

IMPORTING AND EXPORTING:

Except as authorized by this Act or the regulations, an individual cannot import or export any narcotic substance into or out of the United States or Canada. Every individual who has contravened, has been guilty of an indictable offense, and is liable to imprisonment for life, but not less than seven years.

"IMPORT" To bring into the country or cause to have been brought into the country. The offense of importing has been complete when the contraband items have entered the country. However, an accused did not have to have been present, or have carried the items herself/himself at the port of entry; in order for an offense to have been committed, which may also have been committed in whole or in part of more than one location in the country. For example, the offense could have been tried at the place where the accused had made the arrangements for importation; and at the territory where the goods had entered the country.

"SMUGGLING" Refers to illegally having transported steroidal compounds into a country where it had been illegal to possess them. For example, it had been illegal to possess these items in the United States and Canada, but not in the country of Mexico.

"POSSESSION" Illegally having contraband items such as steroidal compounds (in the United States and Canada) within an individual's personal property such as vehicles, residential property, luggage, etc.

"The unlawful possession of anabolic steroids is a misdemeanor under Section 11377(b) H&S, unless there is a prior conviction for the same offense. Possession for sale is a felony under Section 11378 H&S and the illegal sales of anabolic steroids is a felony under Section 11379 H&S. Further, doctors, pharmacists and veterinarians who

sell, furnish, administer, dispense and/or prescribe anabolic steroids for narcissistic body building purposes are violating Sections 11153(a) and 11154(1) H&S felonies."

According to the Canadian Federal Narcotic Control Act; Possession of Narcotic/offense and punishment:

3. (1) Except as authorized by this Act or the regulations, no person shall have a narcotic in his possession.
(2) Every person who contravenes subsection (1) is guilty of an offense and liable.

(a) on summary conviction for a first offense, to a fine not exceeding one thousand dollars or to imprisonment for a term not exceeding six months or to both and, for a subsequent offense, to a fine not exceeding two thousand dollars or to imprisonment for a term not exceeding one year or to both; or

(b) on conviction on indictment, to imprisonment for a term not exceeding seven years.

According to the United States Federal Narcotic Control Act; Possession of Narcotic/offense and punishment:

"Unauthorized possession of prohibited drugs is denominated as a criminal offense in every jurisdiction in the United States, but there are variations among the states regarding classification and penalties".

(a) Knowing or intentional possession of any controlled substance without authorization:

First Offense - A term of imprisonment of not more than one year, a fine of not more than $5,000.000 but must be at least $1000.00.

Second or Subsequent Offenses - A term of imprisonment of not less than fifteen days nor more than two years and/or a fine of not more than $10,000.00.

Third and Subsequent Drug Offenses - Imprisonment for not less than 90 days and not more than 3 years, a minimum fine of $5000.00 but not to exceed $25,000.00.

Alternative Disposition - The minimum sentences imposed by this subsection are mandatory and may not be suspended or deferred. But for those with no prior conviction of any state or federal drug offense, deferred prosecution leading to ultimate dismissal of the charges is possible with the discretion of the court.

"TRAFFIC" has been defined in the Canadian Narcotic Control Act as:

(a) to manufacture, sell, give, administer, transport, send, deliver or distribute, or,

(b) to offer to do anything to in paragraph (a) otherwise than under the authority of this Act or the regulations.

"TRAFFICKING" had referred to the possession (in this case, of anabolic steroids and related substances) for purpose of trafficking/offense and punishment.

According to the Canadian Federal Narcotic Control Act:

(1) No person shall traffic in a narcotic or any substance represented or held out by the person to be a narcotic.

(2) No person shall have in his possession any narcotic for the purpose of trafficking.

(3) Every person who contravenes subsection (1) or (2) is guilty of an indictable offense and liable to imprisonment for life.

According to Section 841(a) of the United States Federal Act:

"It shall be unlawful for any person knowingly or intentionally to distribute a controlled substance". The definition of "distribute" is simply "to deliver (other than by administering or dispensing) a controlled

substance". It is clear that a person who delivers drugs to another is liable as a distributor, but, one who receives drugs for personal use also may face such liability where it is established that the person intended to further distribute the drugs, e.g., by supplying the drugs to guests.

(a) (1) Knowingly manufacturing, distributing, or possessing with intent to manufacture, distribute or dispense any of the controlled substances.

(a) (2) Creating, distributing, dispensing, or possessing with intent to create, distribute or dispense any of the controlled substances or a counterfeit substance.

Penalty:

First Offense - Imprisonment not less than 10 years or more than life, and if death or serious bodily injury results from the use of such substance, imprisonment shall be not less than 20 years or more than life, a fine not to exceed the greater of that authorized by the provisions of Title 18, or $4,000.00 if the defendant is an individual, or $10,000,000.00 if the defendant is other than an individual or both.

Second and Subsequent Offenses - Imprisonment not less than 20 years or more than life, and if death or serious bodily injury results as a result of the use of the drug, imprisonment shall be for life, a fine not to exceed twice the greater of the amount authorized by the provisions of Title 18, or $8,000.00 if defendant is an individual or $20,000,000.00 if defendant is other than an individual, or both.

Alternative Disposition - No probation, suspended sentence or parole eligibility during imprisonment for first, second or subsequent offenders. 5 years supervised release for those with no prior convictions; 10 years supervised release for those with a prior conviction.

MEASURES IN WHICH SOME INDIVIDUALS HAD FREQUENTLY EMPLOYED IN ATTEMPTS TO HAVE AVOIDED LEGALITIES WHEN IMPORTING AND EXPORTING STEROIDAL CONTRABAND ITEMS ACROSS INTERNATIONAL BORDERS:

1. PERSONAL APPEARANCE:

Most gambling athletes had been very conservative in efforts of having hidden their muscular physiques. This had been somewhat accomplished by having worn conservative clothing which had been somewhat concealing. If an athlete had been "shopping" for either clinical or veterinarian pharmaceuticals earlier that day, they had been very careful to have changed their clothing in attempts to have avoided being recognized by a possible description by employed informants. Also, they had always made certain that previous bodyhair which usually had been shaved, had grown within an acceptable length, in attempts to also ward off possible suspicion. Many Federales and other associated Custom agents had been educated in having recognized the shaved arms and legs to be that of a bodybuilder, in particular, a potential steroid smuggler.

2. GETTING THE STEROIDAL ITEMS THROUGH CUSTOMS AT AN AIRPORT:

Many athletes had often employed other less conspicuous figures such as their girlfriends, wives, or "pencil-necks" to have imported their steroidal compounds across the international borders. Custom Agents had been alerted to especially pay close attention to attractive women traveling alone, especially if a muscular individual had similarly traveled alone, and had previously been cleared through Customs. Some athletes had indicated that it had been best if these individuals who had been carrying contraband re-entered their country first, as to not have aroused any unwarranted suspicion. Once this individual had passed through Customs without having been detained, the event of an unlawful search and seizure could not have been established, and no law enforcement body could legally have detained this individual, or the accompanying personal property without suffice probable cause.

In some cases, authorities had asked for permission to have searched personal property under the false pretenses such as searching for weapons; after clearing through Customs. The intimidated athlete or individual, had often consented to the search, which had led to an arrest and jail, if contraband had been discovered. However, individuals who had been aware of their legal rights, had denied the request, which had left the authorities without the opportunity of having searched the suspect. In fact, if the individual had inquired if he/she had been under arrest, and if a negative response had been obtained, this individual had been allowed to leave. According to the law, the authorities had not been allowed to have further examined this individual, once a no arrest situation had been established. Many individuals had kindly indicated that they did not want to appear have been unco-operative, but they had wished to leave; and had been legally entitled to have done so.

3. GETTING THE STEROIDAL ITEMS THROUGH CUSTOMS BY MEANS OF A MOTOR VEHICLE:

Some Individuals had stated that if they had chosen to have ventured back across the border with steroidal contraband, they had been very careful not to have been associated with their vehicle when having purchased the pharmaceutical items. Many pharmacy employees, some veterinarians and other young individuals, often had supplemented their incomes by having provided information to U.S. customs officials regarding potential steroid smugglers. Therefore, without a vehicle description, most individuals had lessened the possibilities of having been exposed as they had attempted to take their physical enhancement contraband items back to their homelands. Sometimes when the athlete had chosen to have utilized the means of a vehicle for transportation, they often had wisely rented a rental vehicle from a neighboring state. This had allegedly warded off some of the potential suspicion often presented by the attention of far-away states, or even provincial license plates. It had appeared that if a vehicle had an out of state license that they had to proceed through secondary checkpoints with some regularity. Often, if an individual(s) had been cleared at one "check-point", it had not necessarily meant that this would have been the case at the next stop, if of course, contraband had been concealed. Most rental vehicles had not been considered to have been high profile, which have continued to have been very popular amongst tourists in Mexico, as opposed to license plates of a distant location which had often been indicative that the possibility of having transported more than the allotted $300.00, had been very likely.

Also, many male athletes had frequently chosen to have been the driver of the vehicle in attempts to have concealed the lower portion of their bodies. This practice had often restricted the agent's view, than what would have been otherwise been obtained as being in the passenger seat. It had also been allegedly beneficial to have travelled with only one other person, ideally, a ladyfriend as opposed to other male athletes, as this had appeared to have drawn the least amount of attention, and if an arrest had been made, there had been less passengers involved.

These individuals had also claimed that having been prepared with their driver's license and/or passport, as well as those of the other passenger(s) at all times, especially when having approached the various check points, had also warded off undue attention. The agents had usually inquired about the citizenship of the driver and passengers, and often had proceeded to question the nature of the trip to Mexico, length of stay, and if any purchases had been made. It had generally been in the best interest of these importing individuals to have claimed souvenir items, in efforts to have made it appear that the trip had been a vacation, as many agents had been accustomed to traveling tourists. Also, it had been important that everyone in the vehicle had the same, consistent stories when having been interrogated by the authorities. Some individuals had claimed that if the Mexican Federales had discovered steroids, they had been detained, and quite often, had been fined the amount of money that they had on their person; otherwise, they had been threatened by jail.

Other individuals, had sometimes selected high profile vehicles such as a van, station wagon etc., with Mexican occupants, as these vehicles usually had contained illegal immigrants, which a majority of border patrol agents had been especially on the alert for. These types of vehicles primarily had been targeted to secondary for inspection, therefore, the chance of a less conspicuous vehicle also having been sent for a secondary inspection had been greatly reduced. Supposedly, approximately 1 out 50 vehicles had been subjected to a secondary inspection, and two consecutive vehicles had been very seldom; unless, of course, suspicious behavior had been noticed.

Custom agents had been very aware of what may appeared to have been inconspicuous hiding places for the concealment of contraband. Door panels, spare-tire rims, false compartments under tire-rims, trunks, hoods, engines, etc., etc., had been usually the first place a suspicious Custom agent had checked. However, trained dogs had not been able to identify steroidal compounds. Therefore, a smuggling individual only had to pass the detection of steroidal contraband, by human Custom agents. If steroids had been discovered, which had not been declared, they had been considered to have been illegally attempted to have been exported. If the individual had been using a vehicle in attempts to have smuggled the steroids, the vehicle had been subjected to seizure; federal or state forfeiture action. Usually, after the smuggler had paid their fine, which had been based on the domestic value of the smuggled merchandise, the vehicle had been returned. However, if large amount of steroids (which would have appeared to have been for the use of trafficking) had been discovered to have been attempted of having been smuggled back from Mexico, it had been very likely that an arrest had been made and felony smuggling charges applied.

4. GETTING THE STEROIDAL ITEMS THROUGH CUSTOMS BY FOOT:

Many individuals had also attempted to have smuggled steroids across the border by having concealed them upon their bodies. However, if this individual had driven through a border site and had been randomly selected for secondary inspection, they had been frequently asked to step out of the car to lean against it, and had been thoroughly frisked. If vials, bottles, or capsules had been taped to the legs, chest, concealed in bras, underwear, and socks, they had been usually detected at this time. Consequently, crossing on foot, had lessened the possibility of having been frisked. Declared souvenir items which had been purchased in Mexico, had often been visually inspected or x-rayed. However, usually, the only time pedestrians had been arrested at the border, had been when they had been identified by an informant.

Supposedly, the best time of the year to have attempted to cross the border with steroidal contraband, had been either on weekend or a holiday; or as a second option, a Friday or Monday; as these days had always been very busy for the Border Patrol agents. Weekends and holidays usually had increased manpower due to the increased traffic at the border. However, the busier the border had appeared, the increased possibility that an individual who had been attempting to have smuggled steroidal contraband, could have passed through undetected.

Consequently, since patrolling the border had been often a first assignment for the majority of the young, partially experienced Custom agents, it had been considered to have been a major accomplishment to have accumulated numerous arrests; which of course, had included individuals who had attempted to smuggle anabolic steroids. These achievements had often resulted in the career advancement, which had allowed the agent to have been relieved of the border duty. One of the best times to have crossed back into the United States, primarily had been near the end of a border patrol shift, usually the 2:00 p.m. to 10:00 p.m. shift, as agents usually had become somewhat torpid; especially towards the end of the shift around 9:00 to 10:00 p.m.

MAILING STEROIDS BACK HOME:

Attempting to have mailed steroids back from Mexico had been very risky for many individuals, as there had been a lot of illicit drug traffic through Mexico, primarily, cocaine and marijuana. Therefore, Custom agents had usually inspected almost everything which came out of Mexico, and had been headed for an United States or Canadian address. If a package which had contained steroidal contraband had been opened and searched by the United States or Canadian Customs, this package had either been confiscated, or delivered, in attempts to have arrested the responsible individual(s). Sometimes, undercover authorities had created a situation in which the delivered package would have required a receipt or a signature; in efforts to have ascertained that this individual had been expecting the illegal package. Upon acceptance of the package, often an arrest had been made, with possible charges of smuggling, as well as crimes against the U.S. or Canadian Postmaster.

PACKAGE SIZE:

Most smuggling individuals had claimed that small packages which had weighed under 1 lb., had the best probability of having dissipated through Customs without having been searched. Other measures such as having written "Happy Birthday" or some other related greeting had often also guised the contraband package.

After having made certain that the contraband packages had been less than 1 lb., the smuggling individual(s) had often employed the following measures in further efforts to have disguised the illegal packages:

1. SMUGGLING INDIVIDUALS HAD NEVER USED THEIR OWN NAMES WHEN ATTEMPTING TO SEND STEROIDAL CONTRABAND BACK TO THEIR HOMELANDS:

When a contraband package had been mailed to an individual(s), the practice of having written someone else's name had always been carefully exercised. This often had persuaded the authorities that this particular package had been misaddressed, therefore, had not been the property of the individual who had resided at the said address.

2. SMUGGLING INDIVIDUALS NEVER HAD ACCEPTED PACKAGES, OR HAD SIGNED FOR ANYTHING WHEN ASKED TO BY A DELIVERY PERSONNEL:

If a postman, courier, or anyone had tried to give a package; or had asked for a signature for a package, most cautious individuals had declined, and instead had informed the delivery personal that they had not been expecting any packages from Mexico. Even if the delivery personal had persisted, these individuals had indicated that the package had the wrong name, which had not been their's; therefore the package had neither been signed for, nor had been accepted. If the package had been left on the individual's doorstep, it often had been taken inside, but not opened as it had been a common practice for some agencies to have hidden a detection device within the package, which had relayed a signal when the package had been opened. Instead, once the package had been taken inside, it had been marked with an ink marker, "Return, Subject not at this address", and then had been conspicuously placed in the closet for minimum of 3 days before any attempt had been made to have opened it. This time allotment had generally allowed sufficient time if by chance, the package had been found and delivered by Customs, (as they usually would have had it retrieved within the first day). After three days, then it had appeared to have been allegedly safe for these individuals to have assumed that the package had arrived unscathed by law authorities.

3. SMUGGLING INDIVIDUALS HAD BEEN SELECTIVE WHEN ADDRESSING CONTRABAND PACKAGES:

Most often, primarily, these packages had been mailed directly to the individual's residence; as opposed to a friend's, relative, or a P.O. Box or a drop box. This practice had allowed for the individual(s) to have assumed the entire responsibility of the package, which had also eliminated any possible chance of a mix-up, which of course, could have unintentionally had lead to a possible arrest. If the use of a P.O. box could not have been avoided, then these individuals had often rented a drop box with the use of a security code, at a 24 hour access independent mail service. Once the package had been retrieved, "Return, Subject not at this address" had immediately been written upon it. Most individuals had usually retrieved these packages at night, when it had been somewhat easier to have identified if they had been followed or not, as the traffic both within and outside the mail service area, had not been as busy. If an uneasy feeling, or the possibility of having been followed had been experienced, most often these individuals had not removed the package from the mail service area. Instead, after having written "Return, Subject not at this address" on it, they had simply dropped it back into the mail. Although in this circumstance, the steroidal contraband had not been collected by the smuggling individual, it had immediately cleared her/him of any steroid possession charges. Consequently, if a particular individual(s) had been targeted as a suspect of having smuggled steroids through the mail, then every package which had been addressed to them from a foreign country had been, and will continue to be searched.

Alert individuals had often concentrated on having observed other occupants and surrounding vehicles, especially those which had magnetic antennas on the trunk or cellular telephone antennas (which could have been anywhere on the vehicle). Often, to have further determined if these individuals had been followed, they had frequently driven for a few blocks, and turned three consecutive left-hand turns in a row, or had elected to do at least two legal U-turns. If an ensuing vehicle had also employed the same measures, then it had been almost undeniable that they had been followed. If this had been the case, these individuals had intelligently elected to have returned to the mail service area, to return the package (as described previously), in efforts to have avoided any legal consequences.

Again, most individuals had left the package unopened once they had returned to their residence. After a day or so had passed, they had often assumed that the package had not been tracked, and that it had been therefore relatively "safe" to have opened it to reveal the contraband contents.

THE INDIVIDUAL(S) HAD MADE IT HOME SAFELY, AND SO HAD THEIR SMUGGLED STEROID SUPPLY

Sometimes, the attempt of having illegally imported steroidal substances had proven to have been a success for the smuggling individual(s). However, even though this contraband had arrived undetected thus far by the law authorities, it had sometimes, not had remained this way. This steroidal contraband had still been considered to have been illegal, and if these individuals had been caught with them, either by possession, or by having distributed them, it had lead to further legal consequences.

In further attempts to have kept the acquired steroidal contraband in the possession of the smuggling individual(s), many had strived to have kept these products in order to have furthered their progress in athletic enhancement. However, sometimes, mishaps had occurred which had led to the arrest of these individuals. Some of the more common situations which had lead to the arrest of several individuals who illegally had steroidal substances had included the following incidents:

1. UNCONTROLLED TEMPER:

Many arrests related to the possession of steroids, had resulted from "domestic disputes", in which the law authorities had been called to disengage conflicts, primarily, between couples. This had often led to the additional charge of steroid possession, as the contraband items which an officer might happen to have noticed while on this particular expedition, had often resulted in the return with a search warrant with the intention of having arrested the residential occupants for illegal possession of narcotics; steroidal compounds. Sometimes, even an angry spouse, girlfriend/ boyfriend had often supplied this clandestine information to the authorities in attempts of having sought revenge against their partner.

2. INABILITY TO REMAIN SILENT:

Intelligent individuals did not inform other individuals of their private "belongings" which they had in their possession and had hidden. This had not been a topic of which to have openly talked about in public areas such as the gym, as an individual(s) could have easily been overheard, and therefore, this newly acquired information could have been reported to the authorities. If an arrest had been made, it had been best that the individual(s) had kept silent, and not had answered any questions, or made any statements without an attorney present. It had been best to have exercised their Constitutional right to have remained silent and to have obtained legal counsel. If the individual(s) had no prior felony convictions, and had been charged with simple possession, a prison sentence had been very unlikely. However, if a written or taped confession, admittance to use, sale, possession, etc., of steroids had been contributed by the individual(s), the possibility of having being fined and having served a prison sentence had been very likely.

3. RELATIVE UNSAFE AND VISIBLE STORAGE AREAS TO CONCEAL STEROID CONTRABAND:

As previously indicated, it had not been a wise idea to have left the illegal steroid substances in plain view for other individuals to have acknowledged. Sometimes, a repairman, neighbor, salesman, etc., had sometimes unintentionally viewed the private illegal items, which had prompted in the notification to the law enforcement. Therefore, cautious individuals who had decided to have concealed their steroids within their private residence, had often avoided having left these items and paraphernalia in plain sight, and also had kept them out of common livings areas such as the kitchen, bathroom and other easily located areas which the law enforcement agents had generally checked. If steroidal contraband had been discovered in these areas, it had allowed the authorities to possibly additionally charge other residential members with possession charges.

Generally the law enforcement personnel often have effortlessly searched a residence, as generally, when some narcotics had been discovered and an arrest had been made, or if the premises had been dirty or cluttered, the interest of the officers assigned to search for items often had diminished. Some individuals had claimed that the best places to have concealed steroidal items primarily had not been easily accessible areas, which would have caused another individual to have become dirty in the process of having searched the surrounding area in attempts to discover contraband.

4. DISPOSING OF EMPTY STEROIDAL PACKAGES WITHIN RESIDENTIAL AREAS:

Cautious individuals had been very careful not to have discarded their empty steroidal (cartons, tablet blisters, bottles, vials, syringes etc.) in with their regular trash, and trash disposal areas. Instead, they had kept these steroidal contraband items separated from the rest of their trash, and had selectively chosen a less conspicuous site such as grocery store garbage bin, carwash trash, convenience store trash, etc., to dispose of their paraphernalia primarily, on a weekly basis. They had also been careful not to have a set pattern or schedule when they had disposed of these items.

This practice had generally kept the law authorities from having associated the steroid contraband items with the individual(s) at their private residences, which had been a common investigative tool which had often been employed by several law enforcement figures.

INFORMANTS

Several law enforcement agencies often had employed individuals generally referred to as *informants*, to help investigate illegal steroid related issues. These informants had often informed the authorities of illegal activity for several reasons such as; possibly if applicable, to have their own charges reduced or entirely dropped in exchange for further information such as who the steroidal contraband had been purchased from, where, other names of other associated individual(s), etc. These individuals had been commonly referred to as a "Suspect Informant or Co-operating Individual".

Another type of an informant had been referred to as a "Mercenary Informant", which had been an individual(s) who had assisted the authorities in exchange for money; and possibly even sometimes had fabricated the truth, broken the law themselves, in efforts to have redeemed their financial rewards.

The "Good Guy" informant had been the least common, as many private citizens usually did not wish to have become involved with crime, therefore, had generally tended to have a blind eye if they had been a witness to a possible misdeed. However, many of these informants had also often reported their knowledge of a possible crime-related incident, in attempts to have possibly eliminated the progression of further illegal activities.

If an "Suspect Informant or Co-operating Individual" had sometimes attempted to have made a case against another individual(s), they generally had been required to have arranged for the delivery or sale of anabolic steroids from one or more of these alleged criminals. This task usually had initiated with a series of telephone calls which had been recorded in efforts to have incriminated the suspect. Therefore, cautious individuals had never done any transactions, or had engaged in any conversations which may have associated them with any illegal activity over the telephone. Instead, they had often chosen to have met in a secluded atmosphere.

If an individual(s) had been convicted of a steroid related offense, and had been required to have served a prison term, they had to also have been cautious of the telephones in which calls had been monitored, and recorded, and of "Jailhouse Informants". These had been individuals who had assisted the law enforcement figures in attempts to have reduced their own charges by having testified against the incriminated individual(s), or by having been paid for the incriminating information. Jailhouse Informants had often befriended other individuals such as arrested athletes in attempts to have gained their confidence; then had utilized the acquired information against the trusting athlete to have further incriminated him/her, and possibly others.

BODY WIRES/TRANSMITTERS

Other forms of having obtained recordings of illegal transactions had included state-of the art transmitting devices such as *cellular telephones, garage door openers,* and body wires, such as the "*Niagra System* and the *System 80*". The latter more common body wire (used 10 to 1) had often been disguised as a pager, or as a leather sunglass case in which the wire had been sewn into the case or into the lining of a hat such as a baseball cap. The body wire guised as a pager did not receive pages and the memory did not have any numbers stored, although it had appeared to have been a standard black digital pager. Cautious commerce individuals had always requested that pagers had been turned off during steroidal item transactions, as this practice had often guaranteed that none of the conversation had been monitored or recorded.

The *Niagra System* body wire had been an older type of body wire which had been approximately the size of a cigarette package, but only half as thick, with two 10 inch wires extending from the top. One of the wires was an antenna, and the other had a microphone on the end, and it had been most commonly either worn by the attachment to the leg area with the cigarette size battery pack secured in a sock, or attached to the stomach area with an ace bandage, with the wires up the center of the chest, secured by duct tape. Although there have been more efficient means of body wires available, the Niagra system had still been largely utilized by several smaller law enforcement agencies.

The *cellular telephone* body wire had not only functioned as a telephone, but also could have recorded in-person conversations as well. Therefore, most athletes had wisely requested that cellular telephones were not allowed at meetings, as similarly, they had practiced not having entered a vehicle in which such devices (also including the *garage door opener)* could have been easily concealed.

Athletes who had warranted suspicions, often had physically searched their newly acquainted business associates. However, if a wire had been discovered, an arrest had generally followed; primarily for the safety concerns of the informant (which had often been an undercover agent), not for any actual crime that had been committed. This arrest had sometimes resulted in minor infractions such as misdemeanor offenses; "Obstructing a Police Officer", and if the athlete had remained silent, and had sought the advice of legal counsel, they had usually been able to have been released.

SEARCH WARRANTS

Entry and Search: A peace officer does not require a warrant to enter and search any place other than a dwelling-house; and may do so, at anytime. A warrantless search can be conducted only where exigent circumstances have rendered it impracticable to have obtained a warrant, such as when the evidence that had been sought had been believed to have been present on a motor vehicle or other conveyance. However, a peace officer had been required to obtain a search warrant to enter and search any dwelling-house which had been under the suspicion of narcotic content in which an offense had been committed.

Warrant to Search Dwelling House: If a justice had been satisfied by the information on an oath which had indicated that there had been reasonable grounds for having believed suspicious narcotic behavior, a search warrant may have been issued. This warrant had allowed a peace officer named therein, to have been able to have entered the dwelling-house and search for narcotics at any time. Probable cause in most steroidal contraband cases had been based on information which had been gathered during the course of an investigation, which could have been as little as items which had been found during the search of disposed items discovered in an individual's trash, or as significant as many undercover purchases of anabolic steroids.

Once a search warrant had been issued, the peace officer had 10 days in which to have served the search warrant and conduct the search. Consequently, most warrants had been served within 24 hours after they had been issued. When the perimeter search had been made entirely on the basis of suspicion, then the search, which had involved having approached the perimeter of the house; attempting to have peered into the residence, had been deemed unreasonable, as there had been no common law right which had allowed a police officer(s) to have trespassed on private property, in attempts to have conducted a search of this kind. The search warrant also had limited the search to specific items of evidence such as of course, anabolic steroids and related substances, syringes, needles, books on the use of steroids etc.

Search of Person and Seizure: A peace officer had been entitled to search any individual encountered in a place entered, may also have seized any discovered narcotic(s), and anything in which the peace officer reasonably had suspected a narcotic had been contained or concealed in. On reasonable grounds, the peace officer may also have obtained any other item, in which had been believed that an offense had been committed, or that may have been of evidence of the commission of such an offense.

Powers Of a Peace Officer: A peace officer may exercise authority in regards to the above three sections, by also having obtained assistance if required, and may also break open any fixtures such as doors, windows, fasteners, locks, floors, ceilings, compartments, plumbing fixtures, boxes, containers etc.

"Knock and Talk" Procedures: This technique had often been employed by several law enforcement agencies as an effective way to have obtained permission to enter and search a private residence without a search warrant. Generally, peace officers had often equipped themselves with body wires and then had approached a suspected individual(s) at their place of residence. If the suspect had answered the door, the law enforcement individuals had identified themselves and asked to have been let in. Cautious individual(s) who had concealed steroidal contraband within their private residences, never under any circumstances, had allowed any law enforcement figure into their residential premises without a search warrant. The law had allowed an officer to have arrested an individual in their residence without a warrant; if the peace officer had seen evidence of a felony crime in plain view.

Plain-View Rule: Law enforcement figures had been allowed to have seized any item which had been accidentally encountered, if they had been legitimately searching for something else when it had been discovered. However, if a search or seizure had been considered to have been "unreasonable", then the acquired evidence; no matter how incriminating or relevant in nature, had been inadmissible.

Consequently, the constitution had guaranteed the right to be free from "unreasonable" searches and seizures, and has been referred to as the exclusionary rule. However, many law enforcement figures have found a way around this obstacle, by having pretended to have searched for other items such as weapons etc., and then had asked for permission to have searched the vehicle, house, suitcase, gymbag etc., to have made sure. If consent to search had been given by the suspect, then the legal right had been given to the officers to search; and if steroidal contraband had been discovered, the officers can seize it and use it as evidence in court; and also possibly use it to build probable cause for a more extensive search. The law had stated that a consent is a waiver of an individual's right to have been free from improper searches; as a search conducted under an individual's consent did not require a search warrant, or probable cause, reasonable suspicion or any other legal basis. Law enforcement figures had been trained to ask for consent even when they had felt that there had been probable cause, or some other legal reasons to have searched. If consent had been obtained, it further had allowed for another way for the authorities to have justified the search, in case the first attempt had proven to have been unsuccessful.

Therefore, if an individual(s) who had steroidal contraband items within their possession, had never permitted a law enforcement figure to have conducted a search, even if it had been under the false pretenses of having searched for other an unrelated object(s), without a search warrant.

If the law enforcement figure(s) had pressured these individuals to let them have searched without first having obtained a search warrant, often the individual(s) had calmly stated that a search could not have taken place until either a search warrant, or an attorney had been present. Sometimes, this had caused the officers to have declined in their attempts to have further examined the individual's property. However, if the officers had believed that they had some other legal reason to have searched, they may have proceeded to have done so without the given consent of the suspect. If this had occurred, then this individual(s) had no alternative but to have allowed the authorities to have conducted their search, as "obstructing" had been a crime in most states and provinces. Consequently, sometimes the practice of not having allowed the officers to have searched without the given consent or a search warrant had often deterred most officers from having further harassed these individuals.

Occasionally, some individuals had ventured and had allowed the law enforcement figures to have searched their private belongings even when they had been concealing illegal steroidal contraband; in attempts to have "bluffed" the authorities. However, once the consent had been obtained, the authorities had always searched suspicious areas and items, and if an illegal item had been discovered, then the individual had been arrested. Often, these consenting individuals had assumed that they could have possibly denied having given the authorities consent to have searched; however, most often, the court had sided with the law enforcement figures and not the arrested individual(s).

INTERVIEW AND INTERROGATION PROCEDURES

It had been quite common for law enforcement agencies to have attempted to further strengthen their cases against an alleged steroid trafficker, by having interviewed or interrogated them in optimism to discover further circumstantial evidence. Unintiminated individuals had often practiced their Constitutional rights, had remained silent, and had asked for an attorney to have been present.

Sometimes, a law enforcement officer had lied in attempts to have acquired incriminating evidence against a particular individual(s). For instance, it had been a common practice to sometimes falsely inform an individual(s), that illegal transactions had been video taped, or recorded on a cassette, which had often led the individual(s) to have believed that his illegal activities had been indisputable, therefore, the only option had been to have either confessed, and co-operate with the law in efforts to have avoided further prosecution. Consequently, some individuals had asked to have seen or hear the supposed taped evidence against them. In the event that this request had been denied, the accused individual had then exercised their rights, and had been free to leave, as apparently, no such evidence had existed.

Another devious method also employed by several law enforcement agencies had been practiced when more than one individual had been arrested for the same crime. In this instance, it had been very common for an officer to have indicated separately to one individual, that a "deal" would have been made to the one who had confessed first, and that the other individual had been contemplating the offer. In the exchange for a confession, the peace officer may also have indicated that he will attempt to have the charges reduced, however, the Prosecutor's Officer had been the only one who had been authorized to have done so. Consequently, if the accompanying individual who also had been arrested at the same time had confessed, then the investigating officers would not have a need to have further interrogated.

Another approach which had also been utilized successfully by the law enforcement agencies had been that of having tested the arrested individual's family morals. This method of fright tactics regarding an individual's family's safety, had often concerned many arrested individuals, therefore, they had been more co-operative. Generally, unless the arrested individual(s) had been arrested for trafficking, or smuggling of steroidal contraband items, the likelihood of a prison sentence had been very slight. Therefore, the concern for the family welfare had often been unwarranted, but had proven to have been a beneficial ploy by law enforcements in having obtained their required evidence.

ENTRAPMENT

It had been a common occurrence, generally referred to as "pro-active" for law enforcement figures, primarily undercover agents, to have actively pursued, and often instigate crime scenes in an effort to have arrested targeted participating individuals. Their rationalization had been that if the individual had been a continuous dealer, then this transaction would have occurred anyway. As a result, this would perhaps have caused the purchaser to also become a nonproductive citizen by having initiated a further crime such as burglary etc., in attempts to have supported the narcotic (steroid) habit.

Two methods that had generally been employed by several undercover agents had been by either having posed as a steroid buyer, in order to have made an undercover purchase from a targeted suspect, or, by the undercover agent actually having sold real steroidal compounds to the suspect. In both cases, once the transaction had occurred, arrests had been made for both purchasing and selling of narcotic items. The latter technique had been gaining in popularity, as the general public have become more tolerant of controversial police tactics; in attempts to have decreased the acceleration of crime.

Unfortunately, many athletes who had engaged in either having purchased or selling of steroidal compounds; had often been arrested by undercover agents who had clandestinely disguised their true identities, and motives. Consequently, although many athletes had interpreted these police measures as "entrapment", this had often not had been the consequence.

In order for an individual to have been able to have claimed entrapment, he/she must have had no prior intention to have violated the law, and had only done so due to the persuasion by the government agents. However, the government had not considered such instances in the same regard, instead, it had merely been viewed as having provided an opportunity for these individuals to have transacted as they might have had anyway.

However, *entrapment* is a defense to a crime, and if the arrested individual could have proven so, then the charges would have to have been dismissed. The entrapment law had often been somewhat difficult to have verified, as the defendant had often had to have proven that "Outrageous Government Conduct" had occurred. This had sometimes been demonstrated by extreme measures and behavior by the undercover agent(s); in their attempts of a conviction. These actions had to have either appalled the conscience of the court, or had stepped out of bounds of decency and fairness of the justice system. The only limitations on what the government could do in order to have set up potential distributors or purchasers; had been the principle of entrapment, and the related notion of Outrageous Government Conduct.

Of course, having avoided interaction of steroidal compounds had been the only absolute guarantee that an athlete would not have to have faced legalities, once the law had been violated. Therefore, athletes should have decided if steroidal physical enhancement products obtained from Mexico, would have been worth a possible criminal record, expensive fines, or possibly prison; if they had chosen to have brought these items back across the border.

HEALTH

THE TOP TEN WAYS TO ENSURE HEALTH RISKS WHEN ENGAGING IN THE ADMINISTRATION OF ANDROGENIC/ANABOLIC STEROIDS:

10. Consume large quantities of alcoholic beverages to ensure more stress on the liver and kidneys, just to guarantee that there will undoubtedly be damage to these organs.

9. Always ingest a high fat content diet, to not only increase blood cholesterol levels which will greatly increase chances of heart disease, but to also add fat to body weight. As all weight is considered to be good for strength increases and bulking up purposes.

8. Gain large amounts of weight in short periods of time. This is an excellent way to put extra stress on the heart and organs, not to mention the perfect way to obtain those desirable stretch marks. However, weight increases, also translates into strength and size increases.

7. Do not consume proper nutritional items, to enforce the prevention of chemical actions of anabolic steroids. Definitely make certain that required amounts of protein, and other macronutrients are not in the diet in order for this to happen. Steroidal compounds do not require other factors in order to produce results.

6. Do not train with weights as anabolic steroids can help reach growing goals just by solely administering them. It has not been proven that the signal which a muscle cell receives from a steroid is not very effective unless the cell itself has been put under great stress by weight training. Nor, that weight training actually tears apart little segments of muscle tissue, and if the tissue is rebuilding itself with the aid of steroids, it will come back bigger and stronger. Always avoid intense training with weights to ensure that muscle mass increases will not develop.

5. Take large quantities of all types of androgenic/anabolic steroids all at the same time. Receptor sites will always be accommodating, and will always continue to function adequately, producing great results in strength and muscle mass gains. Other vital organs will be also not be stressed due to the extra workload generated by steroidal compounds. If one steroid produces a particular result, and another results in a different outcome, then obviously administering an abundant amount of these substances will also result in a great size and strength increase. All steroidal compounds work co-operatively with one another, and there is no need to worry if one compound cancels the other's effect, or increases the possibility of potential side effects, or health problems.

4. Increase the quantity of steroids if appreciable results are not acquired. Or, if desirable results have transpired, take larger dosages to further amplify these increases. If a certain steroidal compound can produce a certain effect, than increasing this amount can only also increase the results, quicker. More, is better.

3. Never, never, stop taking steroids once initiating a cycle. The body's system will be able to function properly on its own in a few years time, after abstinence from steroids is obtained. Development of gynecomastia or virilization effects are just temporary inconveniences, and will completely disappear once the administration of steroidal substances has ended.

2. Ignore all warning signs such as high blood pressure, high cholesterol levels, acne, virilism, mood swings, etc., etc., These are just indications that the steroid compounds are effective in the system, which will soon lead to great athletic achievements. Never obtain routine blood tests or seek the advice of a physician if a particular health concern arises, this is just paranoia from self-administering unknown pharmaceutical compounds.

1. Definitely reuse and share syringes, not only with friends, but with anyone who asks, just simply wipe off the needle with an alcohol swab and this will prevent potential endangerment from

HIV, and other possible deadly diseases. Syringes and needles do not require to be sterile, nor does the steroidal compound which requires injection.

This top 10 list is sarcastically composed, as, if an individual has decided to administer steroidal compounds, and engage in the experimentation of possibly enhancing athletic abilities, then the responsibility of also acknowledging possible health risks must also be undertaken. Most, perhaps even all, side effects can be eliminated, or avoided, if education, proper management, and common sense are applied. Although many side effects are usually just temporary inconveniences, many, if ignored or if left untreated, can develop into more serious health problems and disease. If these factors cannot be considered and practiced, then the use of androgenic/anabolic steroids should definitely not be entertained.

Potential side effects or adverse reactions from using steroidal compounds can be very serious and actually do affect many individuals who use them. Therefore, an athlete should carefully consider and evaluate the risk-to-benefit ratio, when contemplating self-administration of steroids. Even though the media has sometimes unrealistically sensationalized many of these side effects in order to dissuade present and future users, many allegations do hold some underlying realisms.

However, the following information covers many of the common side effects experienced by many athletes who use steroids, and also possible solutions in order to correct these undesired problems.

Again, it is extremely advantageous to seek a physician's opinion and possible examination, if a certain area is of particular concern to an individual. Preventative measures are the best alternative in prohibiting health problems, however, many health problems can be corrected, if diagnosed and caught in early stages, when treatment may retard further amplification of the problem, or even cure it in entirety.

SIDE EFFECTS

ACNE VULGARIS:

Acne is a very common side effect experienced by steroid users, and usually is very problematic for those who have a genetic predisposition for this condition. Acne Vulgaris refers to skin eruptions which often include blackheads, whiteheads (comedones), papules, pustules and cysts, which appear on the facial areas, upper back and/or chest. Sometimes only a certain eruption is experienced, or depending on the individualization, can be a combination of several different eruptions. Females tend to experience acne on their facial areas, much more than males. Males predominantly, suffer acne primarily on their arms, shoulders, and back areas. Anabolic steroids can either provoke acne conditions, or cause existing problems to worsen. Consequently, this condition seems to be selective in potential candidates, as some steroidal compound users will experience severe acne conditions, while other individuals will not.

Acne Vulgaris is caused by bacteria which seems to flourish on the skin, and is usually the result of overactive oil-secreting sebaceous glands, which are abundant in certain hormones, mainly androgens. Whiteheads (closed comedones) are the result of plugs of oil combined with dead skin cells becoming clogged in the skin pores, which prevent it from freely flowing to the surface of the skin. Blackheads (open comedones) result when the plug reaches the surface of the skin, and when it becomes exposed to air, becomes black. Whiteheads initiate under the skin's surface and either result in blackheads or lead to inflammation. Inflammation can cause papules, which are a combination of dead skin cells and inflammatory fluid. A severe form of acne, commonly referred to as Cystic Acne, is small fluid-filled cysts which develop in the skin. Normally, the skin is able to destroy the androgenic hormones which are present in small amounts. However, when anabolic steroidal compounds are used, the androgenic hormones allow the sebaceous glands to produce more oil in the skin, which often exceed the limitation which the skin can normally control, resulting in an exacerbation of the acne condition.

Some steroidal compounds such as Anapolon, Testosterone, and Norandren 50 (veterinary) seem to aggravate or initiate acne problems. This is not only an indication that an individual is entertaining a steroidal cycle, but can also be very detrimental to an individual's appearance, and self esteem.

Solution:

Individuals can avoid strong steroidal compounds which often produce problematic effects, and possibly switch to milder compounds such as Primobolan, Deca-Durabolin, Winstrol and Anavar (the latter two, are currently not available in Mexico), which do not appear to aggravate or initiate acne side effects. Other treatments of acne can include gently frequent wash intervals, two to three times daily, with medicated soap or solution. This includes also shampooing and showering, especially after training, when sweat and a greasy feeling are most evident. Topical solutions such as Benzoyl Peroxide and other preparations can be obtained without a prescription, and should be applied once the affected areas are cleansed. The random use of suntan beds which provide ultraviolet light therapy, can be beneficial in "drying" up the complexion, and lessening the bacteria growth upon the skin. Consequently, too much U/V rays are also harmful, leading to premature wrinkling of the skin, and also darkening pre-existing scars (hyperpigmentation), so that they appear to be more evident. Other remedies such as alpha-hydroxies, or light chemical peels can also be done (depending on the strength of the acid, may be done at home, or may require to be done professionally). This involves a slight "peeling" effect to the top layers of skin, which are dead and need to be removed to prevent clogging of the healthy pores, and consequently, also aid in the appearance of wrinkles. Stronger remedies which require a prescription can include topical agents such as Tretinoin (Vitamin A-Acid Cream or Gel), Clindamycin, stronger strengths of Benzoyl Peroxide, etc., or if conditions persist, oral antibiotics such as Clindamycin, Erythromycin, Minocycline, or Tetracycline may also be prescribed. However, the use of antibiotics can inhibit the effects of anabolic steroids, and desensitize after long durations of use, becoming less effective if they are required for more serious conditions. They may also cause can irregularity in the large intestines. As a last resort, a much stronger, potent oral medication, called Accutane (Isotretinoin) may also be a possibility. However, the use of this compound should be very limited, and blood tests should be done on a regular basis by a competent physician. Pregnancy testing for females will also be obtained throughout the entire course of this prescription. Using Accutane during pregnancy has resulted in very severe birth defects, and if the possibility of a pregnancy is conceivable, *no* physician will prescribe this medication. Accutane is very potent, and sometimes difficult to obtain from a physician due to it's harsh potential side effects. A dermatological visit may be required to obtain this oral compound. This compound can produce problematic effects such as extreme joint pain, gastrointestinal disturbances, intense nasal bleeding, dry, cracking skin, and vertigo.

If acne scars do remain after treatment, there are many techniques currently available to help smoothen the pitted areas. These include laser treatments, which actually plane around the uneven area, to try and achieve more of a smooth appearance. Dermabrasion procedures were previously popular for very severe scarring, however, lasers have since replaced this often traumatic procedure, as recovery time is quicker, and the risks of laser surgery are lessened to those of the previous dermabrasion techniques. Laser surgery must be done by a qualified, licensed dermatologist or plastic surgeon, as if the technique is not properly administered, scarring, and an uneven skin tone, or hyperpigmentation may result. However, these procedures are mostly performed once the acne condition has subsided, and scarring has remained. They do not provide alleviation for current acne problem suffers. If acne conditions are severe, it is best managed by the care and advice of a physician or dermatologist.

For more information on Acne, please contact:
Acne Research Institute
1236 Somerset Lane
Newport Beach, CA 92260
(914) 722-1805 or call (800)-470-ACNE.

ACROMEGALY:

This is a rare, slowly progressive chronic disorder which usually results from an excessive amount of Growth Hormone. Acromegaly may cause thickening of the soft tissues of the body such as the heart, (which may lead to congestive heart failure) and accelerate growth patterns, often leading to a tall height in adolescents. Symptoms include abnormal enlargement of the bones in the head, arms, legs, particularly the jawbones and the frontal skull area. The growth of soft tissues and cartilage usually results in a coarse appearance in the facial features, along with the facial bones becoming prominent, with a protruding jaw, and a possible overbite which may cause a wide separation between the teeth. Overgrowth of the bones and enlargement of cartilage in the joints may result in inflammation with the gradual onset of osteoarthritis. Some individuals may suffer from *kyphoscoliosis*, which is when the spine curves from side to side, and from front to the back. Consequently, compression of the spinal nerves may lead to a variety of other functional abnormalities and discomfort. Other symptoms experienced from this condition include a gradual enlargement of both the hands and feet, abnormal enlargement of the liver, spleen, and/or kidneys, thyroid and/or the adrenal glands, hirsuitism, increased appetite, and the development of a deep and husky voice. Approximately 25% of individuals who have Acromegaly, also develop hypertension; along with possible headaches, abnormalities in vision, (which may progress to eventual blindness), and/or hormonal imbalances, due to abnormal enlargement of the pituitary gland. Also, in approximately 50% of these affected individuals, also have excessive levels of growth hormone secreted by the pituitary gland; which may influence the production of insulin by the pancreas, resulting in elevated levels of blood sugar (glucose). Some may also have an increased metabolic rate, which induces excessive sweating, and/or an increase in the production of oil (sebum) by the sebaceous glands in the skin. Other symptoms which may develop late in the course of Acromegaly, also include muscle weakness, and impaired function of peripheral nerves.

Gigantism refers to an abnormal condition which is characterized by excessive height and size; and typically occurs before puberty as a result of the over secretion of growth hormone by the pituitary gland. Gigantism is associated with enlarged soft tissues and late epiphyseal closure (head of the long bones), which results in excessive growth during childhood; allowing some individuals to reach the height of 7 or 8 feet. Consequently, low levels of Growth Hormone may also be secreted by the pituitary gland later in the course of this disorder, which results in impaired muscle function with low levels of hormone secreted by the ovaries or testes.

Occasionally, some individuals who suffer from Gigantism, may experience tingling and/or burning sensations in the arms and/or legs, which is referred to as *Peripheral Neuropathy*.

Acromegaly may also be caused by the synthetic compound, Human Growth Hormone. This drug is usually clinically prescribed for children with Growth Hormone deficiency such as pituitary dwarfism. However, many healthy individuals with normal levels of growth hormone have also used Growth Hormone to increase potential height (this can only occur in children and adolescents), and to strengthen muscles. However, even administration of synthetic Growth Hormone may also cause the condition of Acromegaly. Previously, *Creutzfeldt-Jakob Disease* developed in some individuals who administered Human Growth Hormone which was derived from human cadavers. This compound has long since been discontinued due to this rapid, progressive, fatal disease, and synthetic versions such as Biotropin, Genotropin, Humatrope, Nanorm, Norditropin, and Saizen were invented, which, to date, are considered to be relatively safe compounds to administer.

Solution:

The best solution to treat the condition of Acromegaly is to actually prevent it from occurring. This of course, can be done by administering the synthetic Growth Hormone compound in conservative amounts, and acknowledging indications of possible occurring symptoms. However, if Acromegaly does result, it is usually treated by the partial or total surgical removal of the pituitary gland. This surgical procedure may also be supplemented by radiation treatment (proton beam, heavy particle, and supravoltage irradiation). Consequently, if the entire pituitary gland requires to be removed, lifelong hormonal replacement therapy will be required. Alternative measures such as Growth Hormone suppressers (drugs which depress the production of Growth Hormone) have been used including the female sex hormones Estrogen or Medroxyprogesterone, and the Phenothiazine derivative, Chlorpromazine. Somatostatin (Sandostatin), which is a natural body substance that inhibits the secretion of Growth Hormone, has also been used as a treatment for Acromegaly, and is effective in 50 to 60 percent of cases. In mild cases of Acromegaly, Dopamine agonists such as Bromocriptine have been found to reduce Growth Hormone levels when used in addition to other drugs.

Investigational treatments of Acromegaly have included a Somatostatin analog (SMS 201-995), known as "selective mini-somatostatin". This compound can significantly lower the mean plasma growth hormone levels when administered preoperatively. SMS 201-995 has recently been approved by the FDA, as it has been able to shrink invasive pituitary macroadenomas and improve surgical remission rates.

For more information on Acromegaly, please contact:
Human Growth Foundation (HGF)
7777 Leesburg Pike
P. O. Box 3090
Falls Church, VA 22043
(703)883-1773
(800)451-6434

ADRENAL GENITAL SYNDROME:

If female anabolic/androgenic steroidal compound users continue to use these substances while pregnant, they will undoubtedly cause birth defects such as male reproductive organs, in their female infants. Although Adrenal Genital Syndrome is rare, this condition may result if a female uses anabolic steroids during critical phases of gestation.

Solution:

In attempts to prevent this from occurring, a female should never take any form of any substance during gestational periods of pregnancy. If a female chooses to become pregnant, she should "cleanse" her system of the effects of substances, by also waiting for approximately a few months to a year, so that this can allow sufficient time for the body to return to a normal state. If the female still proceeds to administer these harmful substances while carrying the fetus, the infant may be required to undergo extensive, expensive sex change surgeries to determine gender.

ALOPECIA/MALE PATTERN BALDNESS/PREMATURE BALDING:

Both female and male athletes or bodybuilders who use steroids which have a high conversion rate to Dihydrotestosterone (DHT), may experience hair loss. Hair loss is exacerbated in individuals who possess a genetic predisposition for balding, and in individuals who use derivatives of DHT in steroidal compounds such as Oxymetholone (Anapolon), Methenolone (Primobolan) injectable, Stanozolol (Winstrol) injectable, (currently, not available in Mexico) and especially Methandrostenolone (Norandren 50 - veterinary), and high-dosage and fast-acting testosterones. Oral compounds of Winstrol and Primobolan, have significantly lower conversion rates; therefore, they do not tend to promote baldness as much as the injectables. The thinning of hair, or actual balding often begins suddenly with oval or round bald patches appearing most commonly on the scalp; sometimes including other areas of hairy skin. Progressively, the affected skin becomes white and smooth, however, the affected skin does not become hard or atrophied. Hair follicles may deteriorate, but oil producing glands in the skin (sebaceous glands) usually only slightly change. New patches may spread by joining previous existing bald patches, and larger bald areas can appear while hair is regrowing in older hairless patches. Loss of hair can be permanent in some cases. Individuals who are concerned with thinning hair or who are already experiencing some balding, will only accelerate these patterns by administering steroids which convert to DHT.

Solution:

Treatment of hair thinning or premature balding is usually directed at producing regrowth of hair. Drugs such as systemic corticosteroids may cause the hair to grow, but long-term treatment may have undesirable side effects. Triamcinolone acetonide suspension may be beneficial, but the effect is often temporary. Other prescription remedies such as Minoxidil (Rogaine) and Ketoconazole (Nizoral) shampoo have been very effective. Nizoral shampoo is actually a prescription dandruff shampoo (available over-the-counter in Canada), which appears to block the effect of androgens on the hair follicles, which results in the lessening of hair loss. It is suggested to wait for approximately two weeks before using this shampoo if topical corticosteroids were previously entertained. This is a relatively inexpensive topical method, and can be obtained for approximately $12.00. Rogaine is an oral prescription remedy which does promote new hair growth. However, it appears that once this compound is discontinued, so is the hair growth, and what may have been acquired, may actually regress. This method can become somewhat expensive, ranging in price starting from $50.00 for a monthly prescription. Aside from avoiding steroids or at least avoiding items which have a high conversion to DHT, Finasteride (Proscar) may be another option, as this compound can lowering the DHT levels in the body. However, this is only with some steroidal compounds that are not DHT-based. Finally, as a last resort, often for cosmetic reasons, wigs and hairpieces may be entertained. There are many possibilities involving hairpieces, and often they are made from actual human hair. These too can range in prices from $50.00, up to $3000.00. A more painful, more expensive, time consuming possibility may also be the surgical intervention of "hair plugs" or a scalp reduction. For more information on these measures, it is best to consult with a qualified plastic surgeon or hair specialist.

For more information on Alopecia, please contact:
National Alopecia Areata Foundation
P. O. Box 15076
San Rafael, CA 94901-0760
(415)456-4644

Or, for further information on Nizoral Shampoo in Canada, please contact:
(800)430-8010.

ANAPHYLACTIC SHOCK:

Anaphylaxis is caused by an individual's extreme hypersensitivity to an antigen (a foreign substance, usually a protein), which can sometimes be a life-threatening allergic reaction to an item which causes the body to release chemicals called mediators from mast cells, and from basophils which are a type of white blood cell. In athletes and bodybuilders, this fatal allergic reaction can also technically occur with the injection of any substance, such as steroidal compounds. Otherwise, Anaphylaxis may be triggered by penicillin, insect venom, pollen extracts, fish, shellfish, nuts, various food additives (particularly sulfites), chemicals, and some medications. This reaction is also known as *systematic anaphylaxis*, *serum sickness* and *septic shock*. Anaphylaxis causes smooth muscles in the airways to contract, which restricts an individual's ability to breathe. Symptoms include abnormal blood circulation, wheezing, extreme swelling, hives, convulsions, fever, joint aches, an extreme drop in blood pressure (shock), unconsciousness, severe pain at the injection site, and if untreated, possible death. This condition manifests when an individual's system becomes hypersensitive to a foreign protein, so that the injection of a second dose, after ten days or more, triggers an onset of an acute reaction; which may be fatal. In some instances the cause of Anaphylaxis is not known (idiopathic), although occasionally, an individual may experience suspicious symptoms upon initial administration, which the body becomes eventually sensitized to. An individual may have a genetic predisposition for certain substance hypersensitivity. However, Anaphylactic reactions are usually limited to serums and not associated with hormone drugs such as anabolic steroids. Consequently, with the abundance of counterfeit steroids on the market, this potential problem is a legitimate concern due to the unknown substances included within an illicit product.

Solution:

Unfortunately, even though a complete allergic history can be performed by a competent physician, this does not offer a guarantee of how an individual will react to substances which the body has never previously been exposed to. It is best to acknowledge discrepancies such as a painful injection, severe swelling, joint pain, etc., and report them to a physician before advancing to the next injection. It is also prudent, not to inject or ingest substances of unknown origin, due to the possibility of harmful, unknown included compounds, which the ingestion of, may prove to be fatal. However, if the reaction is the result of something which is preventable, such as an insect sting, prescriptions are available for treatment kits which contain Epinephrine, which can counteract the action of antigens in the body. These kits must always accompany individuals who are prone to Anaphylaxis, and must be treated immediately if a circumstance arises; followed by acute medical attention. Other possible treatments may include desensitization (allergy shots), which may reduce hypersensitivity to particular substances.

For more information on Anaphylaxis, please contact:
NIH/National Institute of Allergy & Infectious Diseases (NIAID)
9000 Rockville Pike
Bethesda, MD 20892
(301) 496-5717

AROMATIZATION/FEMINIZATION/STERILITY:

Male steroidal compound users sometimes suffer from symptoms which result due to the partial conversion of excessive testosterone, into a female sex hormone, Estrogen. If this occurs, male athletes or bodybuilders will experience feminization characteristics such as the formation of breasts (see gynecomastia), increased tendencies toward fatty deposits, primarily distributed around the lower body area, and extremely soft muscles. These characteristics occur when the estrogen levels have been significantly increased, which is usually experienced after the discontinuance of a steroid treatment, when the male's androgen level is low. Additionally, Estradiol has an inhibiting effect on the male's gonad cycle, and also reduces the natural testosterone production, which inevitably, results in a reduced sperm production. Anabolic/androgenic steroidal compounds also exert an inhibiting effect on the hypothalomohypophysial testicular axis, which often results in a suppression of the normal testicular function. These effects may further result in a reduced testosterone production, decreased spermatogenesis, and a testicular atrophy. High doses of anabolic steroid administration has extreme effects on the male's natural endocrine system functions, which often result in subnormal values in these areas during a cycle. Depending upon the duration of the anabolic steroid use, and the period of time since the last substance intake, percentages of motile and normally formed sperm can also be extensively reduced. However, during the beginning of steroid administration, males may often notice an increased sex drive which, after continuation of these compounds, may descend below normal standards. The elevation of the Estrogen level, the extent of aromatization or feminization, and the degree of suppression, largely depend upon the amount and type of steroids administered. Interestingly, a determining factor appears to be the constitution of the individual, as these characteristics tend to affect some more than others, even when such variables as dosages and substances remain the exact same.

Solution:

The additional administration of anti-estrogenic compounds such as Nolvadex, Proviron, Teslac, or Fludestrin, (the latter two compounds are currently, not available in Mexico), can usually arrest these feminization results. These anti-Estrogens may be constituted within a steroidal regime, or may be administered immediately after the discontinuation of a steroid treatment. These substances are testosterone-stimulating compounds, which are also able to reactivate testicular function. All testes side effects which may have been experienced, are completely irreversible, including the possibility of returning to the original state in regards to gonadotropins, size of testes, synthesis of endogenous testosterones, and spermatogenesis. Sterility appears to be a temporary condition, and can also return to a normal state usually within several months after the discontinuance of steroids. However, sometimes these side effects may slowly regress to some extent on their own, without the assistance of anti-Estrogens, after the steroids have been completely discontinued. If neither of these remedies offer relief from these embarrassing side effects, sometimes surgical intervention may be entertained, especially for the removal of gynecomastia.

BLEEDING:

The administration of anabolic/androgenic steroids may also decrease prothrombin time, which is the time required for blood to clot. A normal prothrombin time is between 10 and 12 seconds; and an increased value indicates that the plasma requires a longer time to clot. Individuals who also ingest acetominophen (Aspirin) in addition to the administration of steroidal compounds can temporarily increase the blood clotting time. However, this may result in a fatal situation if an accidental laceration or internal injury was sustained; as this would conclude in bleeding to death.

The combination of steroids and anti-coagulants is extremely dangerous, and should be avoided. Symptoms of an increased prothrombin time may include a small cut which bleeds excessively for a long period of time, or an exceedingly prolonged nosebleed, which is often also embellished by hypertension.

Solution:

Prothrombin time can be checked by having a blood test by a competent physician. Prothrombin time should be regularly monitored if also administering an anti-coagulant, so that if required, this dosage can be modified to a lower extent during the cycle period. Individuals must exceed caution, and perhaps re-evaluate the risk/benefit ratio, when combining steroids with anti-coagulants.

CANCER:

The association of steroidal compounds causing cancer has yet been proven, with the one exception of the substance, Oxymetholone (Anapolon), which has been linked to liver cancer. Anapolon of course, is a very potent, oral alpha alkylated compound in which the liver, and/or kidney and prostate cancer may prove to be a long term effect from anabolic/androgenic steroid use, which possibly may not manifest until later in life. It is known however, that the liver and kidneys do undergo excessive amounts of stress during the administration of steroids. Consequently, the liver and kidneys are the most susceptible organs to become damaged from steroids as they have to detoxify and cleanse the blood of harmful and unnatural toxins. Together, these organs struggle to maintain mineral balance, and the kidneys especially becomes overly stressed in order to excrete excess minerals in the blood. This excessive exertion often results in kidney stress or enlargement, and in rare cases, may result in requiring dialysis to maintain daily functioning. Another extremely rare condition of the liver is *Peliosis Hepatitis*, in which blood filled sacs actually appear in the liver and disrupt its normal function. This condition may be associate with use of anabolic or contraceptive compounds.

Solution:

To avoid potential risks of developing cancer, it is best to avoid the oral alpha alkylated compound, Anapolon, which has been associated to this etiology. Also, it is always wise to use steroidal compounds in a sensible manner such as dosages in moderation, for short time durations. Although it has not been proven that this substances may cause cancer, it is always best to practice preventative measures.

CARDIOVASCULAR DISEASE:

Heart disease is considered to be the number one fatal disease, occurring more frequently in males, in the Western World. Theoretically, the administration of anabolic/androgenic steroids increases the risk factor of heart disease as these compounds adversely temporarily affect the cholesterol levels. These results have been repeatedly proven on an abundance of lipid profiles which were performed both during and after steroidal treatments; as a common pattern demonstrated a slight increase in total cholesterol and LDL cholesterol, while a decrease in HDL cholesterol was also apparent. High density Lipoprotein (HDL) is considered to be the "good" cholesterol which transports cholesterol from the cells by the blood to the liver. A high concentration of HDL allows for more cholesterol being able to be removed from the arteries. Low Density Lipoproteins (LDL) operates exactly opposite to HDL, as LDL delivers the cholesterol from the liver, to the cells. Therefore, if the LDL concentration is greater than what the cells can handle, the "extra" LDL cholesterol will remain in the blood and eventually attach and form a hardened plaque on the artery walls. This plaque can continue to progressively accumulate and clog the arteries; which often results in a heart attack. Consequently, the accumulation of cholesterol can become more problematic for individuals who also suffer from prolonged hypertension, as this condition causes tears or rugged spots on the arterial walls in which deposits of remaining cholesterol can attach to. Therefore, while administering a steroid cycle, a user amplifies the possibility of risks which may result in the two leading causes of death; hypertension, and hypercholesterolemia. These risks can be even further exacerbated by remaining on a high dosage and long duration steroid cycle. Fortunately, once the steroid treatment has been discontinued, cholesterol levels often return to a previous normal state, prior to the administration.

Solution:

It is wise for individuals to acknowledge that if they desire to administer steroidal compounds, that they increase the potential risk of causing coronary artery disease, and should practice preventative measures to avoid this concern. Regular lipid profiles can be obtained by having a blood test performed by a clinic or physician. Desirable cholesterol levels prior to a steroid treatment should be below the 200 range (200 milligrams per 1 deciliter (3 oz), with a higher HDL level, than a LDL level ratio. If these levels dramatically change while entertaining a steroid treatment, then perhaps precautionary measures such as reducing the intake of dietary cholesterol and saturated fats, and performing regular aerobic exercise, can often retard further elevation. Individuals who practice these methods, often experience lower cholesterol changes which usually within two to four weeks after cessation of steroids, can return to a precycle condition. Medications which can reduce cholesterol levels and the risk of heart disease include Cholestyramine, Colestipol, Gemfibrozil, Lovastatin, and Niacin.

CARPAL TUNNEL SYNDROME:

Carpal Tunnel Syndrome is a condition which is caused by compression of peripheral nerves, and it can affect one or both hands. It is characterized by a sensation of numbness, tingling, burning and/or slight pain in the hand and wrist which initially may be temporary, but eventually becomes chronic. Individuals may be awakened at night with the sensation that the hand has fallen asleep. If this condition is left untreated, muscle atrophy in the hand may develop, although all of the fingers may not be affected. However, weakness or clumsiness in gripping objects may occur if the thumb is involved. Symptoms may worsen with activities which require wrist flexion or prolonged gripping for prolong periods of time. In extremely rare cases, Carpal Tunnel Syndrome may also be caused by tumors of the wrist.

Sports-related causes of median nerve compression may involve a variety of symptoms including wrist tendon inflammation, narrowing (stenosis) of the carpal canal and incomplete or partial wrist dislocation with possible displacement of blood vessels. Athletes or bodybuilders who especially perform a repetitive exercise repeatedly, are at a greater risk of potentially developing Carpal Tunnel Syndrome. Furthermore, inborn muscle, bone, nerve or blood vessel abnormalities may combine with overexertion or injury to also cause Carpal Tunnel Syndrome. Any stress or injury which narrows the carpal canal in the wrist, can inadvertently apply pressure on the median nerve which leads to the hand. Strain or injury involving the hand and wrist, or various other disorders such as wrist fractures or dislocations can induce bone spurs or thickenings, and may cause Carpal Tunnel Syndrome. This disorder can emerge as a symptom of various other diseases, or may occur as a single primary condition.

Solution:

Treatment of Carpal Tunnel Syndromes vary according to the degree of severity, and the persistence of symptoms. Mild symptoms with no muscle atrophy may be treated using steroidal and nonsteroidal medications, or by splinting to immobilize the wrist. Corticosteroid drugs also may be injected into the carpal tunnel, with extreme caution as not to inject the steroid into the nerve. However, if symptoms are severe, and conservative measures do not result in relief from the symptoms, or if there is significant muscle weakness, surgical intervention may be warranted. Surgery involves the decompression of the carpal canal, which allows the blood to flow freely once again. Carpal Tunnel Release Surgery often provides immediate relief for chronic suffers, and may be a covered procedure by some health insurance companies. However, recovery is usually approximately 4 to 6 weeks, which involves complete rest and no use of the affected hand. If pressure on the median nerve has been apparent for a prolonged period of time, recovery may be incomplete. Electromyogram (EMG) studies to test nerve conduction velocities should be obtained before surgery to determine the degree of compression. This test can also increase success rates by ruling out other nerve compression conditions. Carpal Tunnel Release Surgery should be performed by a highly skilled, competent, plastic surgeon.

For more information on Carpal Tunnel Syndrome, please contact:
American Carpal Tunnel Syndrome Association
P. O. Box 514
Santa Rosa, CA 95402-0514
(517) 792-1337

CHANGES IN THE SKIN:

Other changes which are often experienced in the skin are the changes in the skin's appearance and texture. This is especially experienced by females who use androgenic steroidal compounds, as Estrogen which is responsible for smooth, clear skin is suppressed and dominated by Testosterone. An increase in Testosterone levels often produce male characteristics, one of which includes the rough texture and large pores. Once this virilization effect has resulted, it is irreversible.

Stretch marks and skin fissures in the shoulders/chest, on the inside of the upper arms, buttocks, and inner thigh areas, are also often exhibited in steroidal compound users. These conditions as a result of a rapid weight increase, in a short period of time. This applies a great deal of stress upon the skin, and does not allow sufficient time for the skin to stretch, to adapt for this sudden weight increase.

Solution:

Lotion or moisturizing remedies can somewhat soften the acquired rough texture apparent on the body's surface. Large pores however, cannot be reduced or corrected. They can be somewhat camouflaged to a certain degree with camouflaging cosmetics. However, once they have become enlarged, this is a permanent condition, which often also lead to other problems such as acne.

Stretch marks can be prevented by slowly increasing the amount of weight gain in a gradual manner to allow the skin to accommodate for the change. Also, the application of Vitamin E cream to the affected areas, will aid the skin in remaining supple, which may help somewhat in the prevention of stretch marks. However, once stretch marks are acquired, they too are somewhat permanent, and of course, disfiguring. Currently, there are new techniques of laser surgery which can improve the appearance and in some cases, remove unwanted scarring from stretch marks. However, this can be very expensive, ranging from $500.00 to $3000.00, briefly significantly disfiguring, approximately 2 to 3 weeks, time consuming, and one must find a qualified dermatologist, or plastic surgeon to perform this technique.

For more information on laser surgery, please contact:
The American Society of Plastic & Reconstructive Surgery
444 East Algonquin Road
Arlington Heights, IL 60005
(708) 228-8376

DIABETES MELLITUS:

Insulin-dependent Diabetes is a disorder in which the body is unable to produce enough insulin and therefore, is unable to convert nutrients into the energy necessary for daily activity. Individuals who have Diabetes, experience a malfunction in the production of Insulin. Normally, sugars and carbohydrates which are consumed, are processed by digestive juices and turned into glucose. The glucose then circulates in the blood as a major energy source for body functions, and is regulated primarily by Insulin, which is a hormone produced by the pancreas gland that enables the body to use and store glucose quickly.

Individuals with *Type I Diabetes (Insulin-dependent Diabetes* or *Juvenile-type Diabetes)* lack sufficient insulin, therefore, glucose accumulates in the blood to levels which are too high for the kidneys to excrete. The kidneys, in attempts to remove the excess sugar, excrete large amounts of water along with essential body elements, such as occasionally fats and proteins, which result in frequent urination, thirst, and weakness. Hunger and fatigue are also experienced due to the body's inability to utilize foods properly for nourishment and energy. In order to utilize alternate sources of energy, the body refers to its stores of fat and protein, which results in weight loss and the accumulation of acetone and related acids (fat breakdown products) in the blood. These metabolites of fat then produce increased acidity of the blood, quicker than the kidneys are able to excrete them, which transpires into a potentially fatal condition called *Ketoacidosis,* or *Diabetic Coma.* Unlike hypoglycemia, the symptoms of Ketoacidosis develop slowly over a period of days, and without immediate treatment, an individual may go into a state of diabetic coma, which can lead to death. This condition is characterized by excessive urination and thirst, and may also involve loss of appetite, nausea, vomiting, rapid deep breathing, abdominal pain, and drowsiness.

Type II Diabetes (or Non-Insulin-Dependent Diabetes) usually affects individuals over the age of 40, who have normal or even above normal production of Insulin, however, their bodies do not respond efficiently to the Insulin produced. Type II Diabetes is the milder form of the disease.

Diabetes can lead to more serious complications, such as *Diabetic Retinopathy,* which is a condition which results from changes in the blood vessels of the retina, and if advanced, is a major cause of blindness. Less frequent, but just as serious, are several other eye problems which can also arise, including cataracts, glaucoma, and optic nerve disease. Diabetes may cause similar changes in the blood vessels of the kidneys, which may lead to kidney failure and a condition known as *Diabetic Nephropathy.* The nerves may also be affected by Diabetes, which can result in loss of feeling or abnormal sensations in different parts of the body. For the individuals who suffer from serious neuropathy, it can produce problems such as tingling and numbness in the feet, dizziness, impotence, leg pain and double vision. This complication, is known as *Diabetic Neuropathy.*

Diabetes Insipidus is a disease in which the kidneys do not retain enough of the water which passes to them from the blood. An individual who has this disease urinates excessively and becomes extremely thirsty. Diabetes Insipidus is caused by a lack of vasopressin, which is a hormone which controls the amount of water excreted from the body as urine. Vasopressin is produced from part of the brain called the hypothalamus, and is stored in and released by the pituitary gland. However, a disease or injury which affects the hypothalamus or the pituitary gland can also cause Diabetes Insipidus. Consequently, Diabetes can also lead to *Atherosclerosis*, which is a form of arteriosclerosis (hardening of the arteries) which may further cause a stroke, heart failure, or gangrene. Individuals with Diabetes are twice as likely to suffer from coronary heart disease and stroke, and five times as likely to suffer from arterial disease of the limbs, than non-Diabetic individuals.

In most Diabetics, the cause of the disease is unknown, however, high levels of Growth Hormone, may stimulate the production of glucose by the liver, which may lead to Diabetic conditions. Diabetes is also common in some families, but usually most sufferers have no known family history of the disease. There is some evidence which indicates that individuals who develop Type II Diabetes are actually born with one or more inherited traits which predispose them to developing this disease. Also, additional factors such as aging, obesity, or stress, may trigger the onset of Diabetes in such individuals. Many researchers believe many cases of Type I Diabetes also involve inherited traits, which may cause the body's disease-fighting immune system to mistakenly attack Insulin-producing cells of the pancreas instead.

Solution:

Diabetes cannot be cured, but proper treatment can improve an individual's condition. Many Diabetics can live almost as long as those of normal health.

Type I Diabetics require to receive one or more daily doses of insulin, which must be absorbed into the bloodstream to be effective. Insulin cannot be administered orally, as it is destroyed by the digestive system, therefore, it must be injected hypodermically. Portable pumps have increasingly become a popular method to inject Insulin, which permit continuous administration of insulin, as well as additional amounts of Insulin when needed to control the changes in blood sugar level which occurs after meals; as well as the use of pumps which are actually implanted within the body. Pancreas transplants or transplants of the organ's Insulin-producing cells may also be an option in the treatment of Diabetes. A procedure called hemodialysis is frequently used to remove waste products from the blood when the kidneys can no longer perform this function adequately. Diabetics with serious renal disease may also be candidates for a kidney transplant, if a suitable donor organ is available.

Most Type I Diabetics are required to follow carefully planned diets which consist of specified amounts of carbohydrates, fats, and proteins. Many cases of Type II Diabetes can also be controlled by a diet which is low in calories. Many individuals also test their urine or blood one or more times daily for glucose and for acetone, which is a substance produced when the effect of Insulin is inadequate. Therefore, a daily routine of Insulin-injection, controlled diet, exercise to burn off glucose, and testing for blood sugar level is vital in achieving and maintaining good blood sugar control in individuals with Insulin-Dependent Diabetes. Urine testing for glucose spillage had been a standard practice in past years, but has recently been replaced with self blood glucose testing. This involves self monitoring of blood glucose levels by using a single drop of blood which is obtained with a finger stick. This is then placed on a chemically treated pad which is on a plastic strip; and the color change of the chemically treated pad is then compared to a color chart or interpreted by a battery operated portable meter.

A Diabetic must follow preventative, planned diets strictly - except if an *Insulin reaction*, or *Insulin shock* is occurring, which may happen when the effect of insulin is so great, that it causes the level of sugar in the blood to decrease too low. The individual may perspire greatly, become nervous, weak, or even unconscious. This condition can be quickly treated by consuming food which is rich in sugar, candy or even table sugar.

Ketoacidosis can be prevented by careful daily evaluation of insulin needs. Particularly stressful situations such as illness or surgery may require increased amounts of insulin. Most importantly, an individual with Diabetes should never skip or delay an insulin injection and should pay careful attention to proper diet. If required insulin is not taken, the amount of glucose in the blood may become excessive, which may result in Diabetic Ketoacidosis, which may conclude in a Diabetic coma.

Some Type II Diabetics whose condition cannot be controlled by diet alone require Insulin, or the administration of oral drugs which can reduce the level of glucose in the blood. The dosage of Insulin prescribed by a physician is dependent upon an individual's diet and exercising habits.

Most cases of Diabetes Insipidus cannot be cured, however, the disease can be controlled by taking Vasopressin.

For more information on Insulin-Dependent Diabetes, please contact:
American Diabetes Association
National Service Center
1660 Duke Street
Alexandria, VA 22314
(703) 549-1000 or (800) 232-3472.

ENLARGED HEART:

Occasionally, cardiac hypertrophy may develop unknowingly in individuals who administer high dosages in long durations of steroidal compounds. Unfortunately, anabolic/androgenic steroids effects all muscle tissue, including the heart muscle. Although increasing the muscle mass is desired of skeletal muscle, the opposite applies to the cardiac muscle, as enlargement can be very dangerous, and can result in fatality. Possible symptoms which may be experienced include heavy labored breathing, hypertension, and heart palpitations. However, symptomatology is often rare until excessive damage has occurred.

Blood lipid changes associated with increased risk of atherosclerosis are also seen in individuals who administer androgenic/anabolic steroids. These changes include decreased high-density lipoprotein (HDL) and occasionally, increased low-density lipoprotein (LDL). These alterations may be very distinct, which could have a serious impact on the risk of atherosclerosis and coronary artery disease.

Solution:

Administering steroidal compounds in moderation for short time intervals will often retard the possibility of enlarging the heart muscle. However, if this condition does result, it is best to discontinue all agitating steroidal compounds, reduce bodyweight and water retention, perform aerobic exercise, and maintain healthy ranges of blood pressure and cholesterol levels. A chest x-ray or an ultrasound which is performed by the medical profession, can indicate if this condition has progressed or regressed. Occasionally, this side effect may be reversible if proper measures are abided for a certain duration.

ENLARGED PROSTATE:

This is another side effect which only affects males who administer steroidal compounds; as steroidal use has been associated to benign enlargement of the prostate. The prostate is a gland which surrounds the neck of the bladder and the urethra in males. Prostate cancer is a major cause of cancer in males, which may prove to be fatal. Symptoms of abnormalities in the prostate are usually nonexistent, however, as the disease progresses signs of urinary obstruction or bone pain may occur.

Solution:

Regular physical exams by a physician is recommended, in which rectal examination can determine if the prostate is enlarged before it becomes problematic. This condition can be treated and is an area which a male individual should have checked at least once a year. Surgical intervention may be required, which involves resectioning of the portion of the gland which is encroaching on the urethra.

GROWTH DEFICIT/SHORTNESS:

All anabolic/androgenic steroidal compounds, with the exception of Oxandrolone (currently, not available in Mexico), have the ability to induce the maturation of the epiphyseal plates. This results in the termination of bone growth, even if an individual has not reached the intended full growth potential. Therefore, steroidal compounds should not be used by teenagers who usually experience tremendous growth spurt patterns during the adolescent years. Continued administration of steroids will result in a premature closure of the epiphysial cartilage which leads to a growth stunt, and ultimately results in a decrease in the normal predicted height.

Solution:

If young adolescents choose to use steroidal compounds, the height which they initiate steroidal treatment at, will predominantly be the height that they will remain at for the rest of their lives. Further growth is unfortunately impossible, making this an irreversible side effect. Not even the administration of Growth Hormone after this has occurred, will restart the growth of the bones.

GYNECOMASTIA:

This condition can occur naturally in males, but is more commonly experienced as a side effect in male steroid users, due to growth of their mammary glands. A term of "Bitch tits" is a common term used in many locker rooms and gyms indicating the development of "female breasts". Gynecomastia usually occurs when a steroidal compound converts to Estrogen, and the levels become so high that it actually mimics the female hormone patterns, often resulting in the formation of breasts. The first signs of gynecomastia are often painful bumps which are under the nipple area. These bumps gradually grow, with the buildup of fatty tissue around them, causing them not only to be painful, but unsightly as well. It is not understood why some steroid users develop this condition with even the smallest dosages, and others can use massive dosages, and not be effected. Some users do not experience gynecomastia while they are entertaining a steroid cycle, but sometimes, a few weeks after their cycle is completed, can notice these feminization effects. This can often be attributed to slightly elevated Estrogen levels from the cycle which did not dominate until the steroids were discontinued. Aldactone, Aldactazide and Tagamet (the latter two compounds, are currently not available in Mexico), have been associated which the cause of gynecomastia.

Solution:

If these symptoms are caught within the early stages, the use of anti-estrogen compounds such as Nolvadex and Proviron, (please refer to the compound's sector for a full reference), or Teslac, (currently, not available in Mexico), either during a steroidal treatment, or immediately after a steroidal cycle is completed, can usually arrest these feminization problems. However, if the usage of these products does not prove to be successful, then the possibility of surgical intervention may be warranted. Gynecomastia Surgery (Subcutaneous Mastectomy) is also common, and usually presents as a last resort for males who cannot acquire alleviation from these bothersome symptoms. The surgery, involves either local or general anesthesia (depending on the degree of gynecomastia), and the surgery time can usually anywhere from 45 minutes to 1 1/2 long. It can be sometimes done right in the physician's surgical office, but usually requires a operative setting. Most health insurance companies will not cover the expenses for this procedure, but many males will still seek this method for relief from pain and embarrassment. The price range for this surgery can range from $1500.00 up to $3000.00, depending upon the physician. The surgery involves the actual removal of the fatty, breast tissue. This is often done surgically through an incision around the aerola. Liposuction is also usually accompanied, which is the removal of fat cells through a cannula. The scars then fade to be quite conspicuous. This procedure tends to be permanent, as once fat cells are removed, they are removed on a permanent nature. However, in rare incidences, this problem can manifest again in extreme overdoses, as the remaining breast tissue, and fat cells may stretch to compensate for the removed ones. Consequently, if interactions and precautions are complied with, this is very unlikely to result. It is extremely beneficial to obtain the services of a good Plastic Surgeon to perform this technique. It is wise to find one that performs this operation quite often, and is familiar with bodybuilders.

HEADACHES:

Several steroidal compound users suffer from occasional headache pain, which may also be somewhat debilitating. There are several different types of headaches ranging from muscular contraction or *tension*, *exertional*, *vascular*, *cluster*, or of a *migraine* nature. Most of the time, headaches are often a symptom of high blood pressure, which should be regulated by medical intervention. However, more frequently, headaches are usually caused by strenuous exercise or exertion which simply cause muscles in the neck and scalp to excessively contract. Cluster headaches also may occur from spasms, edema or inflammation of the carotid artery in the neck, and are a rare form of a severe disabling headache. These headaches are usually deep, nonthrobbing, extremely painful, and tend to recur in the same area of the face, eye, temple or forehead, each time they occur. The involved eye and nostril tend to water excessively, and the eyelid may also droop. The onset of Cluster headaches is usually during sleep, and most often awaken the individual with severe, one sided head pain. However, the pain sometimes stops, allowing the individual to fall back asleep, but is usually only awaken again with another attack of headache pain. There are two types, cyclic or chronic cluster headaches, which occur together, one to four times in a day for several weeks or months; then suddenly halt. However, they occur again several months or years later, in small occurrences, thus often being referred to as "cluster". Migraine headaches, or *Endocrine* headaches, usually involve only one side of the head, and are usually suffered by individuals who have a genetic predisposition to them. Often associated with these painful attacks are double vision, irritability, nausea, vomiting, constipation or diarrhea, and sensitivity to light. Medical research has suggested the constriction of the cranial arteries may trigger migraine headaches, but the cause of the constriction is not clearly understood. Pain from Vascular, Cluster, and Migraine headaches can all be triggered by a hormonal imbalance. Since anabolic steroids and several other drugs which are used by athletes and bodybuilders, can seriously alter the natural function of the endocrine system, this may be the reason for the occurrence of headache conditions. Some steroidal and associated compounds such as HCG, and Clenbuterol are well-known for causing the onset of headache pain; which can be so severely incapacitating in some individuals, that they cannot tolerate the effects of these products.

Solution:

Most often headaches are treated conservatively, according to their nature of onset, and associated symptomatology. Exertional, Tension, or Vascular headaches can most often be alleviated by termination of the aggravating activity, bedrest, and use of acetominophen, Tylenol, Advil, or other over-the-counter medications for headache pain. Sometimes, chiropractor adjustments can greatly reduce pain without the requirement of painkilling substances. The treatment of Cluster headaches is often delayed because of sudden onset during sleep. Individuals may sometimes be helped by inhaling ergotamine or oxygen. However, sometimes use of the following drugs may prevent the headache from recurring: Methysergide, Lithium Carbonate, Prednisone, Verapamil, or Nifedipine. If hypertension conditions exacerbate headache pain or if relief from headaches does not occur once agitating factors are eliminated, this must be reported to a competent physician or a neurologist, for proper management and care.

For more information on Headaches, please contact:
National Migraine Foundation
5252 North Western Avenue
Chicago, IL 60625
(800) 523-8858 (Illinois)
(800) 843-2256 (outside Illinois).

HYPERTENSION/HIGH BLOOD PRESSURE:

The condition of high blood pressure is a common problem which is often suffered unknowingly by many steroid users. Hypertension is a persistent elevation of blood pressure which is the amount of pressure placed on the walls of the arteries as blood is pumped throughout the body. Hypertension often results in athletes or bodybuilders, due to excessive water or sodium retention accompanied by a rapid increased weight gain due to the administration of several steroidal compounds. In this case, this is referred to *Secondary Hypertension,* as what causes this condition is known. Consequently, *Primary Hypertension* refers to this condition when the cause is unknown, however, it may be caused by kidney disease, endocrine disorders, high sodium intake, obesity, smoking, alcoholism, oral contraceptives, or emotional stress. Unfortunately, there are usually no indicative symptoms of high blood pressure unless it becomes extremely elevated; thus presenting such symptomatology as headaches, vision disturbances, insomnia, and breathing difficulties. Hypertension can lead to a numerous amount of other chronic diseases such as arteriosclerosis, which can further lead to an aneurysm, mini-strokes (transient ischemia attacks), kidney failure and possibly accelerate heart disease.

A normal range of a blood pressure reading is usually considered to be 120/80, but can be anywhere from 100/60 to 140/90. The systolic blood pressure refers to the upper reading which measures pressure when the heart muscle is contracting. The diastolic blood pressure is the lower reading which measures pressure when the heart muscle is at rest. When only the systolic blood pressure is high, it is referred to as systolic hypertension. These readings are often measured by an instrument called a sphygmomanometer, however, there are many monitors currently available which enables much easier, convenient methods of obtaining these readings.

Solution:

Routine checkups by a physician often include the checking of a blood pressure reading. Any elevated reading should result in prompt action on behalf of the individual. Conservative measures which an individual can try to accomplish is to slowly gain bodyweight, and keep the water retention to a minimal amount by controlling sodium intake. Also regular BP readings would also indicate if an elevation of pressure is evident, which should result in immediate recourse. Usually, an individual does not require to change or abandon current steroidal treatments, if monitoring and proper action is taken.

Treatment of hypertension includes the use of diuretics to reduce sodium and water levels in the body and lower blood pressure. Dyazide and Aldactone are diuretic prescription medications which are often prescribed by a physician to help regulate the blood pressure. Beta-blocking drugs which reduce constriction of blood vessels, and vasodilators which are drugs that relax the muscles in blood vessel walls are also commonly used. Also, centrally acting drugs which lower the heart rate by controlling the sympathetic nervous system, and angiotension converting enzyme (ACE) inhibitors which reduce constriction of blood vessels as well as salt and water levels, may be prescribed. Athletes and bodybuilders often prefer to administer Catapres, (currently, not available in Mexico) as this is an antihypertensive compound which in addition, also stimulates the endogenous production the the growth hormones, which tends to have an anabolic effect.

For more information on Hypertension, please contact:
American Heart Association
7320 Greenville Ave.
Dallas, TX 75231
(214)750-5300.

HYPOTENSION/LOW BLOOD PRESSURE:

Orthostatic Hypotension is a condition that is experienced when an extreme drop in blood pressure occurs when an individual suddenly stands up. The blood pools in the blood vessels of the legs, which results in a temporary decrease in the amount of blood which is carried back to the heart by the veins. Subsequently, less blood is pumped out from the heart, which results in a sudden drop in blood pressure. Normally, baroreceptors (specialized cells in the body) quickly respond to changes in blood pressure, which then activate automatic reflexes to increase levels of catecholamin in the body. Increased catecholamine levels can rapidly restore the blood pressure. However, when there is a defect in this relex action, reflex mechanisms may be inadequate to quickly restore the decrease in blood pressure, and therefore, orthostatic hypotension may result. Symtoms of Orthostatic Hypotension which usually appear after sudden standing may include dizziness, lightheadedness, visual blurring and fainting.

A common cause of Orthostatic Hypotension usually results from hypovolemia (a decrease in volume of circulating blood) which can occur from excessive use of medications such as diuretics (which increase urination), or from the use of Nitrate preparations used to treat chest pains (angina pectoris) or heart failure. Other drugs which may cause Hypotension are Quinidine, L-dopa, Vincristine, barbiturates and alcohol, Monomine Oxidase inhibitors and Tricyclic antidepressants, and Phenothiazines. If hypertension medication dosage is too high, Orthostatic Hypotension may also result, or it may also occur as a complication of Diabetes, hardening of the arteries or Addison's disease.

Neurologic disorders which involve the autonomic nervous system may interrupt or damage the automatic reflexes that occur upon standing. Orthostatic Hypotension may also result from neurological damage due to Diabetes, excessive alcohol consumption, syphilis, which can destroy the spinal cord (tabes dorsalis), progressive disease of the spinal cord such as syringomyelia, or numerous other neurological disorders.

Solution:

Treatment of Orthostatic Hypotension is dependent upon the cause. When it is due to a decrease in volume of circulating blood (hypovolemia) due to administration of medications, Orthostatic Hypotension is easily and rapidly reversed by simply correcting the dosage, or discontinuing the medication under a physician's supervision. The drug Ephedrine (currently, not available in Mexico), may be also administered orally, and in some instances, salt intake may be increased, or salt-retaining drugs may be prescribed.

For more information on Orthostatic Hypotension, please contact:
NIH/National Institute of Neurological Disorders & Stroke (NINDS)
9000 Rockville Pike
Bethesda, MD 20892
(301)496-5751
(800)352-9424.

HYPERTHYROIDISM/HYPOTHYROIDISM:

In healthy individuals, the thyroid gland takes up iodine from the blood to form a hormone called Thyroxine, which regulates growth and metabolism. The Thyroid-stimulating hormone (TSH), which is another hormone, causes the thyroid to release the Thyroxine. TSH is produced by the pituitary gland, which lies near the center of the skull.

Goiter which is a condition in which the thyroid gland becomes enlarged, develops because the thyroid gland is not active enough, or because it is too active. The thyroid gland is located toward the front of the neck between the Adam's apple and the top of the breastbone. Most often, a goiter appears as a smooth swelling at the front of the neck. *Hypothyroidism,* refers to the condition when the thyroid is not active enough; therefore, the pituitary gland responds to the low level of thyroid activity by producing more TSH. This excess amount of TSH often causes the thyroid to swell.

Hypothyroidism may be due to a lack of iodine (salt) in the diet, possible defects in the enzymes which produce the Thyroxine, or possibly due to antibodies which attack the thyroid. Other possibilities include congenital hypothyroidism which is inherited as an autosomal recessive trait, which may also be caused by disorders of the hypothalamus or pituitary centers in the brain. Other possible causes may be attributed to disorders which affect control of the thyroid hormone, or from a blockage in the metabolic process of transporting thyroid or iodine in the thyroid gland itself. Even surgery or radiation to the thyroid gland may result in hypothyroidism. Hypothyroidism may also be the result of an auto-immune disorder which are caused when the body's natural defenses against invading organisms such as antibodies, or lymphocytes, suddenly begin to attack healthy tissue. Eventually, the thyroid may be completely destroyed. This is known as a condition called *Hashimoto's Thyroiditis* or *Lymphoid Thyroiditis*, which is the most common cause of the enlarged thyroid gland (goiters). This disease can occur at any age but is experienced more in the third to fifth decades of life, and is more common in women than men.

Patients suffering from Hypothyroidism become physically and mentally sluggish. Their skin becomes thick and dry, and they may gain weight. Symptoms of Hypothyroidism may result in extreme tiredness, enlargement of the thyroid gland, severe constipation, nerve compression in the hands and feet, often resulting in a yellowish discoloration of the skin, a lower than normal body temperature (hypothermia), anemia, poor memory, dull-witted behavior and a change in personality. In some cases a psychosis ("myxedema madness") may develop. The tongue may also become enlarged (macroglossia) due to mucinous deposits. The heart may become enlarged due to a collection of a high protein fluid around it. The lungs and abdominal spaces may also become enlarged also due to fluid accumulation. Infertility may also be experienced by both sexes, and males may also be may affected by impotence.

A condition referred to as *Hyperthyroidism,* occurs when the thyroid is too active. In this disorder, the thyroid cells produce too much Thyroxine, and the thyroid may enlarge to form a goiter. *Grave's Disease* is a rare disorder which is believed to occur as a result of an imbalance in the endocrine system. This disorder causes increased thyroid secretion (hyperthyroidism), enlargement of the thyroid gland (goiters) and (exophthalmos) protrusion of the eyeballs. Common symptoms of hyperthyroidism include nervousness, weight loss, swelling of the legs and eyes, clubbing of the fingers, extreme sensitivity to light, heat intolerance, emotional instability, or hyperactivity, irregular heart beat, and males may develop gynecomastia. Symptoms may occur as a single incident and then proceed into remission, or recurrent attacks may occur.

Solution:

Both Hypothyroidism and Hyperthyroidism treatment is dependent upon the origin of the condition. Individuals who suffer from Hypothyroidism may be prescribed pills containing small amounts of Thyroxine, the use of desiccated thyroid, thyroglobulin and triiodo-thyronine, surgery, or radioactive iodine, which is a form of iodine which can slow down the the activity of the thyroid. However, the administration of a synthetic thyroid hormone, Levothyroxine (Eutirox) or Liothyronine (Cynomel) is the treatment of choice for hypothyroidism. If the administration of drugs is responsible for the suppression of thyroid function, then the drugs may be discontinued to achieve thyroid normality. Agents which reduce anti-thyroid antibody formation, are the treatments of choice for individuals who have developed Hashimoto's Thyroiditis.

For more information on Hypothyroidism, Hyperthyroidism, please contact:
American Thyroid Association
Endocrine/Metabolic Service 7D
Walter Reed Army Medical Center
Washington, DC 20307
(800)-542-6687

IMMUNE SYSTEM SUPPRESSION:

Administration of some steroidal compounds such as Testosterone, seem to provide an improved state of health and recovery, as there appears to be somewhat of a reduction in the occurrence of viral illness. Unfortunately, usually approximately a month after the discontinuation of a cycle, many previous steroid users experience an observable incidence and prolonged duration of viral illnesses. Aggravating colds, infections and possible pneumonia are often experienced, when previous states of health were unmarked. These experiences lead to the probability which implies the possibility of anabolic/androgenic steroids temporarily alter the immune system. The longer duration of administration of steroids, reflects on the greater amount of suppression of the immune system. However, an individual must acknowledge if these symptoms do not seem to alleviate after a period of a few weeks, as other more damaging effects such as Acquired Immune Deficiency Syndrome (AIDS), may actually have transpired from some other etiology.

Solution:

Individuals terminating a cycle of steroids, should try to avoid certain hazards such as becoming tired and rundown, which easily allows the immune system to become less effective in fighting against illness. Ensuring optimal health is crucial, until the body's own immune system has a chance to rejuvenate to ward off infections and illness on it's own. If these ill feeling symptoms do not clear up within a few weeks, it is best to seek medical intervention, and possibly undergo an AIDS blood test.

IMPOTENCE:

This is a side effect which only affects males who administer steroids, who subsequently also suffer from temporary changes in libido patterns. Initially, at the beginning of a steroid treatment, a male's sex drive is actually higher than normal, often accompanied by increased frequency and duration of erections. However, with prolonged steroid use, this desire often lessens to an extent which is considerably below normal, resulting in only a slight capability of maintaining an erection. Occasionally, an individual who administers high dosages of only anabolic steroidal compounds can create a tremendous imbalance between anabolic and androgenic hormones. This often results in androgenic effects which control the ability to maintain an erection to become diluted. Impotence most often occurs after the discontinuation of a steroid cycle, as the exogenous source of Testosterone has been removed, leaving the body's normal blood androgen levels to remain suppressed, until such time when the natural system begins functioning once again.

Solution:

The side effect of impotence is preventable, and also reversible in all instances associated with the use of steroids. Substances such as Gonadotropyl, Gonakor, or Profasi (HCG) can prevent this undesirable occurrence by being administered during a steroid cycle, or, it can also reverse the effects by being administered after the completion of a steroid cycle. The physiological factors which often contribute to impotence, usually include a decreased production of natural Testosterone by the testes as the exogenous steroid overpowers the natural endocrine feedback system. This can be corrected by adding oral Testosterone, or another high androgenic compound to the cycle; in a relatively moderate dosage.

INSOMNIA/DIFFICULTY SLEEPING:

Individuals who administer steroidal compounds often experience difficulty either falling asleep, or remaining asleep throughout the night. This is a common side effect of several substances including steroids, which do produce a slight stimulating affect upon central nervous system. A lack of sleep tends to be problematic as this is necessary for proper recovery in order for maximum muscle growth, and a general well-being. Interruptions in sleep patterns also reflect upon mood, productivity, and energy levels; which also tend to be negatively affected.

Solution:

Normal sleep patterns can easily be obtained once again by terminating the steroid treatment. Occasional use of over-the-counter remedies sleeping pills or Melatonin may offer some relief. However, the use of Melatonin on a continued basis with the use of steroidal compounds is not recommended, due to the possibility of Melantonin's ability to lessen the anabolic effects of steroids.

JAUNDICE:

There are several different types of jaundice; but particularly, this is an indication of possible serious liver disease. Symptoms include yellowing of the skin, eyes, mucous membranes and bodily fluids. Jaundice is caused by the deposition of bile pigment which often results from excess bilirubin the blood, which may be caused by obstruction of bile passageways, excessive destruction of red blood cells, or disturbances in the functioning of liver cells. Jaundice can also be associated with hepatitis, which is an inflammation of the liver in response to toxins or infective agents. Athletes or bodybuilders who have administered high dosages of steroidal compounds for prolonged time periods, may especially suffer from jaundice, which is usually accompanied by fever, gastrointestinal symptoms, and itchy skin. Jaundice can be detected on a blood test by an elevated bilirubin level, or by diagnostic studies such as ultrasonography (u/s), or by computed tomography (CT Scans) to determine etiology.

Solution:

Alleviation from symptoms of hepatitis or jaundice may be acquired simply from the discontinuation of the agitating steroidal compounds, along with medical attention. This condition is very rare in healthy nonabusers of steroids, who administer these compounds in moderation and short intervals.

KIDNEY DAMAGE:

As the kidneys are involved in the filtration and excretion of toxic byproducts, they are under a considerable amount of strain when steroidal compounds are administered. Hypertension, as well as variations in the water and electrolyte balance of the body may often lead to long-term changes in the kidney's function. A rapid growing kidney tumor called *Wilm's Tumor,* which normally appears only in infants and children, has also appeared in certain rare cases in individuals who administer steroids. It is however, unclear if there is an actual connection between the condition and the use of steroids, although several steroid users have experienced dark-colored urine and, in extreme cases, blood in the urine. Symptoms of kidney disorders may include lumbar pain, renal colic, fever, disturbances in urination, presence of blood or pus in the urine, tenderness or swelling in the costovertebral region, edema, enlargement or miminution in the size of the kidney. Some steroidal compounds such as Parabolan, (currently, not available in Mexico), appear to have a toxic effect on the kidney function.

Solution:

The avoidance or limited usage of problematic compounds which place enormous amount of stress upon the kidneys would greatly reduce the possibility of kidney damage. Regular medical checkups involving palpitation, or even a CT Scan can distinguish if possible kidney damage has occurred. If this condition is left untreated, the requirement of dialysis may be a great possibility in order to function in daily life activities.

LIVER PROBLEMS:

Occasionally, individuals who administer androgenic/anabolic steroids, develop *Peliosis Hepatis*. This is a condition in which the liver, and sometimes the splenic tissue, are replaced with blood-filled cysts. These cysts are occasionally present with minimal hepatic dysfunction, therefore, have been associated with liver failure. Peliosis Hepatis is not often recognized until life-threatening liver failure, or intra-abdominal hemorrhage develops.

Liver cell tumors are most often benign and androgen-dependent, but fatal malignant tumors have occurred. However, hepatic tumors associated with androgens or anabolic steroidal compounds are much more vascular than other hepatic tumors, therefore, may also be silent until life-threatening intra-abdominal hemorrhage develops.

Solution:

The development of symptoms of Peliosis Hepatis can usually be retarded by discontinuance of the steroidal compound, which usually results in complete disappearance of lesions. Also, termination often results in regression or cessation of liver cell tumor progression as well. However, large quantities of standardized Silymarin extract (Milk Thistle Seed) can produce a large improvement in liver function, as well as the use of the antioxidant, *Pycnogenol**. The recommended dosage of standardized Silymarin extract is approximately 500 mg per day, while Pycnogenol can be sprayed into the oral cavity, approximately for a total of 8 sprays, 4 times a day.

MUSCLE CRAMPS:

Muscle cramps have usually been experienced at one time or another by every athletic individual due to the distribution of well-developed muscles. These cramps are temporary, excruciately painful, involuntary skeletal muscle contractions, which most often occur at rest, primarily during sleep at night. These cramps initiate when a muscle already in its most shortened position involuntary contracts. The cramp is asymmetric, and usually affects the gastrocnemius muscle and small muscles of the foot. However, sometimes this can occur in just about any possible muscle location, such as the back, upper thigh, and arm areas. Individuals who also suffer from cirrhosis, or in the last months of pregnancy may also experience this type of cramp. Ordinary muscle cramps are not due to fluid or electrolyte abnormality, however, individuals administering certain steroidal compounds often increase the chances of suffering from muscle cramps. Injectable Winstrol-V (currently, not available in Mexico), is notorious for causing very painful muscle cramps. Also, the use of nonsparing-potassium diuretics can also deplete levels of the mineral potassium, resulting in an upset of the intracellular fluid balance, which results in a muscle cramp. These muscle cramps are very intense and usually persist for a few minutes, which seems to be a very long duration when one is being experienced. Afterwards, the cramped area remains to be sore, somewhat similar to a bruised state.

Solution:

The maintenance of a high potassium level will help lessen the possibility of constant muscle cramping. Obviously, avoiding certain compounds which are known to exacerbate muscle cramps may help prevent these muscle cramps altogether. However, if a muscle cramp does present, passive stretching of the involved muscle, rubbing and active contraction of the antagonists will relieve an established cramp. Substances such as Methocarbamol, or Chloroquine may help to relieve muscle cramps. Prescriptions for Quinine Sulfate are no longer obtainable due to the fact that this compound was responsible for the death of 16 people; as it can cause a life-threatening drop in blood counts. This drug still exists as it is still used to treat malaria, however, the FDA will not allow a physician to prescribe it for muscle cramps. However, Taurine, which is an amino acid with Vitamin B6, is one of the three possible nutrients which will help prevent painful muscle cramps (the other two are Magnesium and Potassium). Consequently, Taurine has a more profound effect in alleviating these cramps in most suffering individuals. A general recommended dosage is approximately 1 to 2 grams at bedtime, or several hours prior to a training session.

MUSCLE TEARS:

A common argument of the medical community is that anabolic/ ndrogenic steroids may increase muscle mass; however, this is not a qualitative gain, due to the fact that muscle tissue increases, however, associated tendons and ligaments remain unaffected. Therefore, if the muscle rapidly increases its size and strength, the tendons and ligaments are usually unable to support the increasing demands of the muscle fibers. Interestingly, an increased occurrence of torn muscles has been experienced amongst steroidal compound using athletes and bodybuilders. Muscle tears are considered to be an extremely serious injury, and require surgical reattachment of the muscle. However, surgical intervention cannot guarantee the muscle to regain its original appearance.

Solution:

Rapid increases in muscle size and strength can occasionally cause tendonitis, inflammation, or even a possible tear in the muscle. The best thing an athlete or bodybuilder who chooses to enhance his physique by the use of steroids can do to avoid these problems is to gradually gain size and strength in a planned and progressive pattern.

PALPITATIONS:

Heart palpitations are commonly experienced by several individuals who partake in administration of anabolic/androgenic steroids. These effects often present as premature ventricular contractions (PVC's) which may indicate an elevated level of the central nervous system. Symptoms of palpitations are somewhat alarming as a very abrupt heartbeat is very obvious and usually experienced; indicating that a ventricle of the heart has contracted out of sequence. However, palpitations and PVC's are harmless, if not associated with another health condition. The onset of palpitations frequently occurs during heavy physical exertion, but become greater after discontinuation of the activity, when the heart is returning to a normal beating rhythm. Individuals who tend to suffer from this condition usually have a predisposition for an irregular heart rhythm to begin with. Substances which seem to agitate palpitations often include high doses of caffeine, Spiropent, Novegam, and Ephedrine (currently, not available in Mexico).

Solution:

Although as previously stated, heart palpitations are not dangerous unless they are also experienced with another health disorder. However, preventative measures such as possibly avoiding such substances which are known to have this effect will usually help minimize this condition.

PSYCHIC CHANGES:

This is one of the most controversial side effects in which the media tends to embellish on in order to dissuade potential and current anabolic/androgenic steroidal compound users. However, both females and males who use high dosages and long term durations of androgenic steroidal compounds can develop an intense, sometimes violent, aggressive behavior. However, aggression levels seem to predominantly affect males at a higher rate due to the fact that if androgenic steroidal compounds are used excessively, they tend to transform a considerable amount into Estrogens, which causes a hormonal imbalance in the normal male's system. The only possible advantage of this is that it provides the ability to train harder and more intensely. However, the disadvantages overwhelm the one particular advantage, as the male hypothalamus reacts to the female hormone Estradiol, which tends to aggravate this type of negative behavior. Consequently, a state in which an individual experiences this type of change in behavior, can be physically harmful to the self, or often to others as well. Variances of harm can range from neglect to abuse, death, and may be psychological and/or physical. Some risk factors associated with the misuse of androgenic compounds can include antisocial characteristics such as catatonic or manic excitement, panic states, spousal or child abuse, negative role modeling, rage reactions, developmental crisis, suspicion of others, paranoid ideation, delusions, hallucinations, substance abuse or withdrawal and hormonal imbalances such as depression, psychosis, or mood swings and possible, although very seldom, suicidal behavior. The effects of aggression can be amplified by the use of alcohol particularly.

Defining characteristics may include body language such as clenched fists, facial expressions, rigid posture, tautness which often indicates an intense effort to control. Increased motor activity, such as pacing, excitement, irritability, agitation or anger, repetition of verbalizations, continuation of complaints, requests and demands, self-destructive behavior, or hostile threatening verbalizations; or even boasting of prior abuse, and increased levels of anxiety may also be demonstrated. Overt and aggressive acts such as goal-directed destruction of objects in an environment, such as beating or breaking of items, or seldom the possession of destructive means such as a gun, knife, or other sort of weapon can also become a destructive means of release. All these possible incidences contribute to the coined term of "Roid Rage".

Solution:

In an effort to minimize these frightening, destructive potential side effects, it is best to control the use of androgenic items which can cause the aggressive bouts in particular individuals. It is also important for the athlete or bodybuilder to recognize and acknowledge that this increase in aggression does and can happen. Once this predicament is understood, an individual can lower the susceptibility to this undesirable condition by limiting or discontinuing the problematic androgenic compounds.

STOMACHACHES:

Occasionally, some oral steroidal compounds, particularly, Anapolon, Stenox, Primobolan, Methyltestosterone and Dianabol (the latter two oral compounds are currently, not available in Mexico), can cause abdominal discomfort. These pains can vary from an occasional cramp, to a constant ill-feeling, nausea, and a general soreness.

Solution:

To alleviate these stomach pains which seldom occur, an individual can choose to abandon oral entities of the administered steroids, and possibly switch to injectable versions. Other conservative measures which may offer some relief, include consuming larger quantities of water, over-the-counter remedies for upset stomach, such as Pepto-Bismal, Milk of Magnesia, etc.

WATER/SODIUM RETENTION:

This refers to the puffy, bloated look which most steroid users most often suffer from when administering various types of steroidal compounds. Most steroidal compounds will cause a water and electrolyte imbalance in the body as a result of an increased storage of water and sodium. One disadvantage is an increased water retention in the skin. Edema, which refers to the puffiness and swelling of tissues which often results from excessive water retention, is usually prevalent as a result of sodium retention. Some steroidal compound users actually encourage this side effect, as they believe it is somewhat responsible for the initial strength and weight gains, which are usually felt when starting a cycle. Also, the muscle fibers, joints and connective tissue, can actually benefit from the increased water retention. It is apparent that this side effect allows for a stronger connective tissue, and a "lubrication" of the joints, which often helps in injury-free training.

However, for the majority of users, this side effect of water retention is not appreciated, nor welcomed. It can not only indicate possible health concerns such as potential high blood pressure, as the system is suddenly overloaded with additional water, the heart and blood vessels must transport more fluid than normal through the body. Also, it may also be a sign of an underlying heart or renal disease. Sodium retention seems to occur equally in both men and women users. Cosmetically, water retention can cause the body to look puffy, especially in the facial area, mainly around the cheeks and eye tissues as they become swollen, and often acquire a tight appearance. This is not only somewhat embarrassing to the user, especially to most women who do not appreciate to appear to look heavier than they are, but also in addition to these ill effects, is the implication which identifies that an individual is indeed on a steroid cycle. The degree of the water and salt retention depends primarily on the type and dosage of a particular steroid, and of course, the predispostion of the user.

Solution:

In the possibility of hypertension, it is sensible to discontinue the steroid use or at least control the high blood pressure with medication. For cosmetic purposes, some athletes and bodybuilders engage in the use of potassium sparing diuretics such as Aldactone, or Dyazide, from the thiazide family, in combination with their steroid cycles. This appears to prevent both serious edema and the possible accompanying high blood pressure. If heart or renal disease is apparent, the acquired water retention will not subside with the cessation of steroid use as it does in the average athlete or bodybuilder. It is recommended to seek the advice of a competent physician for proper medical management.

VIRILIZATION/MASCULINIZATION:

Virilization or masculinization predominantly are side effects which result in females who use Testosterone or androgenic hormonal compounds. If high dosages and long duration periods of these types of compounds are entertained, the greater probability of acquiring the characteristics of a mature male will transpire. Adverse reactions include those of hirsuitism, increased facial and body hair, clitoromegaly, hoarseness or deepening of the voice, menstrual irregularities; even cessation of menstrual periods, increased acne, increased libido, male pattern baldness or thinning of the hair, anxiety, depression, mood swings, increased aggression, and changes in the skin texture.

A clear indication that virilization side effects may be developing, is often the indication of a hoarseness, which can inevitably lead to the deepening of the voice. This adverse reaction appears to be irreversible as permanent changes in the larynx take place. Other irreversible effects are those of clitoromegaly, which is the enlargement of the clitoris. This often occurs due to the increased amount of Testosterone, which is characteristic of producing male sexual organs. So in essence, the clitoris in a female, is similar to that of a male's penis, therefore, tends to somewhat experience a growth sensation, to slightly resemble that of a male's penis. Hirsuitism, increased facial and body hair growth is also very commonly affecting females who use anabolic steroidal compounds. Thickened, coarser hair will develop on the female's chin, side of the cheeks and jawline, and under the chin (a beard sensation). Hair may also begin to grow thicker and denser around the nipples, chest, stomach, pubic area, and legs. However, the color of this increased hair growth may or may not be the same color characteristic of the individual. Some females may acquire facial characteristics resembling that of a male, such as a more prominent jawline, and broadening of the nose. Changes in skin are often also encountered, as Estrogen, which is the female's primary hormone is responsible for the softness and suppleness of skin. When Testosterone becomes the dominant hormone, acne, increased pore size, and rough, textured skin becomes apparent. Male pattern baldness or thinning of the hair may be experienced also by women who use DHT characteristic steroidal compounds. Mood swings, anxiety, depression, aggression, as well as fever and illness, may also affect a female using steroidal compounds. These variations in feelings occur due to the variances in hormone levels. Menstrual irregularities, including amenorrhea, which is the cessation of menstrual periods often occur due to the lessening of Estrogen (which is the dominant hormone which induces menses), and the dominance of the androgens. An increase in libido, or sexual desire is also very commonly experienced in females when using steroids, due to the fact that Testosterone is responsible for this characteristic. Therefore, an increase in Testosterone, will also increase the sex drive, to a very great extent. These harsh side effects are generally the reasons why some steroidal compounds such as Anapolon, Norandren 50 (veterinary), Stenox, Testosterones, and other high androgenic agents should be avoided by females, or at least, used in very low moderation.

Solution:

Some effects which may be slightly reversible include hirsuitism, increased facial and body hair growth, clitoromegaly, voice changes, menstrual changes, mood swings, anxiety, depression, aggression, increased libido, acne, and thinning or male pattern baldness. However, these problems may only be slightly alleviated if the problematic steroidal compound is discontinued, and the possibility of using an anti-androgen such as Aldactone is entertained. Consequently, if these side effects become apparent, they will usually remain to some extent, and will never return to the state previous to steroid use. Depending on the duration and dosage administration of the substances, will greatly affect the quantity and quality of side effects suffered. If females have desired to administer steroidal compounds and avoid these ill effects, they have been able to use low doses of some nonandrogenic compounds, including Anavar, Winstrol, (both are currently, not available in Mexico), Novegam and Spiropent, and Primobolans.

Some conservative measures of confronting these acquired side effects may include: Hirsuitism - electrolysis, or individual plucking of each hair. Hoarseness or voice deepening - once this is acquired, it will always be evident. Scraping of the larynx is costly, dangerous, and unsuccessful. Menstrual irregularities - reintroduction to Estrogens and Progesterones, it is best to seek the advice of a competent gynecologist. Clitoromegaly - this too, once acquired, will always remain. Surgical intervention of "trimming" the labia is not recommended, as it is dangerous and very painful. Skin changes - acne can be improved by either oral or topical products. However, large pore skin and coarse skin texture will remain. Psychic changes - may be aided by medication, again, it is best to seek the advice of a competent physician. Increased libido, thinning or balding - often will return to a normal previous state, once steroidal compounds are discontinued. However, sometimes balding patterns may have become permanent, in which case, the use of Proscar, Rogaine, Nizoral shampoo or hair pieces may be required to be entertained. (Please refer to the Balding sector, for further information).

BLOOD, AND ASSOCIATED HEALTH TESTS

One of the most important and easiest ways to practice preventative medicine and protect the system from steroid administration damage, is by obtaining a regular blood screening test. These screenings can often detect if steroidal compounds are increasing the risk of cardiac disease, possibly detect other possible existing aliments which may have become aggravated, and confirm or disprove liver abnormalities.

Occasionally, some athletes refuse to have these essential screens performed due to the desired secrecy of personal chemical habits. Consequently, several individuals often have frequent blood testing of cholesterol and triglycerides, (which of course, include many of the screens which are required for most athletes anyways) to disregard health concerns. However, many individuals choose to have their blood drawn by a clinic or related facility, and retrieve the results to interpret these findings themselves. A physician is however, much more qualified in perceiving these results, and if need be, can diagnose and treat problematic areas which may lead to a serious health condition. It is very important to have an abnormality brought to the attention of the medical profession, so that proper treatment can be provided. Also, it is equally important to abandon the administration of the problematic substances until such a duration when proper health is once again maintained.

Results from various screenings may vary from one individual to another. Therefore, it is very beneficial for an athlete to have a blood screen performed prior to the initiation of a steroid regime, in order to establish a baseline of which future screen results can be compared to. This will indicate a normal range of blood parameters; if no other pre-existing abnormalities are detected. It is imperative for an athlete to have a general knowledge of these tests and the ranges in order to prevent potential health problems by having these periodically checked. It is also beneficial to know which particular tests to have performed, as physicians usually just test for regular bloodwork, which may often omit important tests which may be crucial to an athlete's health. Many physicians do not have the knowledge of the effects of steroidal compounds, therefore many are uneducated on relevant testing. Consequently, it is vital that athletes specify which tests they want performed. The usual blood tests which are requested are SMA-22,or a SMA-25/HDL, SMA-24/HDL, or a Cholesterol/Triglyceride, HDL/LDL ratio. The names of these tests vary depending mostly on the laboratory, location and country. These screenings can indicate which types of stress and/or if possible damage has occurred to organs which are susceptible to the toxicity of anabolic steroids, particularly the liver, kidneys and/or heart.

An initial blood test should be obtained before a steroid cycle is entertained. If the blood tests initially indicate that all values are normal, then another blood test should be performed usually within six weeks of the cycle (as this time allotment allows sufficient time for an accurate reading). It is not recommended that these tests be repeated sooner than six weeks, as many readings fluctuate, then later return to normal a couple of weeks later. If the results indicate something problematic, proper termination of the steroidal compounds should be undertaken to retard further possible damage. If the blood tests return within normal limits, then it is presumably safe to proceed with the steroid regime. It is important to repeat these screenings in approximately a month's time after the completion of a cycle to investigate how the body is recuperating after the steroid cycle. These steps should be repeated each and every time a new steroid cycle is entertained. Several blood tests should be performed approximately one month after initiation of a steroid cycle, two months into the cycle and immediately following the cycle. However, some values are affected by steroidal compounds and therefore do not transpire accurate findings until total abstinence has been obtained for 2 to 3 months.

Liver enzyme values of SGOT, SGPT, and HDL usually rise significantly during steroidal treatments, only to return back to normal ranges either later in the cycle, or after the discontinuation of the compounds. These temporary changes are usually not an indication of subsequent liver damage; and are benign. However, liver enzyme values which remain elevated for a prolonged interval, should be acknowledged that possibly the administered steroid is having a toxic effect on the liver, and should be discontinued and treated immediately to avoid further health problems. This is particularly appropriate if high SGOT is also accompanied by a high Alkaline Phosphatase and/or a high LDH levels.

During the course of administering steroidal compounds, it is very difficult to maintain the crucial low cholesterol and desired HDL/LDL ratio. Consequently, after the discontinuation and during the nonsteroidal duration, it is important that these levels return and remain at a normal range. It is also important prior to the initiation of a cycle, otherwise, the administration of steroids should not be entertained, due of course, to the expedition of potential health problems. Usually, an accurate screening can be acquired by athletes who abandon exercise for 48 hours or more.

Unsurprisingly, athletes do experience some differences in their blood screening results, especially those who intensely train with weights. Occasionally, temporary changes in SGOT and SGPT may be encountered which usually is indicative of some type of liver stress in passive individuals. However, athletes can interpret these changes as exhibitive that muscle tissue has been broken down and that metabolic changes are occurring. This is another valid reason to acquire screenings prior to steroid cycles, which will establish a standard baseline for a particular individual.

In preparation for these screenings, an 8 to 10 hour fast (no solids or liquids) is required which is followed by the acquiring of several 10 mls of blood (this amount will vary depending on the amount of screenings), which is sent to a laboratory for analysis. Screening results can usually be available for interpretation within 48 to 72 hours. Inquiries of duration of screenings and tests should be made at the initial visit, as some may take longer than others.

Blood screening values may also vary as different laboratories use a variety of analytical methods, which often result in different range values than in the following listings. However, the following tables will still provide an illustration of some of these possible screenings, (there are an abundance of tests not included, however, a consulted physician should be able to conduct appropriate testing if inquired, and necessary).

The following listing is a suggested possibility for an athlete to have these particular blood screenings performed to rule out the following abnormalities. This table is not a complete table, as there are many other tests which may be performed to eliminate possible health hazards. These references have been adapted from the *New England Journal of Medicine SI Unit Conversion Guide.*

ANEMIA:	Vitamin B12.
BONES:	Alkaline Phosphatase, Calcium.
DIABETES:	Glucose.
HEART:	Cholesterol, Potassium, SGOT, SGPT, Triglycerides.
IMMUNE SYSTEM:	Globulin.
KIDNEYS:	BUN, Calcium, Chloride, Phosphorus, Potassium, Sodium, Uric Acid.
LIVER:	Alkaline Phosphatase, Bilirubin, BUN, GGT, LDH, SGOT, SGPT.
NERVOUS SYSTEM:	Chloride, Potassium, Sodium.

The following value ranges are derived from plasma, serum:

	Suggested Athlete Blood Screen	
Determination	*Reference Value Conventional Units*	*SI Units*
Alkaline Phosphatase	30-120 Units/L	30-120 U/L
Bilirubin: Total	0.1-1 mg/dl	2-18 µmol/L
BUN (Blood, Urea, Nitrogen)	8-18 mq/dl	3.0-6.5 mmol/L of urea
Calcium: Female > 50 years Male	 8.8-10.2 mg/dl 8.8-10.3 mg/dl	 2.2-2.56 nmol/L 2.2-2.58 nmol/L
Carbon Dioxide Content	22-28 mEq/L	22-28 mmol/L
Chloride	95-105 mEq/L	95-105 mmol/L
GGT	0-30 Units/L	0-30 U/L
Glucose, Fasting	70-110 mg/dl	3.0-6.1 mmol/L
LDH	50-150 Units/L	50-150 U/L

Suggested Athlete Blood Screen Continued....

Lipids:		
Total Cholesterol		
Desirable	400-850 mg/dl	4-8.5 g/L
Borderline High	<200 mg/dl	<5.2 mmol/L
High	>240 mg/dl	5.2-6.2 mmol/L
Triglycerides	40-150 mg/dl	>6.2 mmol/L
LDL		
Desirable	<130 mg/dl	<3.4 mmol/L
Borderline High	130-159 mg/dl	3.4-4.1 mmol/L
High Risk	>160 mg/dl	>4.1 mmol/L
Phosphorus, (phosphate)	2.5-5 mg/dl	0.8-1.6 mmol/L
Protein:		
Total	6-8 g/dl	60-80 g/L
Albumin	4-6 g/dl	40-60 g/L
Globulin	2.3-3.5 g/dl	23-35 g/L
SGOT	0-35 Units/L	0-35 U/L
SGPT	0-35 Units/L	0-35 U/L
Sodium	135-147 mEq/L	135-147 mmol/L
Uric Acid	2-7 mg/dl	120-420 µmol/L

The following charts are included, as there are many areas of which may be of concern to an athlete. Again, these are not complete tables, but may be of particular importance to some individuals. This particular reference is included in the previous table.

The following value ranges are derived from plasma, serum:

	Electrolytes	
Determination	*Reference Value Conventional Units*	*SI Units*
Carbon Dioxide Content	22-28 mEq/L	22-28 mmol/L
Chloride	95-105 mEq/L	95-105 mmol/L
Potassium	3.5 - 5 mEq/L	3.5-5 mmol/L
Sodium	135-147 mEq/L	135-147 mmol/L

***Serum Estrogen and Testosterone*:** Blood screens are obtained by athletes who attempt to accelerate anabolism. These screenings can be performed on a yearly interval, as they are usually not employed to investigate potential health problems. A serum Estrogen screen can be obtained while entertaining a steroidal treatment, while a serum Testosterone screen cannot; as the latter will only be accurate when complete abstinence from anabolic/androgenics steroids has been practiced for approximately 2 to 3 months. Testosterone is an extremely valuable anabolic/anti-catabolic hormone which can indicate in both female and males, libido, training and emotional status. A high Testosterone level combined with a low Estrogen level is ideal for both sexes. If results indicate a high serum Estrogen level in males who administer steroidal compounds, it is often due to the aromatization of Testosterone to Estrogen. Anti-estrogen compounds such as Nolvadex, Proviron, Teslac (currently, not available in Mexico) will also increase serum Estrogen levels, as these will be also be perceived as Estrogen on a blood screening. Consequently, the discontinuance of these compounds is also imperative for an accurate reading.

Depressed levels of Testosterone can generally indicate overtraining; which is often amplified by nutritional deficits. When Testosterone levels are low, an athlete encounters the dangers of actually breaking down muscle, instead of progressing with further gains. Additionally, the ability to store fuel including important creatine phosphate stores and glycogen is also lowered; which are crucial energy components for heavy weight lifting. Natural Testosterone levels become depressed during and after anabolic steroid administration. Values during a steroidal treatment which are below or on the low end of normal, often imply overtraining or emotional stress. Again, it is imperative for athletes to establish individual normal values, even possibly determining personal testosterone cycles. For example, if a high level of testosterone is normal for a particular athlete, it may also appear normal if interpreted in layman context; even though it has decreased from overtraining. Consequently, if an athlete is aware of personal normal values, a decrease in Testosterone may be significant, even though it is still considered to be within typical normal value ranges.

Futuristically, saliva testing has great potential of becoming a very popular technique of acquiring screening values due to it's simplicity and easy accessibility. Small samples of approximately 5 cc's of saliva obtained upon waking can provide efficient results. Unlike blood or urine samples, salvia remains viable for approximately two weeks in room temperature. Consequently, a range which is considered to be normal in young adult males (upon awakening) for salivary testosterone, is 5.9 to 14.9 nmol -1. Values which descend below or at the low end, possibly indicate either too much stress, or overtraining.

Testosterone-Epitestosterone Ratio: This screening is perused to detect steroidal Testosterone administration such as Primoteston Depot, Primosiston, Sten, Sostenon 250 etc., as Testosterone levels increase, while Epitestosterone levels remain the same. Testosterone compound administration will result in a positive finding if the ratio indicates 6.0 or higher. The Testosterone-Epitestosterone Ratio after administration of Testosterone, can remain elevated for approximately 10 days.

The following value ranges are derived from plasma, serum (tissue when indicated) by RIA (radioimmunoassay):

	Estrogen/ Testosterone	
Determination	*Reference Value Conventional Units*	*SI Units*
Estradiol, (as estrogen)		
Female	20-300 pg/ml	70-1100 pmol/L
Peak Production	200-800 pg/ml	750-2900 pmol/L
Male	<50	<180 pmol/L
Estrogen, (as estradiol)		
Female	20-300 pg/ml	70-1100 pmol/L
Peak Production	200-800 pg/ml	750-2900 pmol/L
Male	<50 pg/ml	<180 pmol/L
Estrogen Receptors (Tissue)		
Negative Result	0-3 fmol of estradiol bound/mg of cytosol protein	0-3 fmol of estradiol bound/mg of cytosol protein
Doubtful Result	4-10 fmol of estradiol bound/mg of cytosol protein	4-10 fmol of estradiol bound/mg of cytosol protein
Positive Result	>10 fmol of estradiol bound/mg of cytosol protein	>10 fmol of estradiol bound/mg of cytosol protein
Testosterone		
Female	<0.6 ng/ml	<2 nmol/L
Male	4-8 ng/ml	14-28 nmol/L

Determining Testosterone, Cortisol, and related steroid hormone levels are the most valuable screenings to indicate training and recovery feedback.

Testosterone-Cortisol Ratio: In regards to training programs, this is presumably the most accurate measure of anabolic/catabolic status. If ideal values of this ratio are indicated, rapid increases without interruptions or plateaus are usually acquired. A Testosterone-Cortisol Ratio can be very significant when compared to previous screenings; thus often eliminating estimations regarding progressive effectiveness. Overtraining, injury, illness, or emotional stress can be suggested by a ratio of less than 0.0200.

Cortisol: High levels of Cortisol exert a powerful catabolic effect in muscle, bone, and connective tissue, therefore, anabolic steroidal administration is very ineffective while these levels are increased. Current and progressive increases in muscle mass are radically negatively affected by these high levels. Gradual increases when first initiating a steroid treatment, and gradual decreases when finishing, will help to minimize the elevation in Cortisol (and Estrogen levels). Consequently, high Cortisol levels are also associated with severe psychological disturbances, hypertension and reduced levels of restful REM sleep. If levels of Cortisol are high upon waking, it is usually indicative of overtraining, illness, poor recovery, or excessive emotional distress. The normal range in young adult males in a salivary coritsol screening (upon waking) is 100-300 nmol/L.

The following value ranges are derived from plasma, serum, and urine when indicated:

	Cortisol	
Determination	*Reference Value Conventional Units*	*SI Units*
Cortisol 0800 hr 1800 hr 2400 hr	 4-19 ug/dl 2-15 ug/dl <5	 110-520 nmol/L 50-410 nmol/L <140 nmol/L
Cortisol, free (urine)	10-110 pg/ml	30-300 nmol/d

Steroid Hormone Testing: Presumably, the most sensitive indicators of anabolic and overtraining status, are Testosterone, Cortisol and the Luteinizing Hormones. These hormones can be assessed by either blood or salvia tests. However, most athletes do not entertain these tests mostly due to the requisite privacy of their chemical administration. Administration of steroidal androgens cause natural testosterone release to become restricted through feedback inhibition of pituitary Luteinizing hormone. Spermatogenesis may become suppressed through feedback inhibition of the follicle stimulating hormone (FSH), if large doses of exogenous androgens are administrated.

A supraphysiologic excess of testosterone is experienced approximately 6 to 24 hours after administration of exogenous Testosterone, which for several days after this, is followed by normal physiologic levels, and then concludes with a subnormal level for approximately 9 to 14 days after the injection. The Luteinizing hormone (LH) and follicle stimulating hormone (FSH) levels return to normal by the 14th day, which have become suppressed by Testosterone administration. (These highly fluctuating levels clinically lead to mood swings, and variations in libido levels).

The following value ranges are derived from plasma, serum:

	FSH/LH	
Determination	*Reference Value Conventional Units*	*SI Units*
Follicle Simulating Hormone (FSH)		
Female	2-15 mIU/ml	2-15 IU/L
Peak Production- (Female)	20-50 mIU/ml	20-50 IU/L
Male	1-10 mIU/ml	1-10 IU/L
Luteinizing Hormone (LH)		
Female	2- 20 mIU/ml	2-20 IU/L
Peak Production - (Female)	30-140 mIU/ml	30-140 IU/L
Male	3-25 mIU/ml	3-25 IU/L

Complete Blood Count (CBC): Is another valuable blood screening which indicates white and red blood count levels and other significant findings. Athletes often have elevated Erythrocyte (RBC, red blood cell) levels, which often exceed the normal range indicated below. This elevation indicates an increase of oxygen transporting capabilities of blood, which is beneficial to athletes. Androgens also can stimulate the production of red blood cells by enhancing the production of erythropoietic stimulating factor. When using high quantities of androgenic steroidal compounds, Hemoglobin and Hematocrit values should also be checked periodically to rule out the possibility of polycythemia (an excess of red blood cells). (Again, this is not a complete CBC reference indicated below).

The following value ranges are derived from plasma, serum:

	Hematologic Tests	
Determination	*Reference Value* *Conventional Units*	*SI Units*
Hematocrit (Hct) Female Male	 33%-43% 39%-49%	 0.33-0.43 0.39-0.49
Hemoglobin (Hb) Female Male	 11.5-15.5 g/dl 14-18 g/dl	 115-155 g/L 140-180 g/L
Leukocyte Count (WBC)	3200-9800/mm(3)	3.2-9.8 x 10(9)/L
Erythrocyte Count (RBC) Female	 3.5-5 million/mm(3) 4.3-5.9 million/mm(3)	 3.5-5 x 10(12)/L 4.3-5.9 x 10(12)/L
Platelet Count	150,000-450,000/mm(3)	150-450 x 10(9)/L

Thyroid Hormone Function: Are important indicators of the function of metabolism . T-4 and TSH are manufactured by the pituitary gland, which causes the thyroid gland to secrete other thyroid hormones. T-3 affects body temperature, and the ideal uptake percentage would be 30 to 35 for most athletes and bodybuilders who wish to burn bodyfat and increase anabolism. However, thyroid function tests can be unreliable if substances which interfere with the binding capacity of serum proteins are also administered. Therefore, it is important to have this test performed while an individual is not entertaining a steroidal compound cycle to establish a normal range. Androgenic steroidal compounds decrease levels of thyroxine-binding globulin, which result in decreased total T-4 serum levels and increased resin uptake of T-3 and T-4.

The following value ranges are derived from plasma, serum:

	Thyroid Hormone Function Tests	
Determination	*Reference Value Conventional Units*	*SI Units*
Thyroid Stimulating Hormone (TSH)	2-11 uU/ml	2-11 mU/L
Thyroxine-binding Globulin Capacity	15-25 ug T4/dl	193-322 nmol/L
Total Triodothyronine (T3)	75-220 ng/dl	1.2-3.4 nmol/L
Total Thyroxine by RIA (T4)	4-12 ug/dl	52-154 nmol/L
T3 Resin Uptake	25%-35%	0.25-0.35

Urinalysis: Urine screens are usually very accurate for the detection of administration of particular substances in the system. However, this screen can be inaccurate in claiming some steroidal compounds and other substances due to the ability of other compoundal substances characteristics, or even other combined urine samples which can disguise results. Therefore, this screen is slightly only occasionally accurate, and currently, is not used in sport-related testing, unless there are no other available testing measures available. Consequently, Urinalysis when employed for medical investigations, can still prove to be advantageous in discovering possible health concerns. It can detect proteinuria which is abnormal levels of Albumin and Globulin, which indicates altered renal function; due to the possibility of kidney damage, Diabetes Mellitus or pyelonephritis. High levels of urine (polyuria) can indicate abnormalities such as Diabetes Mellitus, Diabetes Insipidus, nervous diseases, possible kidney disorders, and the use of diuretics. Low levels of urine (oliguria) can indicate acute nephritis, heart disease, fevers, eclampsia, diarrhea, vomiting, and inadequate fluid intake. No urination, (anuria) is very serious, as it usually is associated with Uremia (urinary substances in the blood), acute nephritis, or metal poisoning. There may be several other conditions of urination problems such as dysuria (painful urination), or incontinence (inability to urinate), which may also be signs of related health problems.

The following colors of urine are indicative of:

Bile-Colored:	Possible jaundice.
Blue:	May result from methylene blue or the presence of indigo.
Brown-Black:	Poisoning (mercury, lead, phenol), hemorrhage.
Colorless:	Extremely diluted urine or achromaturia.
Greenish:	Bile pigment, associated with jaundice.
Milky:	Fat globules, pus in genitourinary infections or chyluria or lipuria.
New-mown Hay:	Indicative of diabetes.
Overripe Apple:	Acetonuria or the presence of acetone bodies.
Pale:	Diabetes Insipidus
Orange - Reddish:	Blood pigments, drugs, or food pigments.
Violet:	May be caused by turpentine.

Yellow to amber: Depends upon the concentration of pigment, however, amber usually indicates normal urine.

For a routine urine test, usually a voided specimen in a clean container is sufficient. Cleansing the penis or vaginal area with soap and water prior to voiding a urine sample is advantageous to avoid contamination. A midstream (which refers to the middle portion of urinating) sample should be obtained and can be gathered either at the clinic (or associated facility) or at home. A fasting period is not required for these screens to be effective. Results can be obtained very quickly, as usually they are evident within a few minutes after being analyzed.

***Ketotone Strip*:** Evaluations can indicate ketone levels in the urine. Ketones are the end products of fat metabolism which are an useful indication of whether the body is in a ketotic state. These strips change from a tan to purplish color if unburned ketones are present in the urine. The latter color of purple is desired as this indicates that the body is not converting protein into glucose, but instead, into ketones which cannot be stored by the body or reconverted into regular fats. Burned ketones cannot be detected upon testing. This test should be done upon awakening in the morning as possibly, the color of tan will dominate results if performed during the day due to the likelihood that the body is burning present ketones for fuel and energy. The darker the color purple becomes, the greater amount of ketones are present in the urine sample.

The following value ranges are derived from urine:

	Urinalysis	
Determination	*Reference Value Conventional Units*	*SI Units*
Catecholamines: Epinephrine Norepinephrine	 <20 ug/day <100 ug/day	 <109 Nmol/day <590 nmol/day
Creatinine: Female Male	 14-22 mg/kg/24 hr 20-26 mg/kg/24 hr	 0.12-0.19 mmol/kg/day 0.18-0.23 mmol/kg/day
Potassium (diet dependent)	25-100 mEq/day	25-100 mmol/day
Protein, quantitative	<150 mg/day	<0.15 g/day

Urinalysis Continued...

Steroids:		(mg/day)		(umol/day)	
17-Ketosteroids	Age:	Male	Female	Male	Female
	20	6-21	4-16	21-73	14-56
	30	8-26	4-14	28-90	14-56
	50	5-18	3-9	17-62	10-31
17-Hydroxycortico-steroids (cortisol):					
Female		2-8 mg/day		5-25 μmol/day	
Male		3-10 mg/day		10-30 μmol/day	

Nitrogen Balance Testing: This test detects the difference between the amount of nitrogen that is ingested and excreted. When the intake amount is greater, than a positive nitrogen balance exists, whereas, when the opposite results, a negative nitrogen balance prevails. As nitrogen is a component of all proteins and is extremely essential for the building of tissue, this testing measure is commonly accepted as a scientific standard for evaluating whole body protein/anabolic statuses. Nitrogen balance improves only when there is sufficient intake of proper calories and protein. A Nitrogen Balance Test is not only an optimal standard of anabolic nutrition testing, but also constitutes the foundation for evaluation of protein sources, biological values and others. Estimating approximate Nitrogen balance can be very beneficial to athletes who attempt to foremost balance the intake of food and supplements; and can also indicate potential anabolic trends.

Unfortunately, the metabolic nemesis of dietary protein in the body cannot be readily measured as it contains Nitrogen in a fixed amount of 6.25 grams of protein to 1 gram of nitrogen. However, Nitrogen loss can be detected, by measuring Nitrogen intake against Nitrogen loss. This ratio provides an estimate of the Nitrogen/anabolic status of the body.

Urine Urea Nitrogen (UUN) is a form of which 90% of nitrogen loss occurs in the urine.

Nitrogen Balance studies can be performed by utilizing a test called Nitro Strip II, which measures UUN loss by changing colors. Estimated Nitrogen Balance is detected when measured against protein intake, which yields optimal results when conducted with the first urine stream upon awakening; combined in a series of three attempts to demonstrate a comparative bias.

Other Tests Which May be of Value and Importance to Athletes

Blood Pressure Values: This should also be periodically checked, as it is an important indication that the system may be experiencing some problems, which may further lead to possible health concerns. A BP reading can be easily obtained by a clinic (or related facility), or can be done personally by an individual. Many pharmacies, clinics, etc., can instruct how to obtain these readings, so that they can be performed on a private basis. There are also many other devices available which do not require the knowledge of performing this task, instead, actually only require a finger of the tested individual, which results in an electronic display of the clinical finding. Blood Pressure readings can be performed at anytime, anywhere, and the administration of steroidal compounds do not interfere with accurate readings. They can however, elevate findings which were previously normal. It is very important to keep the blood pressure within a normal range, and to seek medical attention if any abnormality is noted.

Ranges obtained by a sphygmomanometer.

Blood Pressure Ranges:	**Systolic/Diastolic**
Normal	120/80 or less
Borderline	140/90 - 160/95
Hypertension	160/95

As previously indicated, there are many, many tests, screenings, scans, and x-rays available to rule out or detect possible health concerns. It is extremely important if athletes choose to enhance their athletic endeavors by the means of anabolic steroidal compounds, that they also protect their health by applying common sense measures, and obtaining appropriate health screens. If an area is of particular concern to an athlete, it should be brought immediately to the attention of the medical profession, so that pertinent action can be taken.

The following value ranges are derived from plasma, serum.

	Other Possible Blood Screening Tests	
Determination	*Reference Value Conventional Units*	*SI Units*
Coagulation Screen: Bleeding Time Prothrombin Time	 3-9.5 min <2 sec from control	 180-570 sec <2 sec from control
Creatinine	0.6-1.2 mg/dl	50-110 umol/L
Iron Female Male	 60-160 ug/dl 80-180 u/dl	 11-29 umol/L 14-32 umol/L
Lactic Acid	0.5-2.2 mmol/L	0.5-2.2 mmol/L
Prostate Specific Antigen	0-4 ng/ml	
Vitamin B12 Normal Borderline	 205-876 pg/ml 140-204 pg/ml	 150-672 pmol/L 102.6-149 pmol/L

MACRONUTRIENTS:

* **Carbohydrates**
* **Energy**
* **Fats**
* **Fiber**
* **Protein Complex**
  Amino Acids
* **Water**

CARBOHYDRATES:

Carbohydrates are one of the three main classes of nutrients which provide energy to the body; the other two, are proteins and fats. Carbohydrates are also considered to be a macronutrient, which are required in the body in large amounts. They include all sugars; fructose, glucose, glycogen, lactose, sucrose, starches, cellulose and glycogen, which are the main sources of energy.

Carbohydrates are made during photosynthesis, and humans obtain carbohydrates by ingesting plants or other animals, then, this becomes stored for future use and energy. All carbohydrates consist of the chemical elements; carbon, hydrogen and oxygen.

Carbohydrates make up approximately 55% of the total number of calories in a well-balanced diet. Foods which are considered to be high in carbohydrates are bananas, corn, bread, pasta, rice and potatoes. Also, some sources of carbohydrates such as fruits, vegetables and whole grain cereals, also contain important amounts of vitamins and minerals. However, several "junk foods", such as candy, chocolate, and soda pop, may also have a high sugar content, which may be considered to be a high source of carbohydrates, but in actuality, they are only a source of energy for the body, as they do not provide the health benefits.

A deficiency of carbohydrates will result in fatigue. Consequently, an over abundance of carbohydrates can result in fat accumulation, tooth decay, diabetes and heart disease.

Kinds of Carbohydrates:

There are two kinds of carbohydrates, *simple* and *complex.*

Simple Carbohydrates: Have a simple molecular structure. Some carbohydrates can also be broken down into two categories; monosaccharides and disaccharides. These are both sugars; monosaccharides are simple sugars, and disaccharides consist of two monosaccharides.

The main monosaccharides include glucose, fructose and galactose. Among the most important disaccharides are sucrose, lactose and maltose.

Fructose: Is an extremely sweet sugar which is derived from fruits and vegetables.

Galatose: Occurs in food only as part of a disaccharide called lactose.

Glucose: Is a mildly sweet sugar, which is the most important carbohydrate in the blood.

Lactose: Is milk sugar, which makes up about 5% of cow's milk.

Maltose: Or malt sugar, is used to flavor some candy.

Sucrose: Is table sugar.

Complex Carbohydrates: Complex carbohydrates have a complicated molecular structure which consist of simple carbohydrates that are joined in long chains. They are also called polysaccharides, which are made up of many monosaccharides. Polysaccharides include starch, cellulose, and glycogen. A molecule of starch consists of hundreds or even thousands of glucose molecules joined end to end. Polysaccharides are the chief form of carbohydrates which are stored by plants.

Starch:	Occurs in foods such as beans, corn, potatoes, and wheat.
Cellulose:	Makes up much of the cell walls of plants.
Glycogen:	Or animal starch, is the chief form of stored carbohydrate in animals.

Carbohydrates can be further divided into another two groups: *Starchy* and *Fibrous*. Examples of such are:

Starchy Carbohydrates	***Fibrous Carbohydrates***
Pasta	Broccoli
Rice	Cauliflower
Sweet Potatoes	Carrots
Beans	Celery
Yams	Cucumbers
Lentils	Iceberg Lettuce
Oatmeal	Mushrooms
Peas	Tomatoes

(Please refer to the nutrition section for further references).

How the Body Uses Carbohydrates:

Carbohydrates are used by the body as fuel, however, only monosaccharides can enter the bloodstream directly from the digestive system. The body must digest disaccharides and starch in the small intestine before they can be used. For example, sucrose must first be broken down into glucose and fructose, lactose must be broken down into glucose and galactose, and starch has to be broken down into maltose, and then into glucose.

Once carbohydrates have been broken down into simple sugars in the small intestine, the blood transports them to the liver. The liver then changes fructose and galactose into glucose, which is carried by the blood to all of the cells of the body. Glucose is used as fuel by the cells for the muscle and nerves, and also to build and repair body tissues. The liver changes excess glucose into glucogen, which it then stores. If the level of sugar in the blood becomes low, the liver changes glycogen back into glucose and releases it back into the blood. Glycogen is also stored in the muscles as an emergency reserve of energy, and some is changed back into glucose when the body requires energy quickly.

Cellulose, which unlike most of the other carbohydrates, cannot be digested by the human body, therefore, has no food value. However, certain amounts of cellulose are useful as it maintains the health and tone of the intestines, and aids digestion.

Carbohydrates can also demonstrate a "protein sparing" effect, as when the carbohydrate reserves become low, the body will convert protein into glucose for energy. Under normal circumstances, protein exhibits a vital role in the maintenance, repair, and growth of the body tissues, which is referred to as *glyconeogenesis.* Ingesting a sufficient amount of carbohydrates is very important, as if there is not enough for the body to utilize for energy, it will metabolize more protein to compensate for fuel. This will result in muscle depletion, due to the reduction in the body's protein stores. Decreased amounts of carbohydrates can leave muscles feeling and appearing flat, as muscle fullness depends largely upon the glycogen stores within. Similarly, vascularity is also largely dependent upon carbohydrate intake. Ingesting simple sugars prior to a competition often helps bodybuilders achieve vascularity quickly.

Interestingly, a low carbohydrate diet will result in a decreased bodyweight owing to the loss of water weight, due to the fact that every carbohydrate gram which is stored within muscle tissue, is usually accompanied by approximately three grams of water. Therefore, by decreasing the carbohydrate intake, a natural drop in body water will also occur. However, this is only a temporary state, and once carbohydrate ingestion is resumed, the body often rebounds and actually results in retaining excess water. This too, is a temporary state and will dissipate after several days. Consequently, if the carbohydrate intake is too low, the energy levels will also be low, which usually results in the possibilities of overtraining, less energy, and loss of muscle fullness.

ENERGY:

Energy, which is more commonly referred to as calories, is a unit which is used to measure heat energy in the metric system of measurement. A calorie is actually the amount of energy which is required to raise the temperature of one gram of water by one Celsius degree.

Calories are measured by an instrument called a calorimeter, which measures the amount of heat produced by many chemical reactions. One of the most important uses of the calorimeter is to measure the amount of heat which is given off by different foods when they burn. This measurement allows for the measurement of the amount of energy a certain food yields when it is completely used by the body.

Therefore, it is important that the body receives a certain amount of calories a day, as calories are burned for fuel, and the more vigorous the activity or stress, the more calories are required. Caloric intakes however, vary per individual, depending upon their weight categories, male or females, active or inactive, etc. This is also dependent upon other factors such as metabolism and desired weight goals. An average caloric intake can vary from 1500 calories for an average person, but can exceed up to levels of over 8,000 for a bodybuilder; again illustrating that the amount of required calories consumed, can be somewhat individualized. Everything that is ingested into the body and bloodstream, has a caloric value. This includes all beverages with the exception of water; foods, medicines, supplements etc., etc.

A diet deficient in calories will lead to a reduction in weight and fatigue. However, a lower caloric intake will also lower the body's metabolism, making it easier for the body to store fat. Also, if the caloric intake increases at some point, a method of increasing the metabolism will also have to be entertained in order to maintain the desired body weight. Subcaloric diets also do not provide enough food to fuel energy requirements forcing the body to go into a breakdown mode in which muscle (including the heart), tissue is lost. Vital nutrients can also be withdrawn from tissues to fuel the body, which results in depletion of the nutritional reservoirs.

Usually for most athletes and bodybuilders, most of the calories are consumed from food, as well as a certain proportion is obtained from nutritional supplements. For example, a diet may consist of 5,000 calories in a daily total, but approximately 1,700 of the calories may be derived from supplemental intake from protein, carbohydrate powders, MCT oil, vitamins, minerals etc. Beverages also constitute a total of the calories which should be included when calculating caloric totals.

Undereating can very easily place an athlete in an overtrained state. A very fine line exists between losing bodyfat opposed to muscle, while dieting. The ingestion of less calories usually results in decreased bodyfat, however, lowering the caloric intake too much, can cause muscles to sacrifice precious nutrients to compensate for the lacking diet. Consequently, the greater amount of cardiovascular activity that is entertained while on a restricted caloric intake, may also result in a loss of lean body mass, along with the stress hormones which also attack the muscle tissues. Therefore, if low calories are continuously ingested, not only will muscle loss result, but also energy and endurance levels. It is common for an athlete who is calorie deficient, to often credit the loss of energy and strength to overtraining, when in fact, it is due to an insufficient calorie intake.

FATS:

Fat is also one of the three main classes of macronutrients, which also provides required energy to the body. They are composed of carbon, hydrogen and oxygen. Fats are also composed of substances called fatty acids, and an alcohol called glycerol.

Fat has many important uses as it is a concentrated source of food energy for both animals and plants. It is stored under the surface of the skin in humans which act as a protective insulation barrier against heat loss, and cushions against injury in areas such as the eyeballs and other vital organs. Fat transports fat-soluble vitamins through the bloodstream, and helps maintain healthy skin. Certain fats also arbitrate the production of eicosanoids while other particular fats regulate cholesterol. There are three principle forms of fat in the human diet. Fats consist primarily of compounds known as glycerides - principally triacylglycerol or triglyceride, which are made up of one molecule of glycerol, combined with three molecules of fatty acids. Each of these fatty acids is a long chain of carbon atoms with hydrogen atoms attached to them. The fatty acid chains are then linked to the glycerol molecule to finally form a molecule of fat. Triglycerides is the form in which fat is stored for fuel, and is also the most abundant type of fat in food and tissues, which accounts for approximately 95% to 98% of fat ingested through all forms of food. Consequently, the same percentage of triglycerides is also found in human fat.

Triglycerides can also be converted if needed, into one or both of the two other main types of fat found in the human body; *phospholipid* and *cholesterol*. Triglycerides are found primarily in the adipose (fat) cells, where it accounts for approximately 99% of cell volume. Therefore, Triglycerides are able to salvage space, unlike glycogen (the main carbohydrate-storing compound), which has approximately 3 grams of water per each gram of glycogen. Fat also has a characteristic of being less oxidized, which requires more effort in the oxidation process, than carbohydrates. Most triglycerides which are obtained from animal sources such as lard and butter, have many saturated fatty acids; while vegetable triglycerides such as olive and corn oil, contain a large quantity of unsaturated fatty acids.

Phospholipids are mainly found as constituents of cell membranes and myelin sheaths (the coverings of nerves), which also play a part in the production of eicosanoids. Eicosanoids can be further broken down into prostaglandins, leukotrienes, and thromboxanes, which affect and regulate a multitude of other biochemical processes including the production of hormones, and the regulation of blood pressure.

Cholesterol is a main part of the cell membranes, which is required also for the production of bile acids in the liver, and is the precursor for Vitamin D, and steroidal hormones. Cholesterol can be found in all tissues, however, the blood serum cholesterol is what is checked during a blood test screening. A small portion of cholesterol is necessary, however, it is not considered to be an essential nutrient. Too much cholesterol can cause plaque buildup of the blood vessel walls, which can lead to possible atherosclerosis, heart attacks, and strokes. All forms of cholesterol are derived from animal sources, as plants and vegetable oils do not contain cholesterol; therefore, are always cholesterol-free. Unfortunately, not all cholesterol problems arise from consuming foods, as since the liver manufactures it, the process is only partly regulated by how much is ingested; as Triglycerides can be transformed into cholesterol. Therefore, if more cholesterol is ingested, the liver in turn, will manufacture less, and vice versa.

An average individual can ingest approximately 400 to 500 mgs of cholesterol daily, and it is estimated that only 20 to 30% of the population is genetically hypersenstive to the cholesterol that is consumed. Therefore, for the majority of individuals, the amount of cholesterol consumed from food sources, does not directly affect blood cholesterol levels. Instead, it is actually the type of fat ingested, which can have a significant effect on these levels. Consuming quantities of saturated fats can stimulate the production of low-density lipoproteins, which is considered to be the "bad" cholesterol. Saturated fats are fatty acids which carry as many hydrogen atoms as possible, and are usually solid at room temperature, such as lard. They can usually be found in animal meats and byproducts, but palm oil and coconut oils are also high in saturated fats as well. Ingesting animal meats will ensure a proper ratio of saturated fats in a diet. Saturated fats are basically inert, and can only be used as fuel, due to the fact of unavailable space which would normally allow other substances to attach. A saturated fatty acid such as Stearic acid, contains as many hydrogen atoms as possible, that are attached to its carbon chain, which single bond link together the carbon atoms of the chain. However, saturated fats can also raise cholesterol levels, which in turn, can further lead to health problems, primarily heart disease.

Unsaturated fats are fatty acids which have available space to support other hydrogen atoms. Unsaturated fats can be further divided into polyunsaturated or monounsaturated, depending on how many hydrogen atoms are missing. Polyunsaturated fatty acids are fatty acids which contain more than one double bond. All essential fatty acids considered to be polyunsaturated and can be found in corn, safflower or sesame oils. These fats are generally liquid at room temperature and can become rapidly rancid, due to the alteration of the oil properties, which consume the empty hydrogen spaces. To avoid this, almost all oils are processed, which also makes them more saturated. This process is called hydrogenation, which can also change the configuration of a fat from *cis* to *trans*. Oleic acid, which is another unsaturated fatty acid, contains at least one pair of carbon atoms which are joined by a double bond, which in turn, for each combined bond, the carbon chain has a missing pair of hydrogen atoms. These tend to lower the amount of LDL cholesterol in the blood, as the polyunsaturated fats do in fish oils. Monosaturated fats can be found in olive, canola, peanut and avocados, and large quantities of these fats can make an individual fat. However, a small daily quota of monosaturated fats are required, and also appear to have the ability of lowering the LDL cholesterol in the blood as well.

Nearly all natural fats occur in what is referred to as the *cis configuration*. Hydrogen atoms have electrical charges which repel each other, which result in a curve in the molecule. These curves are the characteristic, and the essential shape of the molecule, which in turn transmits signals which enables the body to perform special biological functions. However, this cis formation is destroyed by processing, which causes the atoms to rotate, thereby developing into trans molecules, which no longer transmit the same transmitted messages. The body, still makes an effort to use these unrecognized messages, but unfortunately, when they are incorporated into cell membranes, they can result in abnormal cell function. Most Trans-Fatty Acids start out as unsaturated fats, which are processed by hydrogenation into a more solid form for use in food processing or cooking. Trans-Fatty Acids tend to act more like saturated fats than unsaturated fats in the body, because of this change. This also increases the low-density lipoproteins (LDL), cholesterol, and the risk of heart disease. Consequently, Trans-Fatty Acids are not indicated on most food labels, and therefore, cannot be legally listed as unsaturated fats. However, Trans-Fatty Acids may be identified under the term "hydrogenated vegetable oil", and can be derived by comparing the total fat grams to the sum of the polyunsaturated, saturated, and monounsaturated fats listed; the remaining difference representative of the Trans-Fatty Acids.

Depending on the level of trans fats in the product, processed unsaturated fats may be just as unhealthy in large quantities, as most animal fats. Trans fats can be identified by the words hydrogenated, or partially hydrogenated in the list of ingredients of most products such as margarines or shortenings, which are often processed to allow for a much harder and more stable consistency. Processed oils also contain trans fat, and the more solid the oil, the higher the level of these fats will be found. Even though peanut oil is monounsaturated, most peanut butter products are processed, which changes the monounsaturated cis fats, into the undesirable trans fats. If an individual wishes to consume peanut butter, it is much healthier to consume the natural kind which contains only peanuts and salt, and often requires to be stirred to mix the oil that is floating on top. This type of peanut butter usually can be freshly made at a local health store. Also, peanut oil should be used when cooking, as it will not turn the cis molecules into trans molecules when heated.

Nutritional Importance:

Although fat is an important energy source in the diet, it is a more efficient fuel than either proteins or carbohydrates, due to its high energy content. Fat can produce approximately 4,000 calories of energy per pound (9 calories per gram), whereas carbohydrates and proteins can each produce about 1,800 calories per pound (4 calories per gram); therefore, less than half of the energy is produced by fat. The body can store fat which is almost dry, but large amounts of water are required to store carbohydrates and proteins. The body converts carbohydrates and proteins into adipose (fatty) tissue for storage, then when extra fuel is needed, the body draws on this stored fat. The adipose cells (adipocytes) are found in tissues throughout the entire body, and are often nestled in between muscle and liver cells, where they can aid in supplying immediate energy. The total number of these adipocytes is largely determined in childhood, and overfeeding during this time period, will determine the amount of adipose cells for an individual.

Dietary fats can be divided into two further groups; *Visible* and *Invisible* Fats. Examples of visible fats include fats in meat, butter, lard, margarine, and salad oils, which are also soft at room temperature. An animal or plant fat which is liquid at room temperature, is referred to as an oil. Fats and oil are insoluble in water, however, they can be dissolved in alcohols, chloroform, ether, and gasoline. A fat which is hard at room temperature is beef tallow. Invisible fats are found in foods such as milk, eggs, fish, and legumes; and are finely dispersed throughout many tissues of animals and plants. Many of these fats are also especially rich in essential fatty acids.

A deficiency of fat may result in growth cessation, skin eczema, acne, dry skin or deterioration, dandruff, dry, dull, brittle, or decreased hair growth, nail deterioration, soft, brittle, flaking nails, dry eyes and mouth, diarrhea, allergies, varicose veins, weight decrease or increase, gallstones, decreased radiation resistance, heart disease, cancer, sterility, swollen joints, liver deterioration, fatigue, emotional agitation, decreased immunity, and decreased T-cell blood count. A low fat diet can also become detrimental as certain fats actually improve insulin resistance, which makes it less feasible to store carbohydrates as fat. Fat improves the glycemic index of carbohydrates, which also decreases the possibililty of experiencing an insulin surge, which will encourage fat storage.

Essential Fatty Acids:

Essential fatty acids (EFA's) are necessary for growth and maintenance of the body. EFA's are also known as the foundation for the membranes which constitute the outer border of every cell in the body, and also help form many of the complicated structures within the body cells. The body however, is unable to manufacture EFA's, therefore, they must be consumed. EFA's are especially abundant in brain phospholipid and are consequently, essential for development of brain tissue, the proper development of the retina, and spermatazoa. EFA's also help produce eicosanoids, which partially host several physiological activities, as well as the production of growth-essential hormones, or their precursors, which may be of particular importance to athletes and bodybuilders.

The body can change long chain fatty acids of more than 16 carbons into unsaturated forms, and also lengthen already unsaturated fats by inserting double bonds, which are actually empty spaces. Therefore, the body can manufacture almost all of the different fats it requires, with one exception. The body is unable to produce particular 18-carbon molecules, which it requires for the maintenance of overall health. These fatty acids are referred to as n-6 Essential Fatty acids; linoleic acid is the most common.

Omega n-3 fatty acids, primarily linolenic acid, and two fatty acids which are common in fish oils; eicosapentaenoic acid and decosahexanoeic acid, have recently been included within the category of EFA's. However, the body can produce the latter two fatty acids from linolenic acid, therefore, the only two EFA's which require to be consumed are mainly linoleic and linolenic acids. The ratio of linoleic to linolenic (n-6 to n-3 fatty acids), may be important, as unbalanced ratios may lead to a depletion of n-3 fatty acids in the phospholipids of vital organs. However, a definite ratio calculation has not been clearly decided upon, although a possible 4:10 ratio; which means for every 4 parts of linoleic acid consumed, 10 parts of linolenic acid should also accompany the consumption. This can be achieved by ingesting flaxseed oil, which is high in linolenic acid, however, too much consumption of this can possibly stimulate tumor growth.

Average adults require approximately 1 to 2% of their total daily calories from n-6 fatty acids, and possibly closer to 14% for optimal health. If bodybuilders choose to avoid fat, the probability of acquiring a n-6 deficiency is very likely. Therefore, if a particular restricted, especially low-fat diet regime is being followed, the extra consumption of 1 to 3 tablespoons of flaxseed oil will provide an individual with these required fatty acids. This can easily be accomplished by adding the Flaxseed Oil to meal-replacement drinks divided evenly throughout the day, as a full tablespoon of Flaxseed Oil is approximately 10 grams. This practice will fulfill both the required polyunsaturated fats, and the daily requirement of essential fatty acids at the same interval.

Fish Oil:

Fish Oils have a characteristically high concentration of eicosapentaenoic acid (EPA), and decosahexanoeic acid (DHA), which the body can also produce directly from linolenic acid. Large quantities, up to 24 grams daily of Fish Oil can lower plasma lipids, which can lower cholesterol amounts, as well as inhibit the formation of plaque on the arteries, which may also lower hypertension. However, fish in general, are not usually beneficial sources of EPA and DHA, as some fattier fish such as herring, mackerel, and salmon have high amounts, while other lower-fat fish have lower amounts. Unfortunately, consuming large amounts of Fish Oil can also diminish inflammatory responses, and also suppress the release of particular components of the immune system, which are essential in resisting illness and disease. Fish oils also contain omega-3 fatty acids which encourage the receptor sites on muscles to increase insulin sensitivity, which allows the body to release less insulin, which in turn, tends to limit fat storage as insulin performs its task of channeling the carbohydrates and amino acids into muscle tissue.

A recommended intake consists of approximately 4,000 mgs daily, which would include 640 mgs of EPA, and 480 mgs of DHA.

CLA:

Conjugated linoleic acid (CLA), which is an anticarcinogenic agent found in almost all foods, appears to be much more efficient than Fish Oil, as it may inhibit tumor growth, increase T-cell counts, enhance the immune function, and reduce the incidence of fatty deposits in the blood vessels. CLA may be very beneficial to athletes and bodybuilders who are especially interested in increasing lean body mass while decreasing bodyfat. Although this fatty acid is very similar to linoleic acid, CLA has some very individualized characteristics, and also has a different position and configuration of the double bonds. However, although linoleic acid may stimulate tumor growth, CLA may actually inhibit it in small quantities of 0.1% of a total caloric intake, which also which makes CLA superior to that of Fish Oil, which requires more than 10% of total daily calories, to achieve the same effect. Six to nine grams of CLA consumed daily should be considered as one tablespoon of polyunsaturated fat.

As CLA is still a relatively new discovery, there are many suggestions that this fatty acid appears to yield promising, beneficial results for those individuals who enhance their diets by supplementation of this fat. One theory in particular which may be of special interest to athletes and bodybuilders, implies that when CLA is absorbed into cell membranes, it could possibly change the responsiveness to particular hormone stimulatory and/or inhibitory factors, which are characteristically involved in the destination of the cell's growth and development; or possibly, the effects can be attributed to the counteractive influence on the adverse effects of some catabolic hormones. Nevertheless, CLA potential effects are so significant, that many scientists have recommended to fortify foods with this fatty acid, in attempts to decrease the possibility of developing cancer, and generally, improve overall health.

***Primrose Oil*:**

Is a natural supplement which has been very beneficial to some steroidal compound administrators. A fatty acid, called Gamma linolenic acid (GLA), promotes the formation of prostaglandins, which are hormone-like substances, that cannot be manufactured by the body. However, this can be achieved by the consumption of Primrose Oil, or from the conversion of linoleic acid. Primrose Oil has been used by women to treat PMS for many years; however, those involved with cycling steroids, have discovered that Primrose Oil can actually minimize a number of common anabolic side effects. Reports of consuming Primrose Oil in conjunction with steroidal compounds has resulted in aiding the liver from becoming overstressed and damaged, and it also proved effective in lowering cholesterol levels. Other positive advantages of adding Primrose Oil to a diet is that it can also lower blood pressure, tendonitis aliments, help dry, flaky skin and other complexion problems, and increase appetite and energy levels. The immunity system is also benefited by Primrose Oil, which is usually suppressed by the use of steroids.

Three Primrose Oil capsules are recommended to be ingested three times a day, with or without food. It is most beneficial to ingest these capsules with a full glass of water (as the kidneys will filter anything except for water), and then within thirty minutes after the initial glass of water, three more glasses of water should be consumed.

MCT Oil:

Medium-chained triglycerides, is a dietary fat metabolized in a particular way so that very little is stored as bodyfat when infused in the body. MCT's tend to be used as energy, whereas other fats tend to be used for storage. Therefore, they are also considered to be a beneficial method of adding calories to a diet regime, as it increases the available energy levels which promotes weight gain, however, will be burned as fuel, and the excess will not be stored. For bodybuilding supplementation, the ingestion of MCT's appear to be better utilized for energy than traditional fats, if solely consumed instead of other fats. MCT Oil can be added to the diet orally directly into the mouth, or it can be added to cooking.

Generally, one-third of the fats ingested should be derived from polyunsaturated fats such as flaxseed oil, corn oil, safflower oil, or sesame oil. One-third should come from monounsaturated fats like olive and canola oil, peanuts or avocados, and approximately less than one-third should be obtained from saturated fats such as those contained in animal meats, in fact, lessening the consumption of saturated fats is more beneficial, than detrimental. However, unless an individual is a strict vegetarian, totally eliminating saturated fats from the diet is almost impossible, as this fat is characteristically found in all types of animal meats. Therefore, unsaturated, polysaturated, and essential fatty acids are fats which are beneficial, and the saturated fat is the one to limit in a diet regime.

Many sport experts recommend a diet which derives approximately 30% of its calories from fat. Therefore, if a total daily caloric intake was 1,800, the daily fat intake should be approximately 60 grams. A simple calculation of the total number of daily calories (1800), multiplied by 30%, will result in the maximum amount of fat calories for a daily consumption. For example, 1800 x .30 = 540 total calories, which should be derived from fat, or 540 divided by 9 (fat has nine calories per gram) = 60 total grams of fat. However, fat percentage consumption opinions vary from expert to expert, and can range anywhere from 10% to 30%. However, increased percentages higher than 30% may result in the accumulation of bodyfat, if exercise is not also entertained.

"GOOD FATS":

Flaxseed Oil (Linseed)
Olive Oil
Canola Oil
CLA
Peanut Oil
Fish Oil
Soybean Oil
Corn Oil
Borage Oil
Sunflower Oil
Safflower Oil
Wheat-germ Oil
Primrose Oil
MCT Oil

"BAD FATS":

Dairy Fats
Animal Fats
Palm Oil
Coconut Oils (not MCT)
Fats found in margarine and butters
Olestra

Olestra:

This is a new, "fake fat" which is often used as a fat substitute in order to save calories. However, it may also deplete the body of nutrients, which may lead to deficiencies, and other possible ailments.

FIBER:

Although fiber is also a macronutrient, it is often not classified as a nutrient because it is not absorbed into the body.

Fiber is considered to be somewhat of a "bulk" item which is often able to trick the stomach into experiencing a full sensation, which usually lessens the desire to eat more food. It is also very important to consume large amounts of water with the intake of fiber, as this allows for the expansion of the fiber substance, which results in the suppression of hunger; the increase of the efficiency of the food fiber, and also prevents possible intestinal obstructions. Fiber also acts as a natural laxative and provides relief to constipation. It also helps athletes to control their bodyweight, and stabilize blood-glucose levels by modifying the insulin output. Fiber can be obtained from foods which are in the complex carbohydrate category. Foods high in fiber include fresh fruits such as oranges, pears, bananas, apples, strawberries, prunes, and fresh vegetables such as spinach, peas, corn, broccoli, potatoes, carrots, and green beans. Also, most grain and granola cereals, bran and most bread items are also found to be high in fiber content.

There are two type of fiber, *soluble* and *insoluble*.

Soluble Fiber: Can be digested by the body. These include pectins, gums and mucilages, which are found in such foods as oat bran, barley, oatmeal, beans, psyllium, fresh fruits, vegetables and legumes (nuts).

Insoluble Fiber: Cannot be digested by the body. These include cellulose, hemicellulose and lignin. Such examples of these are found in whole wheat, whole grains, celery, corn, corn bran, green beans, green leafy vegetables, potato skins, and brown rice.

Generous amounts of soluble fiber aid in lowering blood sugar, as it slows down the body's absorption of carbohydrates, and prevents an inordinate rush of insulin. It also helps to lower cholesterol levels by connecting with bile acids and escorting the cholesterol out of the body, as cholesterol cannot be oxidized like fats. Soluble fiber also decreases both the total plasma-cholesterol, and the low-density lipoprotein (LDL) levels, which are very closely linked to the onset of cardiovascular disease. However, fiber intake does not affect the high-density lipoprotein (HDL) levels.

Insoluble fiber helps to move fat out of the body as it is not digestible by the human body. It is able to pass through the digestive track and "pull some fat" along with it, and both the fiber and fat are then eliminated in the stool. Insoluble fiber also supplies the stool with the necessary volume to help prevent constipation, colon and rectal cancer. It is recommended that the diet have a source of natural fiber, as this allows the colon to function smoothly and properly, without the dependency of harsh laxatives which can eventually lead to dependency, and severe colon damage.

The recommended daily allowance (RDA) for total fiber intake is approximately 30 grams per day for average individuals. The American Diabetes Association recommends 40 grams of dietary fiber a day, with approximately 30 grams of soluble-fiber intake daily, to possibly benefit blood-sugar control. Fiber is beneficial to diabetics, as it is able to flatten the glycemic-index curve, which allows for the maintenance of a more stable blood-glucose level.

A diet which is deficient in fiber may result in colon cancer, hemorrhoids, appendicitis, diverticulosis, colitis, ulcerative colitis, chronic constipation, varicose veins, or in a hiatal hernia. Whereas, a diet which contains too much fiber, may lead to stomach discomfort, cramps, excess gas, and/or diarrhea, as the intestinal bacteria ferments the fiber, which often results in these symptoms. The uptake of certain medications such as tricyclic antidepressants, cholesterol-lowering drugs, and thyroid drugs, may be interfered with the consumption of fiber.

Athletes and individuals who administer steroidal compounds may also experience some intervention, as there are possible indications that fiber may possibly also bind to the steroid hormones, which also includes

Testosterone. Several studies have indicated that fiber does bind to various steroids which includes both Estrogen and Testosterone in the intestine, which promotes the excretion of the steroidal compounds. For example, Lignin, is known to increase the sex-hormone-binding globulin (SHBG), which is a blood protein that binds to Testosterone, and makes it inactive. However, these particular studies may have little effect on the free, or total Testosterone levels in men, as these findings were obtained from outside the body, in vitro, which means that they were conclusive from test tubes. Consequently, these results were also most pronounced in vegetarians, as this group were shown to have increased SHBG levels.

However, the physical properties of various fiber sources, definitely demonstrate unconstrained health benefits in healthy individuals.

PROTEIN:

Protein, along with carbohydrates and fats, together make up the main class of food which provide energy to the body. Proteins are essential to life, and exist in every living cell. Proteins can be obtained from food such as cheese, eggs, fish, meat and milk, which are considered to be very high in protein value. However, proteins can also be obtained through "protein drinks, shakes, bars and supplements". Each meal, whether it is an actual meal or a mock meal, should contain a protein to achieve optimal effects of this muscle building macronutrient.

Muscles are able to grow by synthesizing and breaking down protein. The total protein accumulation, or muscle growth, is the resulting balance between the amount made, and the amount broken down. If bigger, stronger muscles are desired, then a significant alteration in the body's existing protein cycle must be made. Therefore, an increase in the rate of synthesis (anabolism), and a decrease in the rate of breakdown (anti-catabolism), must occur. Theoretically, slowing down catabolism can be accomplished by down regulating the several different pathways of protein breakdown inside the cells.

Serious athletes and especially bodybuilders who also train aerobically, place more emphasis on the protein requirements of their bodies. Aerobic exercise if continued over a prolonged period of time, burns not only the stored carbohydrates for energy, but also can dip into the amino acids. The protein requirements therefore, must be increased to avoid a protein deficient state which can lead to sports anemia.

Sports anemia is a condition in which red blood cells and serum levels become reduced. Muscle fibers are damaged during training, and must be repaired following the period of exercise. Therefore, if the protein intake is low, the body will resort to red blood cells, hemoglobin, and the plasma proteins as a source of protein for muscle repair. Sports anemia can possibly occur when this happens, as there is little protein left remaining to rebuild red blood cells at a normal rate.

The Structure of Proteins:

All proteins contain carbon, hydrogen, nitrogen, and oxygen, and some also contain iron, phosphorus and sulfur. Smaller units referred to as amino acids, are the larger complex molecules of proteins which they are broken down into. The amino acids are then linked together into long chains which are called polypeptides. A protein consists of one or more polypeptide chains.

Twenty common amino acids (refer to amino acid section for listing), are arranged into thousands of different proteins. These are required by the human body to assemble the proteins it requires, as the body must have a sufficient supply of these particular amino acids. These are referred to as essential and nonessential amino acids. Essential amino acids are amino acids which either cannot be produced by the body, or if they are, are in insufficient amounts. Essential amino acids must be obtained from various food consumption. Nonessential amino acids on the other hand, can be manufactured by the body, so therefore, do not need to be supplemented by food.

Proteins in the Diet:

It is well known that some of the best sources of protein can be found in foods such as cheese, eggs, fish, meat and milk, as these foods are considered to be complete. Complete proteins contain adequate amounts of all the essential amino acids. Some sources however, may be high in protein, but also high in fat. For example, red meat is high in protein, but also has a high fat content; as opposed to a chicken breast, which is also high in protein, but is much lower in fat. Protein can also be found in cereal grains, legumes, and vegetables. However, these proteins are considered to be incomplete because they lack adequate amounts of one or more of the essential amino acids; but, a combination of two incomplete proteins can provide a complete amino acid mixture! To achieve a complete amino acid, each incomplete protein must have sufficient amounts of the essential amino acids of which the other incomplete protein contains only small amounts of. These foods must be ingested together to provide the correct balance of amino acids. For example, a cereal grain, could be combined with a legume (such as peanuts) to provide such a balance (for example, nuts added to cheerios, *are not only for fun and flavor!!).* However, unfortunately, most breakfast cereals also contain other ingredients which most athletes, bodybuilders and those on a restricted diet must often avoid.

The Recommended Daily Dietary Allowance of protein for the average adult is 0.8 grams per kilogram of bodyweight. This is equivalent to 0.36 grams per pound of bodyweight. The recommended daily dietary allowance of protein for bodybuilders and athletes who want to increase their muscle mass is anywhere from 1.5 to 2.5 grams per pound of bodyweight. For example, a male bodybuilder who weighed 200 lbs, would want to consume approximately 400 to 450 grams of protein per day to increase his muscle mass. This of course, would also be correctly calculated with the proper carbohydrate and fat ratio. Depending of the desired goal, the percentage of protein, carbohydrate intake varies, although the fat intake should always ideally be maintained below 30%. High amounts of protein intake, are not harmful, and will not cause damage to the kidneys, in healthy individuals.

Some examples of recommended food items which are high in protein content and at the same time low in fat content are, some of the more common fish such as white bass, cod, haddock, red snapper, shrimp, scallops, smelt, tuna, perch, catfish; egg whites, turkey breasts, and of course, the ever common chicken breasts (both without skin). *Please refer to the nutrition sector for further protein suggestions.*

Proteins produce approximately 1,800 calories of energy per pound (4 calories per gram), which is the same amount provided by carbohydrates.

Insufficient protein in the diet may cause a lack of energy, possible stunted growth, lowered resistance to disease, and of course restricted muscle growth and strength. Protein deficiencies can also result in alterations in skin and hair pigmentation, nutritional skin dermatosis, fatty infiltration, cell deterioration, fibrosis of the liver, digestion deterioration, emotional agitation, depression, amino acid deficiencies and edema. A diet which is high in protein has also been proven beneficial for the average person who would like to lose weight, as protein can somewhat suppress the appetite cravings.

Another important dietary factor which can cause an athlete to become more susceptible to overtraining, is inadequate protein intake. Protein is a key component to retraining muscle and also providing sufficient amino acids to the amino acid group within the body. Protein is the most important macronutrient to athletes, and especially bodybuilders. Spreading protein consumption over approximately six meals throughout the day will avoid plateaus in increases of lean body mass, which will allow for optimal results of muscle gains.

If a diet is deficient in protein, intense training efforts, even with heavy weights will not result in muscle growth. Instead, in order to encourage the muscles to respond, amino acids must be present to aid in tissue repair, and also muscles have to be maximally stressed with weight resistance. If protein intake is inadequate, recuperation will also be affected, and is also a common reason for overtraining, however, most individuals often mistake overtraining to weight training.

How the Body Uses Proteins:

Proteins not only make up a large part of each cell in the body, but are also important in building, maintaining, and repairing tissues, such as bone cartilage, and muscle.

Chemical reactions are accelerated by proteins called enzymes, which every cell contains. Without these enzymes, the cells could not function, as certain proteins perform specific jobs. For example, the blood also contains proteins such as albumin and hemoglobin. Albumin helps maintain the body's fluid balance by keeping water in the blood, and hemoglobin carries oxygen from the lungs to the body tissues. Antibodies, are proteins in the blood which help protect the body from disease. Hormones, which are chemical substances which many are proteins, control processes such as growth, development, and reproduction.

As previously mentioned, the body acquires most of its energy from carbohydrates and fats. However, the body also uses proteins for energy when carbohydrates and fats cannot meet its energy needs. This should always be avoided, especially if the goal of building muscle mass is desired. In order to avoid this incidence, sufficient amounts of carbohydrates and fats should always be available for the body to burn, so that it does not have to resort to the protein stores. This is commonly what happens in an anorexia nervosa patient who is terribly "skinny", but not lean; as the body has used up all of the energy resources including protein for fuel, as the caloric intake is severely restricted. Therefore, muscle is also "eaten" away leaving a skeletal appearance to the body. Ideally, an adequate supply of all energy resources, especially protein; should be always available for the body, as it cannot store proteins for later use, instead it converts excess proteins into carbohydrates and fats. Therefore, if the body does not receive enough proteins from foods which are consumed, it will use protein from the cells of liver and muscle tissues, and if this continues, can possibly permanently cause damage to these tissues.

Once the proteins have been ingested, hydrochloric acid (which most people have in their stomachs), causes the protein molecules to thicken and clump together (coagulate). The stomach and intestines enzymes then break down the coagulated proteins into individual amino acids. These are then absorbed into the blood and are dispersed throughout the body allowing every cell to assemble the amino acids into the proteins it requires. This process is controlled by DNA, a substance which is in the nucleus of every cell. The DNA does not leave the nucleus to help make the proteins, this is done by RNA, which is a chemical cousin to DNA. RNA is present in both the nucleus and the cytoplasm, and is made in the nucleus of the cell, where protein manufacturing transpires.

DNA's contain "blueprints" for all the proteins which are made in a cell. Each gene contains a blueprint for a specific polypeptide which directs the order in which amino acids will be linked together to form proteins. Proteins are manufactured by initially starting in the nucleus, where an RNA copy of the DNA blueprint for the polypeptide chain is made. The RNA then leaves the nucleus and enters cytoplasm. This RNA, which is called the messenger RNA, then goes to the ribosomes which are the cell's centers of protein production. A ribosome passes on the messenger RNA which interprets the information coded on it. The messenger RNA then acts as a template (mold), to line up the amino acids in the exact order which is called for by the DNA of the genes. Eventually, one by one, the amino acids are linked together to form the polypeptide chain.

In most proteins which consist of more than one polypeptide chain, the chains are manufactured separately, then combined to make the protein. In most proteins which consist of more than one polypeptide chain, the chains are manufactured separately, and then combined to make the protein. The completed protein then starts to do its particular, individualized task. Some proteins are used inside the cell, and others such as hormones and digestive enzymes, are released from the cell to do their work.

Another type of RNA, which is referred to the transfer RNA, collects the amino acids in the cytoplasm and brings them to the messenger RNA ribosomes which are attached to the messenger RNA. For each kind of amino acid, there are specific transfer RNA molecules, which together with the correct amino acid, are brought together with the help of ATP and an enzyme.

During the production of a protein, a ribosome is attached to two adjacent coding segments of a messenger RNA molecule. Each coding segment is called a codon and consists of three nucleotides which specifies one amino acid. The correct transfer RNA, with its amino acid attached, line up on the first codon of the messenger RNA template. Then, after a second transfer RNA and its amino acid have lined up on the other codon, the two amino acids are linked together and the first transfer RNA is then set free to collect more amino acids.

The second transfer RNA holds the growing polypeptide chain to the ribosome which then moves on codon further down to the messenger RNA. The attached amino acid together with the appropriate transfer RNA, lines up on this codon. The amino acid is joined to the first two amino acids, and the second transfer DNA is set free. The ribosome then moves one position further and covers the next codon on the messenger RNA template. This continues until the ribosome has passed over the entire length of the messenger RNA step by step. The last codon on the messenger RNA does not code for an amino acid, instead, it signals that the chain is complete. The protein is complete when the finished polypeptide chain is released.

AMINO ACIDS:

Alanine	**Arginine**	**Asparagine**
Aspartic Acid	**Cysteine**	**Cystine**
Glutamate	**Glutamine**	**Glycine**
Histodine	**Hydroxyproline**	**Isoleucine**
Leucine	**Lysine**	**Methionine**
Ornithine	**Phenylalanine**	**Proline**
Serine	**Taurine**	**Threonine**
Tryptophan	**Tyrosine**	**Valine**

Amino acids are any one of a group of complex organic compounds of nitrogen, hydrogen, carbon and oxygen which combine in certain ways to form the proteins which make up living matter. Some amino acids contain sulfur. Unlike green plants and some microorganisms which produce all the amino acids they require, humans cannot produce all of the 20 amino acids which the body needs to build tissues. Humans require at least nine amino acids which can be obtained from protein foods such as eggs, meat, milk products and some vegetables. The body then breaks these foods down into amino acids, and then links the amino acids to form new proteins.

Amino acids provide another way for the body to ingest additional protein. Many athletes and bodybuilders will increase their usage several months before competition to protect lean body mass, as special amino acid formulations can prove to be beneficial during times of intense training and strict dieting.

Athletes who consume large quantities of protein, should also increase their water and calcium consumption as well. Ammonia is generated by protein metabolism, which is converted to urea, and excreted from the body in forms of sweat and urine. Drinking large amounts of water will allow the kidneys in eliminating these nitrogenous waste, and also dilute calcium salt which could result in kidney stones.

Leucine, Isoleucine and Valine are branched amino acids which are directly involved in building muscle tissue. They assist the muscles in synthesizing other amino acids to promote growth and repair, by carrying nitrogen.

Amino acids are made up of amino groups and certain organic acids, and all amino acids contain one or more groups of one nitrogen and two hydrogen atoms called amino groups. Some simple proteins may consist of only four different kinds of amino acids, however, most of the more complex proteins contain approximately 20 amino acids. Approximately 80 amino acids are found in nature, but only 20 are necessary for human metabolism or growth. Some of these amino acids are supplied by food and the others can be produced by the body. The amino acids which must be provided by food are called essential. Non-essential refers to those amino acids that the body can produce, but are not critically required in the diet. The essential nutrients include water, carbohydrates, linoleic acid (a lipid), eight amino acids, approximately 13 vitamins, and approximately 15 minerals. The human body can make many different types of protein. A single protein may consist of several hundred amino acid units which are linked together by chemical bonds. The order of the amino acids may also vary, producing different proteins; thus these different amino acid sequences determine the functions of the proteins. Some proteins contain all of the essential amino acids, therefore, they are called complete proteins. Milk, cheese, eggs and meat are examples of complete proteins. However, proteins which do not contain all of the essential amino acids are called incomplete proteins. Vegetables and grains are such examples.

Amino acids pass unchanged through the intestinal wall and portal vein into the blood, then through the liver into general circulation. Then, they are absorbed by the tissues according to the specific amino acid needed by that tissue to make its own protein. If these amino acids are not otherwise metabolized, they may be converted and excreted from the body in urea.

There are many forms of amino acids available such as in oral, elixir, intravenously, and injectable.

> ***Essential Amino Acids*:** These are the amino acids which are required for growth and development. The human body cannot produce these amino acids, they must be obtained from food.
>
> ***Semi-Essential Amino Acids*:** These are the amino acids that are sometimes made internally.
>
> ***Non-Essential Amino Acids:*** These are the amino acids which are manufactured within the body, synthesized from essential nutrients. The term "non-essential" merely identifies relative dependence on external sources.

These amino acids are classified as essential, semi-essential, and non-essential.

Essential	**Semi-Essential**	**Non-Essential**	
Isoleucine	Arginine	Alanine	Asparagine
Leucine	Histidine	Aspartic Acid	Cystine
Lysine		Cysteine	Glutamate
Methionine		Glutamine	Glycine
Phenylalanine		Hydroxyproline	Ornithine
Threonine		Proline	Serine
Tryptophan		Taurine	Tyrosine
Valine			

A deficiency in a particular amino acid will result in the following:

Alanine:	Protein decreased.
Arginine:	Impotency, sterility, decreased sperm mobility and formation, immunity and protein decreased, disordered carbohydrate metabolism and delayed sexual maturation.
Aspartic Acid:	Protein decreased.
Asparagine:	Protein decreased.
Cysteine:	Immunity decreased, deterioration of hair and fingernail growth, premature aging and protein decreased.
Cystine:	Protein decreased.
Glutamate:	Protein decreased.
Glutamine:	Decreased I.Q., convulsions, deterioration of alertness, alcohol cravings, retardation, de creased co-ordination, and protein decreased.
Glycine:	Deterioration of growth, liver deterioration, and protein decreased.
Histidine:	Protein decreased, overstimulation, deterioration of myelin sheaths around nerves, hearing deterioration, and diminished sexual arousal.
Hydroxyproline:	Protein decreased.
Isoleucine:	Decreased hemoglobin formation, protein decreased.
Leucine:	Protein decreased.

Lysine:	Fatigue, easily exhausted, nausea, dizziness, deterioration of appetite, decrease in weight, emotional agitation, mental health deterioration, decreased antibody formation, decreased immunity, slow growth, anemia, enzyme deterioration, reproductive systems deterioration, pneumonia, acidosis, blood-shot eyes, decreased Vitamin BT formation, and protein decreased.
Methionine:	Baldness, liver deterioration, toxemia of pregnancy, rheumatic fever, muscles paralyzation, decreased cysteine and cystine production, selenium and protein decreased.
Phenylalanine:	"Nerves", clouded thought, depression, emotional agitation, decreased alertness, sexual interest, insulin, skin melanin, memory and protein decreased, blood-shot eyes, cataracts, increased appetite, depression, behavioral changes, decreased tyrosine formation.
Proline:	Protein decreased.
Serine:	Protein decreased.
Taruine:	Bile salts formation deterioration, decreased cholesterol solubility, protein and vision decreased, epilepsy, decreased potassium in the heart, decreased osmotic control of calcium and potassium in the heart.
Threonine:	Emotional agitation, mental health and digestion deterioration, intestinal malfunctions, increased liver fat, deterioration of nutrient absorption, protein decreased.

Tryptophan:	Sterility, testicle deterioration, decrease in weight, hair decreased, dry skin, blood-shot eyes, slow growth, deterioration of Vitamin B3b production, digestion upsets, decreased clearance of blood clots, nervousness, lack of sleep, memory decreased, aggression, emotional agitation and emotional deterioration, compulsion, hallucinations, depression, schizophrenia, and protein decreased.
Tyrosine:	Paleness and decreased skin melanin, protein decreased.
Valine:	Decreased co-ordination, deterioration of muscle function and mental health, lack of sleep, nervousness, skin hypersensitivity, protein decreased.

WATER:

Water is also included as a macronutrient source. Every living organism consists mostly of water, the human muscles are comprised of over 70% water.

All living things require alot of water to maintain normal life processes, and also must maintain its water supply near normal, or death will occur. Humans can live without food for more than two months, but cannot live for more than a week without water. If the body loses more than 20% of its normal water content, a painful death will occur. Water is the basis of all the bodily fluids including digestive juices, blood, urine, lymph and perspiration. It is involved in nearly every body function including absorption, digestion, circulation and lubrication. Water is also an essential transport mechanism for several nutrients such as vitamins, minerals and even carbohydrates. It serves an important role in all cellular activity.

A diet deficient in water results in thirst, and dehydration. Humans must take in about 2 1/2 quarts (2.4 L) of water daily. This can be in the form of beverages or by water in food. A higher protein intake requires an increased amount of water intake. Overtraining can result if no, or little water is ingested. If the water intake is too low, the ability to transport nutrients can become compromised, resulting in a decrease of muscle fullness, and a toxic buildup of ammonia, urea, uric acid, and other substances, which would begin to accumulate in the body. In fact, if dehydration does occur, constipation may result as water is responsible for moving food through the intestinal track. Also, increased amounts of water should be taken to avoid dehydration when increased activity results in sweating. Sweating is a method which the body utilizes to cool itself down, and in the process, water is lost and requires to be replenished. Water also regulates the body's temperature. However, more than 1 1/2 gallons of water ingested within an hour can be dangerous!

To maintain normal, adequate hydration, a simple calculation of bodyweight, multiplied by .55 will equal the amount of water an individual should drink in ounces on a daily basis. For example, an individual who weighed 200 lbs, should drink 110 oz (200 x .55) of water every day. If more strenuous activities which involve more sweating, such as long-distance running or exercising in extreme heat, the water amount should be increased by multiplying the bodyweight by .66.

How the Body Uses Water:

Watery solutions help dissolve nutrients and carry them to all parts of an organism. Through chemical reactions, the organism can turn nutrients into energy, or into materials it requires to grow or to repair itself. These chemical reactions can only take place in a watery solution. Water is also important for the skin texture and organs to properly function. Water is also necessary to transport waste products, in urine and feces. It can also aid in flushing water-retaining sodium from the system.

Many waters today are bottled to provide better taste, and are actually healthier, as many of the harsh chemicals are filtered out. Water can be acquired from many several sources, and available in several various ways:

Artesian Water:	Water which is drawn from a well, which taps a confined aquifer.
Club Soda:	Is carbonated water with added minerals, including sodium.
Distilled, Condensed, Purified, Deionized, or Reverse Osmosis:	Has been modified to remove minerals. Ingestion of solely distilled water will deprive the body of essential minerals which are usually found in water. Therefore, this type of water intake should be kept to a minimum, but used strictly a week or two before a competition, to avoid intake of unwanted sodium and iron levels.
Ground Water:	Water which is derived from a body of water that is not in contact with any surface water.
Mineral Water:	Water which is derived from an underground source which contains at least 250 parts per million of dissolved solids. Ratings for mineral content are 250 to 500 is considered to be water with a low mineral content, while water with a range greater than 1500, is considered to be high.
Municipal Water:	Water which is derived from town or city water pipes.
Natural:	Has not been modified by either addition or deletion of minerals.
Seltzer:	Is also carbonated water, which sometimes contains minerals, but not with added sodium.
Sparkling:	Is naturally carbonated water.
Spring:	Is actual water which is derived from an under-ground formation from water flows to the

surface of the earth naturally. This water is unmodified by the addition or elimination of minerals and iron. This water has a pleasant taste, and is the most common form of bottled water available.

Sterile Water: All micro-organisms have been removed as per U.S. Pharmacopoeia regulations.

THE FOLLOWING IS A SIMPLIFIED BREAKDOWN OF VITAMIN GROUPS:

Vitamin A Complex

- Provitamin A
- Vitamin A
    - Vitamin A1
    - Vitamin A2
    - Vitamin A Acetate
    - Vitamin A Acid
    - Vitamin A Aldehyde
    - Vitamin A Epoxide
    - Vitamin A Palmitate
    - Monoepoxyvitamin A
    - Neovitamin A

Vitamin B Complex

- Vitamin B
- Vitamin B1
- Vitamin B2
- Vitamin B3
- Vitamin B4
- Vitamin B5
- Vitamin B6
- Vitamin B7
- Vitamin B8
- Vitamin B9 *(commonly referred to as Folic Acid)*
- Vitamin B10
- Vitamin B11
- Vitamin B12 *(only vitamin which contains essential mineral elements.)*
- Vitamin B13
- Vitamin B14
- Vitamin B15
- Vitamin B16
- Vitamin B17

Sub-Vitamin B Complex

Vitamin BC

Vitamin BH

Vitamin BP

Provitamin BP

Vitamin BT

Vitamin BW

Vitamin BX

Vitamin C

Antivitamin C

Vitamin C

Vitamin C2

Vitamin C3

Vitamin D Complex
- Vitamin D1
- Vitamin D2
- Vitamin D3
- Vitamin D4
- Vitamin D5
- Vitamin DC
- Vitamin DM

Vitamin E Complex
- Alpha-Vitamin E
- Beta-Vitamin E
- Gamma-Vitamin E

Delta-Vitamin E
Epsilon-Vitamin E
Zeta1-Vitamin E
Zeta 2-Vitamin E
Eta-Vitamin E
Vitamin E2

Vitamin F Complex
Provitamin F
Vitamin F

Vitamin H Complex
Vitamin H1
Vitamin H3

Vitamin I

Vitamin J

Vitamin K Complex
Vitamin K1
Vitamin K2
Vitamin K3
Vitamin K4
Vitamin K5
Vitamin K6
Vitamin K7
Vitamin K8
Vitamin K9
Vitamin K-S(II)

Vitamin L Complex
Vitamin L1
Vitamin L2

Vitamin Mi

Vitamin MK Complex
Vitamin MK1

Vitamin MK2
Vitamin MK3
Vitamin MK4
Vitamin MK5
Vitamin MK6
Vitamin MK7
Vitamin MK8
Vitamin MK9
Vitamin MK10

Vitamin N

Vitamin P Complex
Vitamin P1
Vitamin P1 Complex
Vitamin P2
Vitamin P3
Vitamin P4

Vitamin Q Complex
Vitamin Q
Vitamin Q1
Vitamin Q2
Vitamin Q3
Vitamin Q4
Vitamin Q5
Vitamin Q6
Vitamin Q7
Vitamin Q8
Vitamin Q9
Vitamin Q10

Vitamin T Complex

Vitamin U

Vitamin U Chick Factor

Vitamin V

Vitamin W

Vitamin X

Vitamin Y.

Various Vitamin Availabilities:

Vitamins and minerals are the micronutrients, which have no caloric or energy value, but are absolutely necessary for good health. Most essential micronutrients are not manufactured within the human body, and must be acquired from food sources, or supplements.

Vitamins: Are complex organic molecules which are essential for biochemical transformations. Vitamins can sometimes fulfill hormone-like functions and aid in the protection of cell membranes. Vitamins can be destroyed by cooking.

Minerals: Are naturally occurring inorganic elements which perform structural and catalytic roles, which include the activation of enzymes and hormones. Certain minerals (such as silicon and fluoride), are nutritionally essential, but not enough research has been performed on their biochemical functions to establish daily requirements. Minerals are not destroyed during cooking.

Accessory Nutrients: There are two types of Accessory Nutrients:

Essential: Are food compounds which have been clinically proven to provide preventive or therapeutic purposes, although they do not provide any demonstrated role in metabolism.

This group also includes PABA and bioflavonoids.

Nonessential: Employs a critical metabolic role. This group includes choline, inositol, carnitine, lipoic acid etc.

The difference between essential and nonessential nutrients is decided upon the basis of bioavailability. Essential nutrients cannot be manufactured by the body itself, although they are absolutely indispensable to human life. The essential nutrients include water, carbohydrates, linoleic acid (a lipid), eight amino acids (plus an additional one for infants), at least thirteen vitamins, and at least fifteen minerals. The term "nonessential" is simply an identifying label for relative dependence on external sources. Nonessential nutrients are manufactured within our bodies, which are synthesized from essential nutrients. For example, a particular amino acid can produce niacin.

Deficiencies in various minerals can result in bone disease, problems with the organs and the nervous system. Consuming a large variety of foods will aid in the accumulation of the essential vitamins and minerals. However, most of these are supplemented by most individuals; and athletes and bodybuilders who often have restricted diet regimes.

If used sensibly, vitamins and minerals can help accelerate recovery time from exercise. Minerals which are the nutrients that are found in organic and inorganic combinations, and are required in greater amounts than vitamins. They are very important to bodybuilders who especially avoid dairy products. A regime which includes a well rounded multi-vitamin, an additional multi-mineral, extra Vitamin C and E, and Creatine Monohydrate can benefit muscles in maintaining hydration, and increasing endurance. After a duration of approximately four months, evaluation of progress will reveal if further additions are required.

Vitamins are available in array of different forms. However, the most popular forms include those of the tablet and capsule variety. Recently, a new method of oral absorbency vitamins has been developed which is truly a renovation in the "pill taking" community.

Oral absorption works by micro-sized beads or droplets of a drug or a nutrient which are taken into the body through the mouth or nose tissue. This proves to be extremely advantageous as the blood capillaries are very close to the surface in these areas, and therefore, the body can readily absorb the nutrients or drugs directly into the bloodstream, which eliminates the normal passages which usual pills have to take. When a medicine or nutrient is sprayed directly into the mouth, a microfine mist flows from the mouth area, directly to the heart. When this leaves the heart, the drug or nutrient should be totally dispensed throughout the body in a matter of *minutes!!!* So, in other words, the effects of these medications or nutrients is almost immediate, and this also eliminate the highs and lows which can be experienced with regular vitamin pills. When a pill begins to dissolve, too much nutrient may be released into the system all at once, therefore, as time progresses, the body experiences a "low" when there is too little nutrient available. If the tablet dissolves too quickly, many possible nutrients may be eliminated in the urine during the high. Spray vitamins are able to maintain the body's energy level and immune systems at a maximum all day, and is 100% more efficient for use of vitamins as opposed to that of a tablet or capsule form. Studies have confirmed that when a drug is taken sublingually, it is released at a controlled rate which allows for full absorption. This is also a reason why heart medication (such as Nitroglycerin) which needs to act quickly, is available in this form.

Science has also discovered that oral or sublingual (underneath the tongue) is the preferred dosage method for many drugs, which eliminates the problem of swallowing large quantities of sometimes, large pills.

MINERALS:

Aluminum	**Antimony**	**Arsenic**
Barium	**Beryllium**	**Boron**
Bromine	**Cadmium**	**Calcium**
Cesium	**Chlorine**	**Cobalt**
Chromium (Trivalent)	**Chromium (Hexavalent)**	**Copper**
Fluorine	**Germanium**	**Gold**
Iodine 131	**Iron**	**Lead**
Lithium	**Magnesium**	**Manganese**
Mercury	**Molybdenum**	**Nickel**

Phosphorus	**Potassium**	**Rubidium**
Selenium	**Silicon**	**Silver**
Sodium	**Strontium 90**	**Sulfur**
Tin	**Titanium**	**Tungsten**
Vanadium	**Zinc**	

Best Time To Take Minerals and Vitamins:

According to most experts, the proper time to take minerals and vitamins is along with food, usually at mealtimes. This allows the minerals and vitamins to be absorbed with the food, which provides the greatest benefits. Mealtime can span from a few minutes before a meal, up to a half an hour afterwards. However, it is recommended that minerals and vitamins be taken immediately after eating, spread out over the day, with meals. This will provide the highest level of vitamins in the system over the longest period of time. Oil soluble vitamins should be taken before meals, and water soluble vitamins should be taken afterwards. Oil soluble vitamins include Vitamins A, D, E, & K, and Water Soluble Vitamins include Vitamin C and B1. Spray vitamins can be taken at any time, anywhere, with or without food!

Do Larger Vitamin Doses Increase Health?:

As often associated with the administration of anabolic steroids, "more is not better" can also be applied with the intake of vitamin supplementation. Large doses of vitamins can be harmful, and if taken in excess amounts, can result in vitamin overdose, toxicity and side effects. Taking large amounts of vitamins is also a waste of money. Vitamins, similar to any substance when taken in large amounts, can cause as many problems as they solve. Again, depending on individual goals, vitamin intake varies, but usually a good multi-vit benefits everyone from the average individual up to the great athlete, and bodybuilder. Differences will also vary in opinions on what is deemed necessary and what is not for specific health issues. Common sense and good judgment strongly applies, as, vitamin supplements are replacing those vitamins deficiencies which lack from a dietary intake. Hence, a proper diet should contain all of the vitamins and minerals required.

ANTIOXIDANTS:

Antioxidants operate at different levels, removing the free radicals as they are produced by different chemical reactions which are constantly occurring in the body. Antioxidants and free radicals seem to be the latest buzz words in the health industry today, and can be found displayed in many health and fitness stores.

All atoms contain a nucleus and electrons which circulate around the central body. Atoms connect to each other to form molecules. This occurs by sharing or exchanging their electrons; and these shared electrons are locked into a stable compound, which are difficult to break down. However, in some compounds, there is what is referred to as a "free radical", which is actually an electron which is not held firmly within the compound, therefore, is free to break away and attach to another compound or body tissue.

Free radicals are formed as the result of everyday metabolism in the body, as it converts food into useful chemical molecule which the body needs for energy and rebuilding. Free radicals however, are also formed by tissue damage, such as excessive sunlight, cigarette smoke, toxic substances in the environment and radiation. The body does possess a number of defenses against these free radicals, however, they may become overwhelmed in times of stress, or as age progresses, and antioxidant enzyme activity becomes decreased.

Antioxidants, are able to capture these free radicals before they attach to vital tissues, and are able reduce the potential damage which may occur. Some of the most studied vitamins are the beta-carotene (a form of Vitamin A), Vitamin E, and Vitamin C. A combination of antioxidants can provide protection which a single vitamin is unable to.

There now is vitamins, anti-oxidants, appetite suppressants, and amino acids available in spray-mists, which are taken orally, as previously described. These are administrated by pumping just 2 short quick sprays into the back of the mouth, approximately four times a day. Due to the degree of simplicity and convenience which is associated with these products, most tablet and capsule forms will become obsolete. Several physicians use these oral methods, and prescribe them routinely. Dr. P. G. Smith reports on one of these sprays, called *Pycnogenol.*

> "I have been using *Pycnogenol** for approximately three months, and have seen amazing results both in my patients and myself. From a personal experience, I have been a Type II Diabetic for the last few years, and just recently on insulin. For the last few years I have been aware of protein in my urine, indicative of kidney damage. Two months ago, I went to an endocrinologist, had an urinalysis and was told that I was lucky I had no protein in my urine, hence no kidney damage!"
>
> -Dr. Paul G. Smith
> Las Vegas, NV
> (702)877-1200.

As these products are so new, there are of course no circumstantial long term studies available as of yet, however, the entity of correcting kidney and liver damage has been well sought by many, especially steroid users who have acquired damage due to heavy or prolonged cycles. Once liver or kidney damage is evident, dialysis is a very probable course of treatment, and thereafter, usually becomes terminal.

**Pycnogenol: Is a concentrate of a special class of water-soluble bioflavonoids that are almost instantly bioavailable in the human body. It also restores equilibrium in capillary circulation, helps restore collagen, and it is the most powerful natural free radical scavenger known.*

THE POWER OF NUTRITION

Alot of emphasis and importance seems to be placed on the proper dosage, administration, and cycling of steroids, as well as proper methods of exercises, recuperation periods, and general aerobic activity. Although each of these areas employ a part of several athletes and bodybuilders curriculums, the truth of the matter is, that proper nutrition is the basis of all success in an athletic endeavor.

The power of nutrition is so valuable, that it is actually the missing link which most athletes and bodybuilders appear to ignore, presumably, due to it's simplicity. Many look to miracle supplements, steroidal compounds, and to certain training regimes, to enhance their potential athletic gains. However, to a certain extent, these will help improve performance, but it is the nutrition factor, which will make or break an athlete or bodybuilder. Similar to anabolic steroids and the combination of stacking, many different diet regimes exist, each producing different results for each participating individual. However, dedication, perseverance, and consistency, will determine the outcome of any successful endeavor, especially those of an athletic nature.

To begin with, proper nutrition can be optimized by spreading calories in a meal evenly throughout the day. Smaller portions of meals at frequent intervals, approximately 5 or 6, consumed 2 to 3 hours apart each day is ideal. Some of these meals can be "mock" meals meaning that they are of a supplemental nature such as a protein/carbohydrate shake, protein bar, etc. Supplemental meals can replace actual meals when it is not convenient to have a "real" meal. These are an excellent way to continue consuming calories throughout the day, and are considered part of the days total caloric intake.

Each meal should include one source of protein and one or two sources of fibrous carbohydrates. This combination of foods provides maximum nutritional benefits as consuming carbohydrates alone allows for a sudden burst of energy which soon diminishes. Protein and fiber however slow down the digestion of the carbohydrates which allows for more consistent energy levels and increased endurance.

Dietary fats can be obtained through a variety of foods. The easiest method of adding fat to a diet is by adding a bit of yolk with egg whites, or by consuming a total of 1 to 3 tablespoons of flaxseed, safflower, linseed, sunflower, or Primrose Evening Oil, divided up throughout the day. This practice will fulfill both the required polyunsaturated fats, and the daily requirement of essential fatty acids at the same interval. However, all meats including chicken and turkey, contain a low fat content, which will add up by the end of the day's total consumption.

It is also beneficial to weigh and portion each meal (in the raw form, before it is cooked). A meal which consists strictly of protein or carbohydrates, is not considered to be a balanced meal. It is important to include proper portions of each, everytime food is consumed. Keeping track of all consumed foods, calories, supplements, etc., will aid in helping to discover which combination produces the best results for individualized goals. Shortly, a feasible combination which provides the greatest results will soon develop, and deletion of the items which are not producing desirable results can transpire.

The following is a general listing of the more popular foods which are considered to be high in evaluation of their chosen heading. These foods are just a brief basic guideline to illustrate how a proper diet plan can be achieved, as there are definitely more food choices which are available and can be implemented into a diet regime. If proper nutrition is not established, nothing else will matter, training, steroid cycles etc., will all be a waste of effort, and money.

The following lists are all based on 100 gram sized portions. One may increase or decrease accordingly by either multiplying or dividing these amounts.

Protein:

FOOD ITEM	GRAMS OF PROTEIN	FAT CONTENT	TOTAL CALORIES
Canned Tuna	20.3	0.5	86
Chicken Breast (without skin)	23.4	1.9	117
Turkey Breast (without skin)	24.6	1.2	116
Egg Whites	10.9	0	51
Round Steak (all visible fat trimmed)	21.6	4.7	135
Catfish	17.6	3.1	103
Cod	17.6	0.3	78
Haddock	18.3	0.1	79
Halibut	20.9	1.2	100
Pollock	20.4	0.9	95
Red Snapper	19.8	0.9	93
Scallops	15.3	0.2	81
Shrimp	18.1	0.8	91
Tuna (not canned)	25.2	4.1	145

These selections of protein are high in protein value, while maintaining a desired low fat percentage. *Please refer to the macronutrient section for further information on protein.*

Fibrous Carbohydrates:

FOOD ITEM	GRAMS OF CARBS.	FAT	CALORIES
Fresh Broccoli	5.9	0.3	32
Frozen Broccoli	5.2	0.3	29
Fresh Cauliflower	5.2	0.2	27
Frozen Cauliflower	4.3	0.2	22
Mushrooms	4.4	0.3	28
Cucumbers	3.4	0.1	15
Carrots	9.7	0.2	42
Green Peppers	4.8	0.2	22

Starchy Carbohydrates:

FOOD ITEM	GRAMS OF CARBS.	FAT	CALORIES
Oatmeal	68.2	7.4	390
Frozen Peas	12.8	0.3	73
White Potatoes	8.5	0.1	76
Uncooked Brown Rice	77.4	1.9	360
Uncooked White Rice	80.4	0.4	363
Sweet Potatoes	26.3	0.4	114
Yams	23.2	0.2	101
Tomatoes	4.7	0.2	22

These selections of carbohydrates also provide optimal choices of this particular macronutrient. *For further information on carbohydrates, please refer to the macronutrient section.*

Fatty Acid Composition of Oils and Fats:

Source	*Polyunsat. %*	*Monounsat. %*	*Saturated %*
Beef fat	2	44	54
Butter	4	37	59
Chicken fat	27	29	44
Coconut oil	2	6	92
Corn oil	60	26	14
Egg yolk	14	51	35
Olive oil	15	69	16
Palm oil	10	37	53
Peanut oil	35	45	20
Safflower oil	78	11	11
Soybean oil	58	15	15
Sunflower oil	70	12	12

QUICK CALCULATION GUIDE TO DETERMINE PROPER MACRONUTRIENT INTAKE AMOUNTS:

To arrive at the proper ratio for the amount of protein, carbohydrate, calories, water, and fat content of a diet, follow these simple calculations:

Carbohydrates Calories which do not come from either protein, dietary fats, or supplements should come from natural complex carbohydrates. To achieve this amount, simply add the total amount of required protein and fat which should be consumed, and subtract this amount from the total daily calories. The remaining amount will indicate the amount of carbohydrates which should be consumed. For example, a 200 lb bodybuilder who's protein requirement was 500 grams, (2000 calories) and fat requirement was 166.67 grams (1500 calories), 2000 + 1500 = 3500 calories. Total daily calories for this individual is 7500. So, 7500 - 3500 = 4000. The total carbohydrate consumption in this example should be approximately 4000 calories of the daily total caloric intake.

Energy (Calories): To determine how many calories are required on a daily basis, first figure out how many calories are typically consumed in an average day. For a week, take note of all the food ingested, weigh it and write down each calorie content. Then at the end of the week, take each day's totals, and divide by 7 (days). For example, Monday 1800, Tuesday 2300, Wednesday 2350, Thursday, 2000, Friday, 2600, Saturday 3000, Sunday 1800 = 15,850 total calories consumed in one week. 15,850 calories divided by 7 days = 2265. This amount will indicate what an individual's average calorie consumption is on a daily basis. Obtaining bodyweight counts every morning before breakfast and documenting these amounts along with total calories per day, will aid in calculating desired caloric goal intakes. To achieve weight and mass increases, and an average gain of 1 1/2 pounds per 100 pounds of bodyweight each week, is not achieved, consume an additional 300 to 500 calories. Increase calories until desired goal weight is reached. As the bodyweight increases, the caloric intake needs to also increase to support the additional pounds and to continue to grow. These calculations will work also for those individuals who wish to lose bodyweight, however, simply reverse the process from increasing, to decreasing.

Fats: Calories from dietary fats should total ideally around 20%, but no more than 30% of total dietary intake. To help determine the maximum number of calories which should be consumed from dietary fats, take the number of daily calories and multiply this by 0.20 or (whatever your chosen amount is) and this will give you your maximum amount of fat calories for the day. For example, a muscle building diet regime may consist of 7500 calories, so 7500 x .20 = 1500 which equals 1500 calories of dietary fat, or 1500 divided by 9 (fat has nine calories per gram) = 166.67 grams of fat.

Protein: For protein consumption take the bodyweight and multiply it by how many grams of protein desired to be consumed. This can vary from 1 gram up to 2.5 grams and possibly even higher. For example, a bodybuilder who weighed 200 lbs who wished to build muscle mass may wish to consume 2.5 grams of protein. So, 200 lbs x 2.5 = 500 grams of total protein, or 500 multiplied by 4 (protein has 4 calories per gram) = 2000 calories of required protein consumption per day, to acquire this individual's potential muscle building goal.

Water: To stay adequately hydrated, take the bodyweight and multiply it by .55 - which is approximately how much water which should be drank in ounces every day. For example, a bodyweight of 200 lbs; should drink 110 oz (200 x .55) of water every day. If exercising in extreme heat or in intense training, multiply the bodyweight by .66.

GLOSSARY

GLOSSARY OF ATHLETIC, MEDICAL, AND ASSOCIATED SLANG DEFINITIONS:

ABDUCTOR: A part of the body which is pulled by a muscle from its normal position by the trunk or main axis. For example, the deltoid muscle located in the shoulder is an abductor which raises the arm outward and upward.

ABSCESS: Refers to a collection of pus in the tissues of some part of the body. This sometimes is common in an injection site where an abscess results from an infection, which usually produces a painful sore, which often is accompanied by swelling or inflammation.

ABSORPTION: The process by which nutrients, or chemical substances enter the bloodstream for use by the body by passing through the intestines.

ACCELERATE: Refers to causing anything in process to move faster or speed up. For example, accelerating metabolism, can be achieved by performing an aerobic exercise upon rising, before eating breakfast.

ACTH: Is an abbreviation of the chemical substance Adrenocorticotropic Hormone. The pituitary gland which is a pea-sized organ which lies at the base of the brain, is where this hormone is produced, stored and released into the blood. ACTH is necessary for the function and normal growth of the adrenal glands, which are two organs that are located on the top of the kidneys. ACTH stimulates the adrenal glands to secrete various hormones, including a group called glucocorticoids, which regulate the use of digested food and help the body adjust to stress. Normally, the pituitary releases high levels of ACTH in the morning, and low levels at night. Mental or physical stress or disruption of normal sleeping habits can easily change this pattern. Physicians use ACTH in the treatment of inflammation and certain illnesses. ACTH used for medical purposes is obtained either from the pituitary glands of animals, or synthetically.

ADDUCTION: Refers to the movement of a limb toward the body, such as returning an extended arm, back to a resting position, such as alongside the body.

ADP: Is an abbreviation for Adenosine Diphosphate, which is an important cellular metabolite involved with energy exchange within the cell. The chemical energy is then conserved in a cell by the phosphorylation of ADP to ATP, mainly in the mitochondria, as a high energy phosphate bond. ADP with CP combined, forms ATP (Adenosine Triphosphate), which is a useable fuel for the contractions of muscles.

ADRENAL STEROIDS: The outer layer (cortex) of the adrenal gland produces cortisol, corticosterone and small amounts of cortisone. These steroids help regulate protein and carbohydrate metabolism. Physicians use adrenal steroids to reduce inflammation (swelling and redness), and to provide treatment for allergies, arthritis, and other diseases. An individual may die unless they are continually treated with steroids; if the adrenal glands are surgically removed.

AEROBIC: This refers to a system of exercises based on a correlation of oxygen consumption and physical fitness. This is designed to promote the supply and use of oxygen by the body. Aerobics are very beneficial for the desired loss of body weight, as this activity speeds up the body's metabolism, which in turn, accelerates the body's ability to consume calories. Recommendations for aerobic activity vary, depending on the reason for activity. For example, if the reason for participation in aerobic activity was for the maintenance of health and fitness, it is recommended that the activity period be performed at least three times a week, at 30 - 45 minute intervals. However, for bodyfat loss purposes, it is recommended daily for at least 30 - 45 minutes in the morning, and then again in the evening. Aerobic activity is also very beneficial for cardiovascular and a general state of well-being.

AGONIST: Is a muscle which is directly involved in contraction, therefore, is primarily responsible for movement of a body part.

ALDOSTERONE: Is a steroid hormone produced by the adrenal cortex, which is responsible for the regulation or electrolyte balance. Aldosterone increases the kidney's reabsorption of sodium, and excretion of potassium.

ALOPECIA: (male pattern) refers to hair loss which usually begins in the frontal area, and proceeds until usually only a horseshoe area of hair remains in the back and temples. The presence of the androgenic hormone testosterone is usually what the loss is dependent upon.

ALPHA ALKYLATED 17: This refers to the addition of an alkyl substitute on the 17 carbon position or a C-17 position, of the steroid molecule. This was discovered to greatly increase the life of the oral steroid in the body. Most oral steroid combinations without this adjustment, would be left inactive after first pass through the liver. Toxicity is the highest of any steroids, however, this adjustment makes oral steroids much more effective.

AMENORRHEA: Refers to the absence or abnormal discontinuation of the menstrual cycle in females. This may be a temporary, or a permanent condition. Amenorrhea is a common virilization side effect sometimes experienced from the use of certain steroidal compounds.

AMINO ACIDS: Any one of a group of complex organic compounds of nitrogen, hydrogen, carbon and oxygen, which combine in certain ways to form the proteins which make up living matter. Some amino acids contain sulfur. Unlike green plants and some microorganisms which make all the amino acids they require, humans cannot produce all of the 20 amino acids that their bodies require to build tissues. Humans need at least nine amino acids which can be obtained from protein foods such as eggs, meat, milk products and some vegetables. The body then breaks these foods down into amino acids, and then it links the amino acids to form new proteins. Amino acids are made up of amino groups and certain organic acids, and all amino acids contain one or more groups of one nitrogen and two hydrogen atoms called amino groups. Some simple proteins may consist of only four different kinds of amino acids, however, most of the more complex proteins contain approximately 20 amino acids. The human body can make many different types of protein. A single protein may consist of several hundred amino acid units which are linked together by chemical bonds. The order of the amino acids may also vary, producing different proteins; thus these different amino acid sequences determine the functions of the proteins. There are many forms of amino acids available such as in oral, elixir, intravenously, and injectable.

AMPHETAMINES: Is one of several drugs which increase physical and mental activity, decrease appetite, and prevent sleep. Many users can become psychologically dependent on amphetamines and some scientists believe that these drugs can also be addictive. Most individuals use amphetamines for energy or pleasure. These drugs can be taken orally, through injection or by sniffing.

AMPULE: Is a small glass container which is sealed and the contained liquid is sterilized. Most ampule lids must be broken off, and are usually intended for singular usage.

ANABOLIC: This refers to the promoting of anabolism; the actual building of tissues, mainly muscles, which may occur through synthetic chemical reactions in metabolism, or by constructive means.

ANABOLIC STEROIDS: Is defined as any of a group of synthetic hormones which increase the size and strength of muscles, that are often used by athletes during training. Testosterone is a hormone that occurs naturally in the body and controls many functions, one of which, is the promoting of anabolism. Steroids copy this natural occurring event and have the ability to do so at an accelerated rate. There are two classifications which anabolic steroids can be divided into; anabolic and androgenic. Anabolic or androgenic features are determined to what degree it is effected, by the type and concentration of androgen receptors found within an organ or tissue. Anabolic steroids also inhibit the amount of cortisol which is a catabolic hormone that is considered also to aid in muscle growth. Both types, anabolic and androgenic steroids are considered to be advantageous, as anabolic steroids are not totally separated between the two. For example, Deca-Durabolin can give both anabolic and androgenic results. So, unfortunately, dramatic gains in muscle size and strength is not usually obtained without having also obtaining undesirable side effects. Females desire anabolic effects as most do not enjoy the androgenic effects such as hirsuitism and the deepening of their voices. Males on the other hand, do not seem to notice, or even mind, as it actually provides more to their "masculinity".

ANABOLISM: Refers to the production of complex compounds by combining simpler molecules. During anabolism, cells combine amino acids to form structural and functional proteins. The body repairs and replaces tissues with structural proteins, and functional proteins perform specific tasks which include enzymes that speed up chemical reactions;

antibodies which fight disease, and many hormones, which regulate various body processes. During anabolism, the cells convert glucose and fatty acids to energy storage compounds. The cells in the liver and the muscles combine molecules of glucose to form a storage compound called glycogen. To form body fat, the cells in the body's fatty (adipose) tissues combine fatty acids with glycerol. By a complex series of reactions, the excess glucose and amino acids can also be converted into body fat. Once anabolic steroids are in the blood, they bind to androgen receptor sites which enter the cell, much like the endogenous hormone would, and then alter the function of that cell. After changes in DNA and RNA patterns, there is an increased rate of protein synthesis. One belief is that this increase of protein synthesis is thought to occur simultaneous to increased nitrogen retention; and another belief is that it is secondary. Retention of nitrogen is actually a sign that muscle tissue is being deposited.

ANALGESICS: Relieve pain without diminishing other senses, or causing unconsciousness. For example, an analgesic may relieve a toothache, but will not eliminate the sensation of feeling hot or cold, or from being able to taste food. There are two types of analgesics: Narcotics and Nonnarcotics. Narcotics often produce drowsiness, and often a feeling of well-being, and are obtainable through a physician, while Nonnarcotics are usually less "potent", and can be obtained off the shelf (OTC), at a local drug or grocery store.

ANDROGENIC: This refers to a classification of Testosterone which is responsible for male secondary sexual characteristics; development of the male sex organs, sex drive, body hair and the deepening of the voice. Androgenic effects are sometimes favored as there is an increase in aggressiveness, strength and a high retention of glycogen. Androgenic steroids result in favorable size and strength gains, but in the long run, also produce many undesirable side effects. This alone often warrants caution to avoid androgenic steroids as much as possible.

ANEMIA: Is a condition in which there is a deficiency of hemoglobin in red blood cells, or sometimes the red blood cells are abnormal in size; or both.

ANTAGONIST: Is a muscle which counteracts the agonist, therefore, relaxes when the agonist muscle contracts.

ANTERISERUMS: These are similar to vaccines and globulins, as they also prevent certain infectious diseases. However, unlike vaccines, these drugs contain antibodies rather than substances which cause the body to produce antibodies. Antiserums only provide temporary protection to prevent infection, as they are able to act more quickly than vaccines. This drug is often prescribed by a physician after an individual has been exposed to an infectious disease, and is not vaccinated.

ANTI-ANXIETY DRUGS: Refers to substances which reduce tension and worry by altering the nervous system. Examples of such include tranquilizers, sedatives, and alcohol.

ANTIBODIES: These are proteins which are found in the blood to combat disease.

ANTI-CATABOLISM: Is basically trying to find a way of slowing down the breakdown of protein in the body, thus altering the body's protein cycle. This is desirable as this would enable the muscle cells to have a chance to grow bigger and stronger. There are many different ways of anti-catabolism including the counter regulatory hormone, cortisol. Researchers have been performing studies on reducing cortisol levels which has had a major effect on protein retention. Weight-lifting or training causes cortisol levels to rise, which increases muscle catabolism (the breaking down of muscle tissue in response to exercise).

ANTICOAGULANTS: Refers to chemical substances which are used to prevent the normal clotting (coagulation) of blood. There are two main categories: Drugs which slow clotting in an individual's bloodstream; and substances which prevent the clotting of blood in a test tube. Anti-coagulant drugs are used to treat and prevent blood clots. Examples of anticoagulants are Heparin and Warfarin.

ANTIHYPERLIPIDEMICS: Refers to drugs which lower levels of cholesterol and other blood fats (lipids) in the treatment of atherosclerosis. Examples of these include Lovastatin, Gemifibrozil, and Pravastatin.

ANTIHYPERTENSIVES: Are used in the treatment of high blood pressure (hypertension). Examples of antihypertensives are vasodilators, which lower blood pressure by causing the muscles in the walls of the small blood vessels to relax enabling the blood to flow at a lower pressure. Other antihypertensives act differently, and quite often, more than one kind is prescribed.

ANTIOXIDANT: This refers to a special class of nutrients which combat "free radicals". Free radicals are a group of cells which damage otherwise healthy cells. Antioxidants are currently the latest trend in health and fitness, and many scientists have discovered that strenuous exercise may increase the number of free radicals roaming around in the body. Therefore, an increase antioxidant supplementation in athletes and bodybuilders has been recommended by many experts. Most antioxidants can be found in local vitamin stores.

ANTI-TUMOR DRUGS: Destroy cancer cells, which injure normal cells as well. Nolvadex is an example of a potent nonsteroidal anti-estrogen which is used in estrogen dependent tumors such as breast cancer.

AROMATIZE: This is a term which refers to a reaction in the body where excess testosterone or androgens are converted into estrogen (female hormone). An example which is most common of aromatizing amongst male athletes, is the development of breast tissue. This is referred to as gynecomastia or "bitch tits". Development of the breast tissue can be an experience which can be both emotionally and physically painful to the male. Prevention of aromatizing would involve limited or correct usage of Testosterones, and other associated steroidal substances. Correction can be obtained by either counteracting the Testosterone with anti-estrogen substances such as Nolvadex, HCG, Proviron, APL, Teslac, (the latter two compounds are currently not available in Mexico), or in extreme cases, surgery.

ARRAY: This is another term which is often referred to as "stacking". This possibly refers to a selection of steroidal compounds being used in a certain combination or cycle.

ARTERIOSCLEROSIS: Is a disease of the arteries which is often referred to as "hardening of the arteries" because it involves hardening, thickening and loss of elasticity in the artery walls.

ATAXIA: Refers to irregular muscle action or failure of muscle co-ordination.

ATHEROSCLEROSIS: Initiates when certain fatty substances, particularly cholesterol in the bloodstream, form deposits on the inner lining of the arteries. Over a period of years, these deposits enlarge and thicken to form plaques which have rough edges which irritate the smooth lining of the arteries. This causes the cells to die and scars to form. The accumulation of dead cells, calcium, and scar tissue in the plaques makes the arteries hard and narrow, which decreases the flow of blood. The rough surface of the arteries may cause a blood clot (thrombus) to form on the arterial wall, which can suddenly block an artery. Atherosclerosis can occur in many parts of the body. For example, in the legs, it may cause pain while walking, skin sores or gangrene (death of tissue). In the heart, decreased blood supply can produce severe chest pain, or a complete blockage can result in a stroke or a heart attack.

ATP: This is an abbreviation for Adenosine Triphosphate, which is an intermediate high energy compound which releases chemically useful energy upon hydrolysis to ADP (Adenosine Diphosphate). Oxygen and glucose contribute to the formation of ATP and can be thought of the actual fuel which enables muscles to move. ATP is generated during the breaking down of muscle tissue in response to exercise, and utilized during anabolism.

ATROPHY: Refers to a state of deterioration, or a decrease in size and functional ability of bodily tissues or organs, which usually results from lack of use.

BASAL METABOLIC RATE: Refers to the energy which is needed for internal or cellular work, that is required by the body at rest (not asleep). In other words, it is the speed at which the body is able to burn calories, while it is at complete rest. It is expressed per unit of time, per square meter of body surface area.

BASEMENT DRUGS: Is a slang term for which many athletes refer to as counterfeit, designer or fake drugs.

BETA-BLOCKERS: Can reduce the rate and force of the heartbeat, lower blood pressure, and also lessen the workload of the heart. This is very beneficial in the treatment of various heart problems.

BIOAVAILABILITY: Refers to how well vitamins and minerals are absorbed from the foods that are ingested, or medically, refers to the efficacy of a drug at the site of disease or malfunction in the body.

BIOCHEMICAL INDIVIDUALITY: Refers to physiological differences which exists in every human being.

BIOLOGICAL DRUGS: Refers to drugs which are made from animal or human substances, including serums, vaccines and drug products derived from human blood.

BITCH TITS: Another slang term for which many refer to for gynecomastia. Gynecomastia is a condition where male breast tissue begins to grow, mainly because of aromatizing of certain drugs such as Testosterones, Anapolon and Norandren 50. Again, these side effects can be reversed either by lowering the doses of the above drugs, or by counteracting these drugs with Nolvadex, HCG, Proviron, APL, Teslac, (the latter two are currently, not available in Mexico), or in extreme cases, surgery.

BLACK MARKET: This refers to counterfeit, or drugs which are purchased other than from a physician or pharmacy. Most steroids which are obtainable today are from the black market, as they have been banned by several governments, and mostly can only be obtained illegally. Some of these drugs are legit, being stolen from the pharmaceutical company or the pharmacy directly, but many are counterfeits containing ingredients other than what is desired. The black market industry is quite diverse, ranging from large suppliers who distribute to wholesalers, who then distribute to dealers, then finally to the purchaser. Other sources can range from physicians, veterinarians, farmers, or anyone who has easy access to these drugs. Currently, most steroids are smuggled from countries where they are legal, into countries where they are not. As a safe measure, individuals should pass the opportunity of purchasing products from unknown origins, or sellers, as chances are, the items are counterfeits.

BLOCKING AGENT: This refers to a class of prescribed medications which can prevent the excretion of steroids from the kidneys into the urine. Many athletes use blocking agents to temporarily test negative for anabolic steroids while they are still on a cycle. Committees and Federations which do not allow anabolic steroids, also disallow the use of blocking agents. Some blocking agents include Carinamide, Anturane, and Probenecid.

BLOOD COMPOSITION HORMONES: Healthy blood contains fairly exact levels of several chemical substances and if these chemicals increase too high, or decrease too low, the body can become harmed.

BLOOD PRESSURE: Is the measurement of the force of blood when it presses against the wall of a blood vessel. Systolic refers to the pressure of the blood during the pumping action of a heartbeat, and diastolic refers to the pressure after the beat, when the heart is filling with the blood. Systolic is the above number in a blood pressure reading, and the diastolic is the number on the bottom. For example, 120/80, 120 is systolic, and 80 is diastolic. 120/80 is considered to be a normal blood pressure reading.

BLOOD TEST: Blood tests are recommended for those individuals who experiment with steroidal compounds. These tests can ensure that blood components are within "healthy" limits, and if not, can alter present regimes to accommodate proper health management. Blood tests may be obtained by request at any local health facility or physician.

BODY COMPOSITION: Refers to the ratio of lean mass (muscle) to bodyfat. For example, a female who weighs 117 lbs, her total measurement totals 90.00, her bodyfat % totals 20.77, her fat lbs equals 24.30, and therefore, her lean mass totals 92.70. So, of her weight of 117 lbs, according to her caliper measurements, she has a total lean mass of 92.70, and 24.30 lbs of her weight is listed as bodyfat. 24.30 + 92.70 = 117 lbs. If she was wanting to lose more bodyfat, she would have to increase her lean mass, and decrease her bodyfat total.

BRANCHED CHAIN AMINO ACIDS: The abbreviated form is BCAA's, which refers to three amino acids, Leucine, Isoleucine, and Valine, because of their interlocking methyl groups and their chemical structures. BCAA's are burned as fuel at the end of sustained high intensity training when the body requires protein for as much as 20 percent of its energy requirements.

BRONCHODILATOR: Refers to any of a group of drugs which open up the small breathing tubes in the lungs called bronchioles. Bronchodilators relax the muscles in the bronchioles thereby expanding the tubes and making breathing easier, relieving such symptoms as coughing and wheezing. They can be taken orally as a tablet, capsule or syrup, or sometimes they are injectable. Sometimes, a canister holds bronchodilators in the form of a liquid or a fine powder, and this can be administered by pushing on a spring on the top of the canister, and while inhaling, the drug enters the bronchioles. Bronchodilators can also produce several side effects such as increased heart rates, blood pressure, and possibly restlessness or dizziness. Some examples of bronchodilators which are used by bodybuilders are Epinephrine, Clenbuterol, Spiropent and Novegam. Bodybuilders commonly use these drugs as they experience a type of "buzz" and also it is felt that these also have an effect on the acceleration of burning bodyfat, and muscle mass increases.

BUCCAL: Or what can be referred to as sublingual, refers to medication or steroidal compounds which are absorbed in the cheek mucosa, by placing between the cheek and gum, or placed under the tongue to dissolve. Drugs that are either buccal or sublingual should not be swallowed, as they have approximately twice the potency of oral drugs. These drugs are fast acting and take as little as 30 to 60 minutes to fully dissolve, and absorb into the bloodstream much faster, and are not as hard on the liver. While taking drugs either sublingual, or by the cheek mucosa, it is important not to eat or drink, but after the tablet is fully dissolved, to either brush or rinse the mouth thoroughly. Normal activity such as talking or swallowing will not disrupt anything. Currently, there is now nasal insuflation drugs which are sprayed into the back of the throat into the mucosa, which are easier to take, extremely effective and are absorbed much quicker than tablets. They are also absorbed nearly 100%, as opposed to tablet forms, which are approximately 20% absorbed.

BUFFED: Slang term referring to an excellent state of physical condition, often accompanied with good muscle size, tone, and definition.

BULKING PERIOD: Refers to a period in the off season, often when a bodybuilder tends to gain body weight by adding muscle, fat, or a combination of both.

CALORIE: This refers to a measure of a unit of energy. For example, a piece of cheesecake may be loaded with calories, but the nutritional value is lacking. Calorie intakes can be adjusted to produce desirable results, such as, increased caloric intakes will usually result in a weight gain; as a decrease in calories, will result in a weight loss. Foods high in calories may not necessarily also be high in nutritional value.

CARBOHYDRATES: Refers to a food group which serves as an energy source for the body. There is varied opinions upon the proper distribution of carbohydrates for a diet, ranging anywhere from a low carbohydrate intake to that of a high intake. For bodybuilding, it is recommended that the carbohydrate intake should be a little higher than the protein intake, but definitely alot higher than the fat intake. Again, depending upon the goals, carbohydrate intake vary and can even change as the demands of the diet change. There are also many carbohydrate supplements available, mainly powders and drinks. It is recommended that some carbohydrates be also ingested in a complete meal, to help synthesize the breakdown of protein. There are also different types of carbohydrates such as starchy and fibrous.

CARDIOVASCULAR ACTIVITY: Sometimes referred to as aerobic activity, but this is any activity which involves accelerating the heartrate for a period of time to increase fitness levels and general health. Bodybuilders engage in cardiovascular activity to speed up metabolism levels, in attempts to burn bodyfat more readily.

CARCINOGENS: Agents that cause cancer.

CARNITINE: This is an amino acid which is found in every living tissue. It is a water-soluble nutrient which is synthesized in the liver from Lysine and Methionine. Carnitine plays a role in the metabolism of fat, as it increases the amount of Carnitine in the diet. It does help transport fatty acids across the cell wall and into the cell's powerhouse (mitochondria), which then enable muscle cells to utilize essential fatty acids for energy metabolism. However, this has only been proven when there has been an extreme deficiency of Carnitine in the present diet regime.

CARRYING HORMONES: Refers to organs called endocrine glands, which produce hormones and releases them directly into the blood. When a hormone reaches a part of the body it regulates, it may affect growth, reproductive processes, how the body utilizes food, or possibly, some other function.

CATABOLIC: This refers to the breaking down of muscle tissue in response to exercise, which is the opposite of anabolic. A negative nitrogen balance most often accompanies catabolic states and is often the reason why athletes who train intensely with weights, also inflict catabolic states upon themselves. Anabolic steroids reverse the catabolic state and actually work more effectively on muscles which are in this condition, which supports why the intensity of workout can contribute to the effectiveness of these drugs.

CHEMICAL NAME: Of a drug, describes it's chemical structure. It is the only name which identifies a drug precisely. Trade names are often also given to drugs because the chemical names are often long and hard to pronouce. For example, the chemical name for Anapolon 50 is Oxymetholone. It is also important to realize however, that certain trade names for drugs may change and be called a different trade name in another country, but the chemical name will always remain the same. For example, Anadrol is called Anapolon in Mexico, but it is known by the chemical name of Oxymetholone worldwide.

CHOLESTEROL: Refers to a fatty substance found in some foods and are manufactured by the body for many vital functions.

CHROMIUM PICOLINATE: Is a trace mineral which plays an important role in carbohydrate and fat metabolism. Again, this is another substance that works well on the average person who is borderline obese, or is chromium deficient, thus bodybuilders seldom receive effective results from this mineral alone.

CHRONOBIOLOGY: The study of time and cycles in the body.

CLANDESTINE: Refers to being arranged or made in a stealthy or underhanded manner, secretive, or concealed, and contrary to the law. For example, many black-market labs can be referred to as clandestine, for making counterfeit drugs.

CLEAN: Refers to an athlete or bodybuilder has tested negative for anabolic steroids. This sometimes means that either the individual has not taken certain steroidal compounds for a certain period of time; therefore, they were undetectable upon testing, or that possibly these substances were never used.

COENZYME: Is a small molecule which works with an enzyme in order to promote the enzyme's activity. Coenzymes are usually vitamins.

CONGESTIVE HEART FAILURE: Refers to a condition where the blood backs up in the veins; which is accompanied by fluid accumulation in various parts of the body. This usually occurs due to insufficient pumping of the heart muscle.

COUNTERFEITS: Refers to products which are not real pharmaceutical drugs. It is sometimes difficult to distinguish between legitimate drugs and counterfeits, as counterfeits are usually very close to the actual product. An experienced user may even possibly second guess, but usually, the real pharmaceutical company include some sign which is difficult to copy for the counterfeiters. Although, it is estimated that approximately 90% of the obtainable steroids on the black-market today are counterfeit, many are still bought by athletes in the hopes that there may possibly be some "hint" of the real product within. Without heeding caution, many of these athletes have terrible responses and side effects, and even become quite ill. It is extremely important to be educated about steroid products as there are several substances available that indeed, are very dangerous.

COLOSTRUM: Is a supplement which is considered to be useless to bodybuilders as the digestive tract destroys all of the powerful immune boosters and growth factors found in it. Colostrum is rich with Insulin-like Growth Factor-1 (IGF-1), and nutrients which boost the immune system and accelerates growth in newborns; as it is found in the mother's milk the first few days after delivery. Unfortunately, colostrum only appears to be advantageous to newborns, at this point.

COMPLETE PROTEIN: Is protein which contains all the essential amino acids, such as an egg.

CONCENTRIC CONTRACTION: Refers to muscle contraction which results in the shortening of muscles.

CONJUGATED LINOLEIC ACID: The abbreviated form, CLA, is actually a fatty acid which is a totally new type of supplement available. It is not a drug, and appears to be completely nontoxic with no known side effects, if consumed in normal dosages. It is currently difficult to find this supplement, but so far is available in oil form, and soon there will be available in gel caps. CLA allows for weight gain without gaining body fat.

CP: Is the abbreviation for Creatinine Phosphate, which is an inorganic phosphate molecule which binds with ADP (Adenosine Diphosphate) to form ATP (Adenosine Triphosphate). It is a common belief that some steroids may increase the availability or production of Creatinine Phosphate so that more ATP can be available to the muscles which increases strength and endurance.

CREATINE: Refers to a substance in the bloodstream which is used for supplementary energy transport in certain body systems. ATP is the main immediate source of usable energy in the body, however, the brain, heart and muscle cells require enormous amounts of energy which creatine aids in supplying. Creatinine is produced in the kidneys and liver. The chemical is absorbed into cells and then picks up the high-energy phosphate group from excess ATP at cellular bodies, called mitochondria. It then shuttles back and forth to other cells to supply the energy. Creatine has received alot of recent attention in the athletic and bodybuilder world lately. It is usually supplemented in a powdered form and has been reported to increase both muscle mass and strength. Creatine is used by natural athletes and bodybuilders, and is not banned from most athletic federations and organizations.

CROSS-LINKING: Refers to a reaction in cell membranes which are thought to be responsible for the hardening of the arteries, skin wrinkling and cataracts.

CRUCIFEROUS VEGETABLES: Refers to vegetables such as broccoli, cauliflower, cabbage, and watercress, which contain indoles, which are compounds which seem to protect against cancer.

CUTTING UP: Refers to the reduction of bodyfat, so that muscle definition and striations become more apparent. Cutting up usually occurs before competition, and at an extremely low bodyfat percentage.

CYCLE: This refers to, in bodybuilding terms, a certain time period containing a certain drug regime is taken for. For example, Testosterone Cypionate and Deca may be taken for a period of four weeks, then exchanged for Testosterone Enanthate and Anavar for a period of six weeks. Again, cycles vary for individuals, females and males, athletes, bodybuilders, powerlifters, and for the desired results.

DART: Is another term used for a syringe, which is used to inject several types of waterbase or oilbase steroidal compounds.

DEFICIENCY: This refers to a condition in which a nutrient or a group of nutrients is lacking. For example, a diet deficient in protein will not build muscle mass.

DEOXYRIBONUCLEIC ACID: "DNA" ia a complex protein which is present in the nuclei of cells. DNA is the chemical basis of heredity, and also decides the programming of the cells per individual.

DESIGNER DRUGS: This term refers to drugs which are counterfeit but may not necessarily be fake. They are usually given a different trade name, and may possibly contain one or more domestic steroidal preparations. Examples of designer drugs are Blasterone, Dihydrolone, DMU, Exelon, and Nordyethylene.

DIGESTIVE SYSTEM: Refers to the group of organs which break food down into smaller particles for use in the body. This breakdown allows the smaller digested particles to pass through the intestinal wall into the bloodstream which are then distributed to nourish all parts of the body. Fats, proteins and carbohydrates in foods consist of very complex molecules which must be broken down, or digested. When digestion is completed, proteins are digested to amino acids and peptides, carbohydrates are broken down into simple sugars, and fats are digested to fatty acids and glycerol. All of these broken down substances are the digested foods that can be absorbed into the bloodstream. Such substances such as vitamins, minerals, and water do not require digestion.

DIHYDROTESTOSTERONE: The abbreviation is DHT, which is a hormone which naturally occurs in the body, and is a parent compound of a number of steroid preparations. DHT plays a major role in the augmentation of skeletal muscle and is also responsible for several of the androgenic effects of testosterones such as facial hair, male reproductive organ development and genetic balding. A high percentage of endogenous and exogenous testosterones are converted to DHT in the body, which may result in the actual building of muscle tissue. Acne and accelerated balding are common undesirable side effects of DHT. Anapolon has a notorious reputation as a DHT, of causing hair loss.

DISACCHARIDE: A type of simple sugar constructed of double molecules of glucose.

DISPENSABLE AMINO ACIDS: Refers to 11 amino acids which the body can synthesize on it's own. The other nine amino acids, humans must obtain from food sources such as eggs, meat, milk products and some vegetables.

DIURETICS: Is either a drug or a substance which increases the amount of urine which is discharged by the kidneys. Most diuretics especially increase the amount of sodium and chloride which is discharged in the urine. In certain diseases, the kidneys do not produce enough urine which results in fluid, salts, and waste build up in the body. Diuretics correct this condition by causing the kidneys to produce more urine. Some natural substances such as water, coffee, tea, beer and sugar solutions, have a diuretic effect on the kidneys. Some drugs can reduce the volume of blood in the body, and are used as diuretics to lower blood pressure in individuals with high blood pressure. Diuretics may cause a loss of potassium and other important substances in the body, and if these losses are not replenished, they may cause seizures, or heart, or blood problems. Bodybuilders often use diuretics in an attempt to remove subcutaneous water to allow muscles to appear more defined. Diuretics may work well for some bodybuilders, but often it leaves the muscles drawn and flat.

Sometimes, severe muscle cramping is experienced when there is too much of a loss of potassium. Diuretics have also been rather controversial in the bodybuilder secture, as they are often blamed for dehydrating contestants to an extreme, and possibly, resulting even in death for certain individuals. Diuretics have been banned by many athletic events and competitions, as athletes have used diuretics also to dilute urine samples (often these organizations have also banned the use of steroids). There are different kinds of diuretics which also range in strength. Potassium-sparing diuretics such as Aldactone are considered to be somewhat of a milder prescription compound. While thiazides such as Dyazide, and loop-agent diuretics such as Lasix, are more potent prescription substances.

DMSO: Stands for Dimethyl Sulfoxide, which is a compound obtained as a by-product of paper manufacturing. It is a controversial drug which is used to treat such conditions as arthritis, bursitis, and sprains. The drug is quickly absorbed through the skin into the bloodstream, when applied externally. There have been many reports that DMSO has a remarkable effect in relieving pain and reducing inflammation. However, the United States Food and Drug Administration (FDA) has not approved the drug for external use on human beings. The FDA will only allow the drug to be used internally to treat interstitial cystitis, which is a bladder condition. DMSO was widely used until 1965, when the FDA banned it as a human drug as reports were produced that it caused eye damage in experiments with animals. Although there have been no reports that there has been eye damage in humans, there have been minor side effects such as bad breath, headaches, nausea and skin rashes. Many people still use DMSO for many ailments, and even obtain industrial DMSO, even though it may contain harmful impurities. DMSO is also used in combination with certain steroidal compounds, to quickly administer these agents via the skin's surface, which eliminates the first pass of the liver.

DRUG: Can be considered as all chemicals which affect living things. There are many kinds and classifications of drugs. For example, they can be grouped according to their form, such as a solid, gas or liquid, or according to the way they are take, such as by swallowing, inhaling or injection. Drugs can even be grouped according to their chemical structure. However, most pharmacologists generally classify drugs according to the major beneficial effect they have on the body. Many of the most widely used drugs belong to one of several dozen groups, which four especially important groups are: Drugs which fight infection, Drugs that prevent infectious diseases, Drugs which affect the heart and blood vessels, and Drugs that affect the nervous system. However, all drugs affect the body in more than one way. For example, a drug may be taken to act on the nervous system, but may also affect the heart. Therefore, the action of this drug on the heart is considered to be a side effect.

DYSPNEA: Is hard or heavy breathing.

EDEMA: Refers to swelling, or the presence of abnormal quantities of fluid in intercellular tissue spaces within the body.

EFFICACIOUS: This refers to producing the desired effect. For example, reducing one's caloric intake can prove to be efficacious in weight loss.

ELECTROLYTES: Refers to minerals which are responsible for maintaining the fluid balance inside and outside cells.

EMBOLISM: Is the obstruction of a blood vessel by foreign substances or a blood clot.

ENDOCRINE CONTROL HORMONES: Affect the production of other hormones including FSH and LH, which are the anterior pituitary hormones which regulate the secretions of the gonads.

ENDOGENOUS: This refers to naturally occurring things in the body. For example, there are steroids which are endogenous steroids, as they are produced in the body for daily functions.

ENDOMORPH: Refers to a heavy-set individual with a predominantly round and soft physique.

ENDORPHINS: Are brain chemicals which naturally reduce pain. D, L-phenylalanine, which is an amino acid, can intensify and prolong these natural painkilling effects.

ENZYMES: Refers to a protein which brings about chemical changes, without being affected itself.

EPINEPHRINE: Is a hormone that is secreted by the adrenal glands, which is also called adrenaline. Epinephrine helps the body adjust to sudden stress, such as when an individual becomes angry or frightened, the adrenal glands release large amounts of epinephrine into the blood. The hormone causes changes in the body to make it more efficient for "fight or flight" response. Epinephrine increases the strength and rate of the heartbeat and raises the blood pressure; it also provides energy to the muscles by speeding up the conversion of glycogen into glucose. Epinephrine can be be chemically synthesized, or be extracted from the adrenal glands of animals. The drug stimulates the heart, and relaxes muscles in the air passages into the lungs. Physicians use Epinephrine to treat severe allergic reactions and to restore the heartbeat in patients who are suffering cardiac arrests. Now, however, Epinephrine is not used as much to treat asthma attacks, as there now are other drugs available which will not excite the heart.

EPIPHYSIS: Refers to a portion of bone which calcifies before it unites with the major part of the bone.

ERGOGENICS: Refers to the study of ergogenesis or muscle performance. Anabolic steroids, which can enhance muscle performance, are often referred to as an ergogenic aid.

ERYTHROPOIESIS: Is the formation of red blood cells.

ESSENTIAL FATTY ACIDS: The abbreviation, EFAs, are vitamin-like substances which have a protective effect on the body. They are called essential because the body cannot manufacture them; they must be obtained from food.

ESTER: Is a product which results from the combination of an acid with an alcohol.

ESTROGEN: Is any of a group of chemically similar hormones that cause the growth and development of female characteristics in human beings, and influence the female reproductive cycle. In both women and men, small amount of Estrogen's are produced in fat tissue, muscles, and many other parts of the body. The drug industry produces synthetic Estrogen's for use in birth control pills and for certain medical therapy.

EXERTIONAL HEADACHES: Refers to headache pain which is often experienced from a variety of exercises or daily functions requiring strenuous physical activity.

EXOGENOUS: This term refers to substances originating outside of the body. Synthetic steroids are exogenous steroids, as an individual must inject this substance for it to be a source of that particular hormone.

FAMINE/FAT ACCELERATION: Refers to a physiological defense mechanism involving the buildup of fat by the body following a period of caloric restriction.

FATIGUE: Refers to a general feeling of being "tired". Muscles can also become fatigued. Generally, rest helps both of these instances. Fatigue often occurs when a repetitive motion is continued for a certain period of time.

FATTY ACIDS: Refers to components of either dietary fat, or bodyfat, which is used as fuel for muscle contractions.

FIRST PASS: All oral steroids must go through this event where a compound goes from the stomach or intestines, to the liver where it is either destroyed or passed through into the bloodstream, before they can get into the blood and bind to cells where they exert their functions. The first pass of an oral steroid is rough on the liver, and destroys a majority of the substance.

FLATUS: Is the medical term for the expelling of gas from a lower body orifice.

FLEXION: Refers to the bending movement of a joint in contrast to extending; or to decrease the angle between the bones which form a joint.

FORCED REPS: Refers to requiring assistance in order to perform repetitions when a muscle can no longer complete an exercise on its own.

FREE RADICALS: This term refers to cellular aberrations, formed when molecules somehow result with an odd number of electrons. These cells destroy healthy cells by robbing them of oxygen, therefore, weakening the immune system. Free radicals are normally not a problem because they are captured by the body's own army of antioxidants. However, trouble often arises when free radicals outnumber the antioxidants (a situation which results from aging and exposure to pollutants and toxins). Unchecked, free radicals roam the body, scavenging for oxygen and ultimately creating the type of cell damage associated with arthritis, cancer, heart disease, and other degenerative diseases.

FRUCTOSE: Is a sugar which is produced by nearly all fruits and by many vegetables. It is also known as levulose, and fruit sugar, and is nearly twice as sweet as table sugar (sucrose). Foods which use Fructose to sweeten their taste, have less calories. Fructose is produced commercially as a liquid, powder, or tablets.

GALACTOSE: Galactose occurs in food only as part of a disaccharide called lactose. It is a white, crystalline monosaccharide found in combined form in lactose, pectins, gums and certain other substances.

GC/MS: This is an abbreviation for gas chromatography and mass spectrometry, which is an analytical method for testing urine samples, and for doing substance analysis. This is the most accurate method used to detect anabolic steroid use. GC/MS not only detect extremely low levels, but can also differentiate one compound from another. Gas chromatography is first used to isolate each individual component for analysis by the mass spectrometry, as a drug extract can contain hundreds of constitiuents. In the mass spectrometry, a beam of electrons shatters the drug's molecules into a distinct pattern of molecular fragments, its mass spectrum. This method is much more accurate than the radioimmunoassay screens, but is also much more expensive to perform.

GENETICS: Is the passing on of characteristics of living organisms from one generation to the next; heredity.

GLUCAGON: Is a hormone which is secreted by the pancreas which raises the blood sugar level by stimulating the breakdown of glycogen to glucose. It is a hormone which is responsible for unlocking fat stores.

GLUCOSE: Is the most important carbohydrate in blood. Glucose is a mildly sweet sugar, also referred to as blood sugar. The liver changes fructose and galactose into glucose, which is carried by the blood to all the cells of the body. The cells then use glucose as fuel for the muscles and nerves, and also to build and repair body tissues.

GLUCOSE TOLERANCE: Refers to the ability to transport blood glucose into cells for use by the body.

GLYCOGEN: The liver changes excess glucose into glycogen and stores it. When the level of sugar in the blood is low, the liver changes glycogen back into glucose and releases it into the blood. Glycogen is also stored in the muscles as an emergency reserve of energy. Some of this glycogen is changed back into glucose when the body needs energy quickly.

GLYCOLYSIS: Refers to the anaerobic conversion of glucose to lactic acid, which produces some energy in the form of ATP.

GYNECOMASTIA: This condition can occur naturally in males, but is more common as a side effect of male steroid users, when their mammary glands begin to grow., resembling that of a female's breasts. This can occur when a steroid converts to estrogen, and the levels become so high that it mimics the female hormone patterns, thus begins the formation of breasts.

HALF-LIFE: Refers to the time required by the body to metabolize or inactivate half of an amount of a substance which was administered. This is an important consideration in determining a suitable amount and duration of administration of substances.

HDL: Is the abbreviation for high density lipoprotein, which is a type of cholesterol in the blood which has a protective effect against the buildup of plaque in the arteries.

HEME IRON: This is Iron which is found in animal protein.

HEMORRHOIDS: Refers to a mass of dilated, tortuous veins in the anorectum, which involve the venous plexuses of that area. There are two kinds of hemorrhoids, internal and external. Hemorrhoids are suffered by some athletes and bodybuilders due to the strenuous strain exerted when lifting heavy weights. This most often occurs when performing an exercise commonly referred to as a squat.

HEMOGLOBIN: Refers to the pigment which transports oxygen in the blood. Hemoglobin is in the red blood cells and gives blood its red color. Hemoglobin combines with oxygen when the red cells file through the air sacs of the lungs, to form a compound called oxyhemoglobin. When the red cells travel through the rest of the body, they give up the oxygen to the tissues, the hemoglobin takes up the carbon dioxide, and then releases it in the air sacs of the lungs. The carbon dioxide is then exhaled. Hemoglobin is also a complex molecule which includes iron and a protein called globin. An individual's hemoglobin type is inherited.

HEPARIN: The prevention of blood clotting by a mucopolysaccharide.

HOMEOSTASIS: Refers to the body's regulatory mechanism which tries to maintain an equilibrium of body temperature, fluid volume and electrolyte concentration.

HORMONES: Refers to any of a number of chemical substances produced within an animal or human, which are secreted in bodily fluids and carried to organs to produce specific metabolic effects. A hormone is produced in one part of an organism, but it causes an effect in a different part, therefore, they serve as a means of communication among various parts of an organism. In humans and animals, hormones control such body activities as growth, development, and reproduction. Hormones regulate a variety of body functions. They may be grouped according to the functions they control such as the way the body uses food; growth; sex and reproduction; the regulation of the composition of the blood; the reaction of the body to emergencies; and the control of hormones themselves. Some hormones can even be synthetically produced such as estrogen and testosterone.

HYDROSTATIC UNDERWATER WEIGHING: This is an accurate test for measuring bodyfat. It involves being immersed underwater, and calculating the body composition by using a certain formula.

HYPERKALEMIA: Refers to a high percentage of potassium in the blood which is abnormally high.

HYPERPLASIA: Is a normal increase in the number of cells within a particular tissue.

HYPERTENSION: The medical term for high blood pressure, which usually results from a high degree of water retention, or a quick increase in a vast amount of bodyweight. Hypertension can be controlled with medication.

HYPERTROPHY: In bodybuilding terms, it refers to the increase in size or the bulk of a muscle, and is usually the goal of every bodybuilder who trains with weights.

HYPODERMIC: Refers to a method of injection of a substance. Hypodermic subcutaneous injections refer to those which are administered under the skin. Other methods include intracutaneously (into the skin), intramuscularly (into the muscle), intraspinally (into the spinal canal), or intravascularly (into a vein or artery).

HYPOGLYCEMIA: Is a condition which occurs when the blood does not contain enough sugar (glucose), to provide energy for the body's cells. Symptoms of hypoglycemia man include hunger, headaches, nervousness, rapidly pounding heartbeat, and sweating. More severe hypoglycemia sufferers may show confusion, amnesia, poor coordination, and slurred speech, and in advanced cases, may lose consciousness and have convulsions. In rare cases, brain damage or death can occur. There are two groups of hypoglycemia; organic and functional. Organic is much more severe than the functional condition, and it results from a physical abnormality. Functional hypoglycemia is reactive hypoglycemia, which is simply an exaggeration of the body's normal reaction to eating.

IMMUNE SYSTEM: The immune system is composed of many parts which work together to fight infections when pathogens or poisons invade the human body. The immune system reacts to foreign substances through a series of steps referred to as the immune response.

IMPOTENCE: Refers to the inability of a male to achieve or maintain an erection of the penis. This may be a short-term, or a long-term side effect which may result from certain steroidal compounds.

INDISPENSABLE AMINO ACIDS: Refers to amino acids which are derived from animal sources of protein.

INDOLE: Refers to compounds which are found in cruciferous vegetables which have cancer protective effects.

INJECTABLE: Refers to a method of transporting medicines or substances via a needle and syringe. Injections are administered to secure a prompt action of a substance when it cannot be taken either by mouth, or when it may not be readily absorbed in the stomach or intestines; as it may be changed by action of the gastric secretions. Primosiston and Sten are examples of injectable drugs. Certain drugs are made to be injected either subcutaneously (below the skin surface), intravenously (into a vein), and others are made to be injected intramuscularly (into the muscle). It is important to make certain which way is the correct way, for full effect.

INJECTION SITE: This refers to the area where the injection of a substance will take place. Three acceptable sites for intramuscular injections are in the buttock area, the lateral surface of the thigh, and in the deltoid region. Again, depending on the drug, will depend on the administration site chosen.

INSULIN: Is a hormone which regulates the body's use of sugar and other foods. Insulin also affects the body's use of protein, fat, and potassium and phosphate (mineral products). Pure insulin is absorbed rapidly by the body and its effect lasts only for a short period. Drug companies manufacture various insulin preparations to prolong the hormone's effect by combining insulin with proteins or by modifying the hormone's chemical structure.

INTRAMUSCULAR: Within the muscle. Intramuscular injections are intended to be injected into the muscle. Most intramuscular injections are given in the upper gluteus maximus region, just below the iliac crest.

These types of injections are used when a drug is not easily absorbed orally, or when there is a large amount of liquid to be used.

ISOKINETIC EXERCISE: Is an exercise which is combined with resistance.

ISOMETRIC EXERCISE: This refers to when muscles maintain a constant length, and the joints are immobile, when a contraction occurs. An example of an isometric exercise would be such as pushing against a wall.

ISOTONIC EXERCISE: This is a type of exercise in which there is a change in the length of muscle and weight, while the tension remains constant. An example of an isotonic exercise would be the lifting free weights.

ITEM: This is what dealers refer to as for selling their "supplements". Dealers will very seldom, if at all, use the term "steroids".

KETOSIS: Refers to when there is too much acetone in the body. Ketosis occurs in diabetes and acidosis. It also results from incomplete metabolism of fatty acids, generally from carbohydrate deficiency. It is a metabolic state which occurs when the glucose in the blood is low (below 50 mg/dl) in which case, most of the fatty acids in the bloodstream are converted into a derivative called ketones. A degree of ketosis may be experienced when on a high protein, low carbohydrate diet. Bad breath and a dry taste is also often experienced when one is in a ketotic state.

KETOSTEROID: Refers to any one of a group of steroid hormones which originate in the adrenal glands and testes. Their presence in urine is used to determine the functioning conditions of these organs.

KREBS CYCLE: Refers to a complicated series of reactions in which the components of carbohydrates, fats and proteins are completely broken down in order to release energy required for the formation of ATP. All nutrient metabolites which are involved in energy production pass through this final common pathway, where more than 90% of the body's energy is generated.

LACTIC ACID: Is a byproduct of glucose combined with glycogen which metabolizes in muscle energetics, which even in small amounts, can result in muscle fatigue and pain. Lactic Acid obstructs muscle contraction.

LACTOSE: Also referred to as milk sugar, makes up about 5% of cow's milk. A molecule of lactose consists of a molecule of glucose and a molecule of galactose. It is a crystalline sugar which is usually obtained by evaporating whey and converting it into hard white crystals. Lactose is an isomer of common table sugar. Lactose intolerance refers to individuals who have difficulty in digesting milk sugar, as they fail to produce the enzyme lactase, which is required for the breakdown of lactose in the body. There are aids now available that one can take before hand, to digest lactose products without suffering from associated ill effects.

LAXATIVE: Refers to a medicine or substance which speeds the emptying of the intestines (bowels). Mineral oil is a laxative that lubricates the bowel contents and helps empties the bowels. Phenolphthalein, which is the active ingredient in chewable and chocolate laxatives, has a direct effect on the intestine; but how this exactly works, is unclear. Some other laxatives, including Epsom salt, provide bulk in the form of retained water, which increases the bowel contents and forces the bowels to empty. Castor oil, and some other laxatives, act by irritating the walls of the bowel. Laxatives should not be taken continually over a long time period, as the bowels become lazy and fail to function on their own. Other harmful side effects can also occur in other parts of the body, and should never be taken by individuals who have abdominal pain. A much safer method of relieving constipation (difficulty in emptying the bowels), can be obtained by drinking ampule amounts of water, and by eating fibrous foods including cereals, whole fruits, and leafy vegetables.

LCT: This is an abbreviation for Long Chain Triglycerides, which is another name for bodyfat and conventional dietary fat such as salad oil and margarine.

LEAN, FIBROUS VEGETABLES: This refers to a type of complex carbohydrate which is high in fiber and minerals, and low in calories. There is a wide variety of vegetables to choose from, including cauliflower, broccoli, mushrooms, spinach, zucchini, etc.., etc.

LEAN MASS: Refers to the amount of actual muscle on an individual's body. Lean mass plus bodyfat together, provide a total body weight.

LEUKOCYTES: Are a type of white blood cells which play a major role in warding off infection by destroying bacteria and eating cellular debris at inflamed areas, among other functions.

LIBIDO: Refers to an individual sex drive, which can be conscious, or unconscious. Certain steroidal compounds can either increase or decrease levels of libido.

LIGAMENT: Is connective tissue which is a strong, fibrous band which supports and strengthens a joint by connecting bones or cartilages.

LIPID: Refers to a family of fats which include cholesterol, phospholipids and triglycerides.

LIPOLYSIS: This refers to the release of stored fat in the body for the use of fuel.

LIPOPROTEINS: Are large molecules in which both cholesterol and trigylcerides are carried through the bloodstream. There are two main types of cholesterol-carrying lipoproteins, low-density lipoprotein (LDL), and high-density lipoprotein (HDL). Cholesterol in blood can be identified as either LDL or HDL cholesterol, depending on which lipoprotein carries it.

LIPOPROTEIN LIPASE: The abbreviation, LPL, refers to an enzyme which governs fat storage. More bodyfat is produced and stored as a result of repetitive low-calorie dieting, which causes the body to produce more LPL.

LIPOTROPICS: Refers to certain supplemental nutrients which assist the body in the mobilization and metabolism of fat. If lipotropics are used as part of a supplement program, they should be taken with meals. Examples of Lipotropics include Biotin, Chromium Picolinate, Choline, Inositol, L-Carnitine, and Betaine.

LOW DENSITY LIPOPROTEINS: The abbreviation LDL, refers to one of the types of cholesterol-carrying lipoprotein in the blood. High levels of LDL contribute to coronary heart disease.

LYMPHOCYTES: Refers to a type of white blood cell formed in the lymphatic system. Lymphocytes make up about 20 to 30 percent of the white blood cells in the body. They also have a key part in the body's immune system by recognizing and responding to specific viruses, bacteria, and other invaders. There are two major types of lymphocytes, B-cells, and T-cells. B-cells produce antibodies and release them into the plasma, where they circulate in the form of globulin proteins; which fight infection. T-cells, release substances which control B-cell activity, and also produce substances which activate monocytes to help destroy harmful organisms.

MACRONUTRIENTS: Refers to nutrients which the body requires in relatively large amounts; such as protein, carbohydrates, fiber, fat, and water.

MACROPHAGES: Refers to cells that are involved in the production of antibodies.

MALTOSE: Or malt sugar, remains after the brewing process, which is a disaccharide found in plants during the early stages of germination. It is used to flavor some candy. One molecule of maltose consists of two molecules of glucose.

MCT OIL: An abbreviation for Medium Chain Triglyceride Oil, is a dietary fat metabolized in such a way that very little is stored as bodyfat. MCT Oil can be added to the diet as a supplement. It can be taken orally, or it can be added to cooking. It is also considered to be a beneficial method of adding calories to a diet regime, as it increases the available energy levels which promotes weight gain.

MESOMORPH: Refers to an individual who has a powerful musculature, low bodyfat percentage, and a heavy skeletal structure. Most bodybuilders tend to have a mesomorph physique.

METABOLIC HORMONES: Regulates the various steps in metabolism, the process by which the body converts food into energy and living tissue.

METABOLIC OPTIMIZERS: Refers to a class of supplemental nutrients which enhance athletic performance such as an increase of lean muscle mass, improved strength, and enhanced endurance. Some examples of popular metabolic optimizers are, Aspartates, Branched-chain amino acids, Desiccated liver, MCT oil, and Supplemental Amino Acid Growth Hormone Releasers.

METABOLIC RATE: Refers to the speed at which the body is able to burn calories.

METABOLIC ROLL: This term refers to the condition in which the metabolism runs efficiently enough to burn fat.

METABOLISM: Refers to the physiological process which converts food to energy, in order so the body can function. The higher the metabolism rate is, the more calories and in turn, more bodyfat can be burned. Aerobic activity is an excellent way to increase metabolism. An aerobic session before eating breakfast, then again after the last meal at night has proven to be the most effective way of increasing metabolism.

MICRONUTRIENTS: Refers to nutrients which the body requires only small amounts of; such as vitamins and minerals.

MINERALS: Refers to inorganic nutrients which are required by the body for a wide range of enzymatic and metabolic functions. They are important for the formation of body structures such as bones and tissue, and are involved in many physiological processes such as metabolism and energy production. Certain minerals which are referred to as electrolytes, are responsible for maintaining the fluid balance of the body. The main electrolytes in the fluid outside of cells are sodium, calcium and chloride; potassium, magnesium and phosphorus are found inside cellular fluid. Electrolytes provide a life-sustaining environment for cells, and must be kept in constant balance to maintain good health. Nutrients are often lost through perspiration, and low levels of minerals and electrolytes can result in fatigue and other ill effects. Some minerals can be obtained through foods, or by supplements, and should always be taken with meals for the best results. There are 96 more minerals, than vitamins, present in the body

MITOCHONDRIA: This is the part of a cell where nutrients are converted to energy.

MOCK MEAL: Can also be referred to as a supplemental meal, refers to a beverage, or substance, which consists of both a carbohydrate and a protein supplement. Mock meals are also a great convenience when time is restricted, and a regular meal cannot be eaten, but can allow for a quick ingestion of required calories.

MONOSACCHARIDE: Is any one of a class of simple sugars such as glucose, fructose and arabinose, which occur naturally or are formed by hydrolyzing polysaccharides or glycosides. In other words, it is a type of simple sugar which is constructed of a single molecule of glucose.

MORTAR: Is a dish or something similar, which has a smooth interior, in which crude drug compounds can be crushed with a pestle.

MUSCLE TONE: Refers to the degree of a muscle's resting tension.

MYOFIBRIL: Filaments within muscle fibers which cause contraction. The greater amount of myofibrils will result in increased strength.

NARCOTIC: Refers to substances which have a strong depressant effect upon the human nervous system. They cause an insensibility to pain, stupor, sleep, or coma, depending upon the amount taken. Narcotics produce an analgesic effect by interacting with specific nerve cells called receptors, in the central nervous system. Although narcotic drugs are extremely beneficial in medicine, they also have dangerous side effects, and large doses can even cause death. The careless use of opium and substances made from it to relieve pain, has often caused drug habits. Examples of narcotics include opium, codeine, morphine and heroin. Physicians and pharmacists must document certain facts and keep records of narcotics. Most steroids are currently included on the narcotic list; therefore, are illegal to possess, trade, transport, export, or sell.

NATURAL: Refers to athletes who have not used anabolic steroids for a certain period of time. Most often, competitions for natural athletes are open to those who have not used illegal ergogenics aids or steroids for a period of no less than twelve months. Severe penalty or suspension can be imposed on those who do test "positive" in natural competitions.

NEUROTRANSMITTERS: Refers to chemicals which relay nerve impulses. This is released at the end of one nerve cell when a nerve impulse arrives there, it diffuses across the gap to the next nerve cell, and then alters the membrane of the cell in a way so that it becomes more or less likely to fire, or actually does fire. In the brain, some amino acids work as neurotransmitters.

NITROGEN: This is an important constituent of many cells, such as protein. Nitrogen distinguishes protein from other substances.

NITROGEN BALANCE: This refers to a state in which the daily intake of nitrogen from proteins is equivalent to the daily excretion of nitrogen. In other words, it is a measurement of whether there is a loss or a gain of lean muscle mass. A negative nitrogen balance occurs when the excretion of nitrogen exceeds the daily intake; and a positive nitrogen balance occurs when the amount of nitrogen ingested is greater than what is excreted. Some feel that an indication that muscle acquisition is occurring when the using steroids, as they are often in a positive nitrogen balance. Nitrogen is excreted mainly as urea in urine, and as smaller amounts in ammonia, creatine and uric acid.

NONHEME IRON: Refers to a type of iron found in plants.

NORTESTOSTERONE 19: This is a parent compound of a number of steroid preparations. Derivatives of Nortestosterone 19, exhibit minimal liver toxicity, and related side effects. Metabolites of this drug can be measured as late as 12 months after administering, therefore, they are easily detectable on drug tests.

NUTRITION: Refers to the use of food for growth, development and health. It is understood that nutrition is very important not only for the maintenance of good health, but also the key factor in all types of athletic ability and performance. Eating a daily balance of the five food groups usually suffices for good nutrition. However, athletes and bodybuilders need much more nutritional value than this, and therefore, have to accommodate to suit their nutritional requirements. Proper nutrition is the basis for all bodybuilders.

OMEGA-3 FATTY ACIDS: Is a type of EFA (essential fatty acid), which is found in fish, which helps to prevent blood clots and plaque buildup on arterial walls. Omega-3 fatty acids also appear to increase white cell activity, thus boosting the body's defense against disease. All fish provide a certain amount of the Omega-3 fatty acids, but halibut, salmon, and rainbow trout, which are cold-water fish, tend to be higher.

ORAL: Refers to a method of which substances or drugs are taken; which is by the mouth, intending to be swallowed. Medications and substances which are to intended to be swallowed, should not be placed under the tongue or in the cheek mucosa, as they are made to be ingested through the gastrointestinal tract. Oral steroids are subject to first pass before they get into the system and then must go back through the liver before they are eliminated. Usually, the entire dosage is eliminated in less than a day, as they are usually fast to enter and leave the system. Often, multiple dosages are necessary throughout the day in order to keep a constant level of the drug in the blood. Oral compounds such as the 17 alpha alkylated group which includes Anapolon, and Stenox are hard on the liver.

OVER-THE-COUNTER: Refers to drugs and substances that can be sold without a written prescription from a physician, dentist or veterinarian. These drugs must be safe for use without medical supervision, and label directions and warnings on over-the-counter drugs, must be clear and easily seen so that they can be used safely and effectively. Most vitamins, minerals, and some drugs can be obtained this way. They can be found in pharmacies, convenient stores, or even grocery stores.

OVER-TRAINING: This refers to the possibility of "over-exercising". Particularly, over-training is apparent when an exercise is performed to an abundance, and no gains are recognized. At this point, it is recommended to take a rest, and possibly re-evaluate the training regime. It is also recommended to take "days off" when heavy training with weight, in order to let the muscles recuperate. Over-training may be also experienced if an individual's diet is lacking particular components, and calories.

OXIDATION: This term refers to a chemical process in which oxygen combines with another substance which is then changed to another form.

PARENTERAL: This refers to injectable liquid drugs which can be intravenously (into a vein), subcutaneously (under the skin), or intramuscularly (in the muscle). Most anabolic steroids are intended for deep intramuscular injection.

PEAK CONTRACTION: Refers to when a cramping sensation is experienced when exercising a particular muscle, by using shortened movements.

PHARMACY: Refers to a place where the profession is concerned with the preparation, distribution, and use of drugs. Most pharmacies, are often called drugstores, also sell a variety of other products in addition to drugs. Pharmacies can be found most anywhere, and many offer many services for convenience such as 24 hour access, delivery services, drug interaction information, etc., etc. Pharmacies in Mexico are called Farmacias.

PIN: Another name which refers to a syringe.

PLACEBO: A substitute substance which often replaces the real compound; which although worthless, will not produce any ill effect.

PLANNED CHEAT: This refers to planning to eat a treat on a certain day, at a certain time, without eating on impulse. Obviously, this is most beneficial in a restricted diet regime.

PLATEAU: This refers to a point in either a training or steroid cycle, where the effectiveness is no longer apparent. With steroids, this most often occurs because steroid receptor sites are no longer recognizing the exogenous androgens. This is of no benefit to the administrator as the steroid is binding to the necessary target cells, and therefore, is not producing results. Plateaus can occur after as little as three weeks of a particular use, but more often are apparent after six or so weeks. To overcome steroid plateaus, sometimes increasing the dosage of the drug is beneficial; this is effective for a short time, but it soon reaches dosages which exceed the risk-to-benefit factor. Another approach may be to cycle the steroids by taking a number of different steroid each for three to six weeks. By taking steroidal compounds in short intervals, the receptor sites usually do not shut down. Another possibility, is to abandon taking steroids altogether for a few weeks, and then restarting a new cycle. This proves to be advantageous for some, as the steroids appear to be more effective. Others find that they do not reach plateaus, as they limit their usage of steroids to two or more compounds. This is often practiced after receptor mapping is obtained, and there is confidence in the selection of steroids. Training plateaus most often occur because the muscles become use to the exercise being performed. It is ideal to change the exercise performed, to continuously shock the muscles, so that they are not used to a particular exercise, on a particular day. This practice will disallow "plateauing". Also, sometimes overtraining is a factor. When this happens, it is beneficial to take a rest, and allow the muscles to rest.

PLYOMETRICS: Refers to a method of training where either an apparatus such as a medicine ball, or the ground is used as resistance to develop muscle tissue elasticity, and also to stretch reflex threshold for quick starting and explosive strength.

POKE: Yet another term which refers to a syringe.

POLYPHARMACY: Is a term that is used when the use of several drugs are used at the same time interval.

POLYSACCHARIDE: This refers to a multiple number of sugar molecules which are linked together in a long chain. An example of polysaccharides would be complex carbohydrates.

POLYUNSATURATED FAT: Is a fatty acid which lacks four or more hydrogen atoms, and can be found in fish and most vegetable oils.

PRESCRIPTION DRUGS: These are dangerous drugs to use, unless they are taken under medical supervision. (Legally) they can only be obtained by a physician, dentist, or veterinarian, who writes a prescription for them.

PROGESTERONE: Is a steroidal hormone obtained from the corpus luteum and placenta. It is also synthetically produced to treat menstrual disorders in women, such as amenorrhea, dysmenorrhea, and threatened abortion.

PROSTAGLANDINS: Refers to any one of a group of hormone-like substances which are produced in the tissues of mammals, by the action of enzymes on certain fatty acid, found in high concentrations in seminal fluid of the prostate gland. They are thought to have a variety of important functions in reproduction, nerve-impulse transmission, regulation of blood pressure, metabolism, and muscle contraction. In other words, they are hormone-like substances which regulate nearly every system in the body.

PROTEIN: Exists in every cell and is essential to plant and animal like, and is one of the three main classes of food which provides energy to the body. Humans obtain proteins from foods such as cheese, eggs, fish, meat and milk. Protein can also be obtained through supplements such as a "protein powder". Protein is important in building, maintaining, and repairing tissues in the human body, especially bone cartilage, and muscle. Proteins produce about 1,800 calories of energy per pound (4 calories per gram). If more lean body mass is desired, it is important to increase the protein intake. It has been recommended that approximately 1.5 to 2 grams of protein be taken per body pound, to increase muscle growth.

PROTEIN QUALITY: Refers to a rating based on the number of indispensable amino acids that are present, digestibility, and absorbability.

PUMPING IRON: Slang for lifting or training with weights.

PURE: Refers to an athlete who does not, or has never used anabolic steroids.

RADIOIMMUNOASSAY: The abbreviation of RIA, refers to a method which is used for the detection of anabolic steroids. It is rarely used as it can produce a number of false positive and negative readings. Instead, the GC/MS, which provides accurate readings, is much more commonly used.

REBOUND: This is a condition which seems to be the greatest following a HCG administration, where athletes experience a rebound state which often incurs the best strength and size gains, shortly after a steroid cycle. This may be due to an over production of testosterone by the testes upon the termination of exogenous steroid use.

RECEPTOR MAPPING: This refers to a useful technique for athletes which determines how much of a steroid is required to be beneficial. As it is well known that each individual reacts differently to different dosages of the same drug or substance, mapping is performed in effort to individualize dosages so that the maximum gains can be obtained, while minimizing the side effects. Mapping initiates with the recording a number of aspects of a cycle. To begin with, all the steroids taken must be documented carefully everyday. Then, graphs of weight and strength gains should also be recorded on a weekly basis. Documentation of any side effects such as acne, gynecomastia, water retention, aggression etc., should also be recorded at least three times a week, as well as other variables such as appetite, energy levels, mood swings, and sex drive. The dosages during a cycle should be increased steadily, while monitoring the side effects. If the side effects are occurring at the same time that weight and strength gains are being experienced, then the dosage should be lowered to see if the gains outweigh the adverse reactions. The other variable readings will indicate as to whether that particular drug or substance is working. Such clues that they are working will be indicated by a high energy level, appetite and sex drive. Although following the graphs can be the most beneficial way to use receptor mapping, this method may also have some flaws. For instance, a person may not have taken a long enough period off of a cycle, possibly is not training correctly, or possibly the nutrition is incorrect; all these possibilities are not taken into consideration. Therefore, many resort to common sense as a form of receptor mapping. Mapping is more accurate when doing one drug at a time. Receptor mapping has proven to be very beneficial for personal information; however, it is not considered to be an exact science.

RECOMMENDED DIETARY ALLOWANCES: The abbreviation of RDA, refers to the amount of nutrients which should be taken in by average individuals to prevent illness and possible disease.

RECONSTITUTION: Refers to returning a substance to it's approximate original state, before it was altered for preservation and storage.

RECUPERATION: This refers to a time period required for muscles to recover from training, in which subsequent muscle growth can also result.

RENAL: Of, or pertaining to the kidneys.

RIPPED: A slang term referring to a defined, muscular state, accompanied by a low bodyfat percentage.

RISK TO BENEFIT FACTOR: This method can be used to analyze the amount of benefit which is obtained by using additional quantities or additional items in an anabolic steroid stack. Of course, common sense strongly applies, and the risk to benefit factor should always be more on the beneficial side, to justify the additional use of anabolic steroids. For example, if increasing the dosage of a drug or substance up to ten times, because of the logic "more, is better", may not always necessarily be beneficial, as the side effects would outweigh the possibly gains. Therefore, a slight increase in gains is not worth the undesirable side effects. If common sense is used, then anabolic steroids can be prove to be beneficial, while minimizing health risks.

'ROID: A slang term for anabolic steroids.

SATURATED FAT: Refers to a fatty acid which carries the maximum number of hydrogen atoms. At room temperature, saturated fats are a solid. Saturated fats are found in meats and dairy products, but ingesting too much, can lead to coronary heart disease.

SERUM: Is the fluid portion of blood which is left remaining after clotting.

SEX STEROIDS: Refers to progesterone, estrogen (female sex organs), and to androgens (male sex organs). Progesterone and estrogen are responsible for the female's smooth, soft skin, high-pitched voice, and the development of breasts. Androgens are responsible for the male's beard, large muscles and deep voice. Small amounts of androgens are also secreted by the sex glands in females, as male sex glands produce small amounts of Estrogen's in males. An example of a powerful synthetic form of progesterone can be found in birth control pills, some of which may also contain estrogen.

SIDE EFFECTS: Refers to unwanted, or uncontrollable effects which may occur when taking certain drugs or substances. Some side effects which may occur may not bother certain athletes or bodybuilders. For example, many anabolic steroids have been known to increase the appetite, sex drive, and aggression. Most male athletes actually welcome these effects as they consider it beneficial to their training and masculinity. However, side effects such as mood swings, hair loss, and gynecomastia are unwelcomed, and caution in dosages should always be considered to avoid all side effects. Testosterones when taken by female athletes produce very masculinizing characteristics, which women definitely do not want. Therefore, females should stay away from certain androgenic steroids to avoid virilization.

SIMPLE SUGARS: Refers to a type of carbohydrate which is constructed of either single or double molecules of glucose. There are six simple sugars found in food, which often provide food with the sweet taste.

SKINFOLD CALIPERS: Refers to a device which measures the thickness of a fold of skin with its underlying layer of fat. Skinfold calipers have springs which exert pressure on the skinfold which allows for an accurate scale to measure the thickness in millimeters. By measuring skinfolds at different allocated areas, it is possible to calculate an individual's body composition, which includes bodyfat, and lean body mass. Next to the hydrostatic underwater weighing method, skinfold calipers are considered to be one of the best methods for an accurate reading.

SPECIFIC DYNAMIC ACTION: This refers to the ability of certain foods to increase the metabolic rate after a meal is consumed. Protein has a high specific dynamic action on metabolism. A high carbohydrate meal boosts the metabolic rate about four percent; while a high protein meal raises the metabolism about 30 percent above normal, usually within one hour after a meal, and can last for as long as three to 12 hours.

STACKING: This refers to a term which applies to the use of anabolic steroids which two or more are taken at the same time interval. This method is quite effective as multiple steroid receptor sites are saturated, therefore, lower dosages may be used. The lower dosages result in less possible side effects. Some stacks may include two or more injectables, orals, or a combination of both. Manufacturers pre-stack some drugs such as Primoteston and Sostenon. Other drugs are stacked by the user's comprehension of the effects; for example, Deca-Durabolin and Norandren 50, along with the intermittent administration of Nolvadex. Stacking may be done on an experimental basis, but it is beneficial to know the properties of each drug, so that full benefits are obtained, and one drug is working with another, not against each other. Most stacking is done through the advice of other users, and what they had found worked for their gains.

STAGGER: This refers to "overlapping", which can refer to the use of several anabolic steroids. Fluctuating the dosage of a steroidal compound can also be a part of the staggering pattern.

STARCHY CARBOHYDRATES: Refers to a natural complex carbohydrate. Starchy carbohydrates are natural, unrefined whole grains such as brown rice and oatmeal, beans and legumes such as kidney beans, lentils and peas, and tubers such as potatoes and yams. More energy is required for starchy carbohydrates to be digested, absorbed and used by the body. Starchy carbohydrates should always be eaten with a source of lean protein as the rate of glucose release is delayed even more, and the energy levels are more steady as a result.

STEROIDS: Refers to any of a class of chemical compounds important in chemistry, biology, and medicine. Steroids play a key role in the processes of living things, are alike in basic chemical structure. Each steroid has a slightly different arrangement of atoms, and therefore, have different effects on living things. Steroids are produced naturally by plants and animals, and are also made commercially. Individual organisms may react differently to the same steroid. Steroids include sterols, such as cholesterol, bile acids from the liver, adrenal hormones; sex hormones, and poisons in certain toads. They influence the body's metabolism, which is the process by which the body changes food into energy and living tissue. Anabolic steroids are produced by chemical methods, or synthetically, from testosterone (the male hormone).

STRIATED MUSCLE: Is a muscle which is characterized by a banding pattern of cross-striped muscle fibers. Striations in muscles are most apparent when bodyfat percentages are very, very low.

STIMULANTS: Certain drugs or substances are used to increase the activity of the nervous system. Stimulants include caffeine, cocaine, and synthetic drugs which are known as amphetamines. Common names for amphetamines include, speed, uppers and wake-ups. Stimulants create a false sense of well-being, as well as increasing mental and physical ability. However, once this effect wears off, a feeling of depression and uneasiness is experienced. Therefore, stimulant users often become dependent to maintain a state of well-feeling.

SUBCUTANEOUS: Refers to below the skin's surface.

SUPPLEMENT: This is not a food, but a preparation which is either a tablet, powder or liquid form. Supplements can also be referred to as minerals, and vitamins; any substance which will give the body an extra "boost" of a certain requirement. Supplemental meals are an excellent way of keeping metabolism high when it is inconvenient to have a "food meal". These may include a protein/carbohydrate drink, shake, or bar, and may be considered as a "meal" for the daily caloric and nutritional intake.

SYNERGISTIC: Refers to an action which is created when agents co-operate with one another, and enhance or multiply the effectiveness of another. Steroids and Growth Hormone are believed to be synergistic. Another example would be the digestion of protein with a carbohydrate.

SYNTHETIC: Refers to artificial substances such as anabolic steroids and growth hormone which are produced to mimic the actual entity.

T-CELLS: Refers to a type of lymphocyte which attacks foreign bodies directly, which destroy them chemically. T-cells are derived from the thymus gland and distinguished from a B-cell by its relatively smooth surface. T-cells are otherwise known as T lymphocytes, the T stands for thymus derived. In other words, T-cells are white blood cells which destroy invading agents.

TENDON: Are bands of strong, fibrous tissues which connects muscles to the bones.

TESTOSTERONES: Refers to a hormone which stimulates sexual development in male human beings, and belongs to a family of hormones called androgens. Anabolic steroids are produced by chemical methods from testosterone. Side effects of high dosages and a long duration of testosterone, may include liver damage, high blood pressure, aggressive behavior, and the appearance of male physical characteristics in females (virilization).

THERMOGENESIS: Refers to the production of body heat, which is a process which increases oxygen consumption and therefore, accelerates the metabolic rate.

THROMBOSIS: Refers to the formation, development or existence of a bloodclot or thrombus within the vascular system.

THYROXINE: One of the two hormones which is produced by the thyroid gland which helps to control the rate at which the cells use food to release energy.

TOXIC REACTIONS: Result from drug poisoning which damages cells, and may be fatal. All drugs can have a mild toxic effect, therefore, a large amount or an overdose may produce a severe toxic reaction.

TRACE MINERALS: Are vital to health, but is an element which is present in small quantities in food.

TRADE NAME: Is given to a drug by the company which manufactures it. A number of manufacturers may sell a particular chemical, however, each company may give the drug a different trade name, or market the drug under the drug's generic name. One drug may have several trade names, and in another country for example, one drug may not be available under one trade name which may be familiar, but does exist under another trade name. Although there may be several trade names available for a particular drug, the CHEMICAL NAME always remains the same. For example, Anadrol 50 made by Syntex in the United States, is known by the trade name Anapolon, made by Syntex in Mexico. So, it is very important to also be familiar with the chemical names of drugs, especially when traveling abroad.

TRIGLYCERIDES: Refers to fats which circulate in the blood until they are deposited in fat cells. They are any fatty compound of a group formed when three acid radicals replace the three hydrogen atoms of the hydroxyl groups in glycerol.

TRIIODOTHYRONINE: One of the two hormones which is produced by the thyroid gland which also helps to control the rate at which the cells use food to release energy.

ULTRASONOGRAPHY: Is the use of an ultrasound to produce an image or photograph of an organ or tissue. Ultrasonic echoes are recorded as they strike tissues of different densities. Ultrasound is also used in therapy to break down scar tissue which usually results from an injury.

UNITED STATES ADOPTED NAME: Commonly referred to as the generic name, is usually an abbreviated chemical name, which provides a hint about a drug's chemical structure. However, the USAN does not fully describe a drug, even though it is shorter than the chemical name, and is easier to use. Pharmacists and scientists in other fields, select all the USAN's, and make up the USAN Council.

UNSATURATED FAT: These fats contain essential fatty acids (EFA's), which have specific roles to play in maintaining health. These fats become liquid at room temperature. There are two types of unsaturated fats; monounsaturated, and polyunsaturated. Monounsaturated fatty acids lack two hydrogen atoms and are found in such foods as olive oil, olives, avocados, cashew nuts and salmon, mackerel, halibut and swordfish (cold-water fish). Polyunsaturated fatty acids lack four or more hydrogen atoms and are found in fish and in most vegetable oils.

VASCULAR: Of, or pertaining to blood vessels, or veins. An individual's vascularity is most apparent, when the bodyfat percentage is very low.

VIRILIZE: This term refers to attaining the characteristics of a mature male, as all anabolic steroids contain some degree of androgens. Females who use steroids risk the possibility of virilizing effects. These include deepening of the voice, clitoral enlargement, amenorrhea, changes in skin texture, changes in facial characteristics, male pattern baldness, increased sex drive, possible depression and anxiety, facial hair growth, and possible fever and illness. Many of these side effects are irreversible, therefore, women should discontinue the steroid use, and possibly re-evaluate the items that she is using if virilization becomes problematic. Some females can handle moderate amounts of androgens, others cannot. Sometimes, using an anti-androgen like Aldactone may arrest the virilizing affects from steroid use.

VITAMINS: Refers to organic substances which are found in food which perform many vital functions in the body. They are essential to good health, and can easily be obtained by eating a well-balanced diet. Lack of vitamins in food causes general poor health, and even diseases such as rickets and scurvy. Vitamins can also be obtained through pills, capsules, spray mists which are sprayed into the mouth, and injections.

WATER-INSOLUBLE FIBER: Refers to a type of fiber which supplies bulk to keep foods moving through the digestive system.

WATER-SOLUBLE FIBER: Refers to types of fibers in grains, legumes, and carrots which has been proven to reduce cholesterol and slow the release of glucose into the bloodstream.

BIBLIOGRAPHY

Anabolic Reference Guide, (5th Issue) 1990, W. N. Phillips. Mile High Publishing, Golden CO.

Anabolic Reference Guide, (6th Issue) 1991, W. N. Phillips. Mile High Publishing, Golden CO.

Anabolic Reference Update, Backset Collection 1988 - 1991, W. N. Phillips. Mile High Publishing, Golden Co.

Canadian Pharmacy Law, 1995, Marie Berry

Cecil Textbook of Medicine, (19th Edition), 1990, James B. Wyngaarden, and Lloyd H. Smith, Jr., Editors; W. B. Saunders Co.

Cluster Headache Pain Vs. Other Vascular Headache Pain; Differences, Revealed With Two Approaches To the McGill Pain Questionnaire, July, 1988, Issue 34 (1), A. Jerome, et al.; Pain.*Human Growth Hormone and Creutzfeldt-Jakob Disease*, Sept 1990; 83(9), S. Zekauskas; J Okla State Med Assoc.

Commission of Inquiry into the Use of Drugs and Banned Practices to Increase Athletic Performance, 1990, The Commission; Commissioner: C.L. Dubin, Ottawa, Ontario.

Compendium of Pharmaceuticals and Specialties, 1996, 31st Edition; C. K. Productions, Toronto, Canada.

Compendium of Veterinary Products, 1993, 3rd Edition, North American Comp. Ltd. Hensal, Ontario, Canada.

Complete Drug Reference, 1996 Edition, The United States Pharmacopeial Convention, Inc., Yonkers, New York.

Defense of Narcotics Cases, 1992, David Berhnheim, Matthew Bender.

Drug Facts and Comparisons, 1996, 50th Edition; Facts and Comparisons, St. Louis, Missouri.

Hyperprolactinemia, Infertility, and Hypothyroidism. A Case Report and Literature Review, March 1988, Issue 148 (3), J. H. Fish, et al.; Arch Intern Med.

Lean Bodies, 1995, Cliff Sheats, First Warner books Printing, New York, New York.

Martin's Annual Criminal Code, 1997 - 1996, Canada Law Book Inc., Aurora, Ont.

Merck Index, 1989, 11th Edition; Merck & Co., Inc., Rahway, NJ.

Med-Line Search, 1991 - 1995.

Med-Line Search, 1996.

Merck Manual, 1982, Volume 1, 14th Ed.: Robert Berkow, M.D., ed.-in chief; Merck Sharp & Dohme Research Laboratories.

Merck Manual, 1992, 16th Ed.: Merck Research Laboratories, Rahway, NJ.

Muscle Media 2000, 1994 - 1996, Various Editions From # 37 to # 54, Bill Phillips, Muscle Media 2000 Inc., Golden, CO.

Muscles Pinpointed as Site of Diabetic Defect, September 1990, Issue 14 (9), Collins, J., Research Resources Reporter.

New England Journal of Medicine SI Unit Conversion Guide, 1992, Laposato, Michael. NEJM Books. Boston.

Nutrients Catalog, 1993, Newstrom, Harvey. McFarland & Co. Inc. Publishers Jefferson, North Carolina, and London.

Orthostatic Hypotension, June, 1988; Issue 37 (6), J. Susman; AM Fam Physician.

Parrillo Performance, 1992, John Parrillo. Cincinnati, OH.

Physician's Desk Reference, 1996, 50th Edition; Medical Economics Company, Montvale, NJ.

Sports-Related Extraarticular Wrist Syndromes, January 1986, Issue 202, M.B. Wood, et al,; Clin Orthop.

The Complete Book of Food Counts, (3rd Edition) 1994, Corinne T. Netzer, Dell Publishing, New York, New York.

The Family Doctor, (3rd Edition) 1994, Allan H. Bruckheim, M.D., Multimedia Corporation, U.S.A.

The Nutrition Desk Reference, 1985, Robert H. Garrison, Jr. and Elizabeth Somer, New Canaan, Connecticut.

The Steroid User's Steroid Survival Guide, 1996, Kent Brown, Rhino World Publishing, Reno, Nevada.

Underground Steriod Handbook for Men and Women, 1993, Daniel Duchaine, U.S.A.

World Anabolic Review, 1996, P. Grunding/M. Bachmann, M. B. Muscle Books, M. Bodingbauer, D-Selm.

World Book Medical Encyclopedia, 1988, Erich E. Brueschke, M.D., et al., eds: World Book, Inc., Chicago, IL.

World Book Multimedia Encyclopedia, 1996, World Book, Inc., Chicago, IL.